Genital Dermatology

Genital Dermatology

Peter J. Lynch, M.D.
Professor and Head
Department of Dermatology
University of Minnesota Medical
School—Minneapolis
Minneapolis, Minnesota

Libby Edwards, M.D.
Chief of Dermatology
Carolinas Medical Center
Charlotte, North Carolina
Associate Clinical Professor
Department of Dermatology
Bowman Gray School of Medicine
of Wake Forest University
Winston-Salem, North Carolina

Churchill Livingstone
New York, Edinburgh, London, Madrid, Melbourne, Milan, Tokyo

Library of Congress Cataloging-in-Publication Data

Lynch, Peter J., date
Genital dermatology / Peter Lynch, Libby Edwards.
p. cm.
Includes bibliographical references and index.
ISBN 0-443-08885-3
1. Skin—Diseases. 2. Generative organs—Diseases. 3. Genital warts. 4. Sexually transmitted diseases. I. Edwards, Libby. II. Title.
[DNLM: 1. Skin Diseases—diagnosis. 2. Skin Diseases—therapy. 3. Genital Diseases, Female—diagnosis. 4. Genital Diseases, Female—therapy. 5. Genital Diseases, Male—diagnosis. 6. Genital Diseases, Male—therapy. WR 140 L987g 1994]
RL72.L96 1994
616.6′5—dc20
DNLM/DLC
for Library of Congress 94-19068
CIP

Distributed in the United Kingdom by Churchill Livingstone, Robert Stevenson House, 1–3 Baxter's Place, Leith Walk, Edinburgh EH1 3AF, and by associated companies, branches, and representatives throughout the world.

Accurate indications, adverse reactions, and dosage schedules for drugs are provided in this book, but it is possible that they may change. The reader is urged to review the package information data of the manufacturers of the medications mentioned.

The Publishers have made every effort to trace the copyright holders for borrowed material. If they have inadvertently overlooked any, they will be pleased to make the necessary arrangements at the first opportunity.

Acquisitions Editor: *Kerry Willis*
Copy Editor: *Lorono K. Johnson*
Production Supervisor: *Sharon Tuder*
Cover Design: *Jeanette Jacobs*

Printed in Singapore

First published in 1994 7 6 5 4 3 2 1

I would like to express my gratitude to Eduard G. Friederich, Jr., Raymond W. Kaufman, and Donald J. Woodruff. Their role in helping me to understand genital disease in women cannot be overestimated. They have in addition served as valued colleagues, important mentors, and warm friends.

Peter J. Lynch, M.D.

To all my mothers: my real one, Ta Fisher; my aunt, Libby Murrill; my grandmother, Lane Temple. Your love, patience, and support have given me my foundations.

Libby Edwards, M.D.

Preface

Genital disease represents an extremely multidisciplinary area of medicine. Patients with genital diseases or concerns about their genitalia may consult generalists, dermatologists, gynecologists, urologists, or physicians trained in the care of sexually transmitted diseases. Heretofore, information regarding these problems was fragmented among the various textbooks peculiar to each of these specialties. For this reason we concluded that there was a real need for a fully illustrated, comprehensive, single text that would cover the dermatologic aspects of anogenital disease in both men and women.

Genital Dermatology is an attempt to fill this need, combining approximately 180 clinical color illustrations with a text based both on our own extensive clinical experience and a comprehensive review of the relevant English language literature. Our book is designed to be user-friendly due to the following four elements. First, its problem-oriented diagnostic format is based on clinical description. This approach, as explained in chapter 4, allows for rapid and accurate identification even of diseases that are unfamiliar. Second, we have included sufficient dermatologic information regarding diagnostic techniques and basic therapy to make the text usable by those who have not been trained in dermatology. Third, at the conclusion of each chapter we have included not only standard bibliographical references but also annotated citations to review articles for those who wish more detailed information. Fourth, to save time and confusion, we have listed American trade names alongside the generic nomenclature for all medications discussed.

This book would not have been possible were it not for the superb assistance of our publisher, Churchill Livingstone. We would particularly like to acknowledge the encouragement and support offered by Toni Tracy and the excellent guidance through the publication process as provided by Kerry Willis.

Peter J. Lynch, M.D.
Libby Edwards, M.D.

Contents

Section VI Ulcers

Section VII Pruritus and Pain

Section VIII Special Issues

I Basic Principles

1 Anatomy

FEMALE ANATOMY

In general, women have only vague concepts of their anatomy and little knowledge of medical terminology. Thus, many women refer to all genital symptoms as vaginal, and their physicians may accept these descriptions as literal.

The *vulva* refers to that area of the skin encompassing the hair-bearing portion of the labia majora to the hymen (Fig. 1-1). It is bordered laterally by the crural folds, anteriorly by the mons pubis, and posteriorly by the perineal body. The labia majora enclose the vulva and are covered with clinically hair-bearing skin over the lateral aspects. The medial surface, although moist from mucus secreted by vestibular and cervical glands, is also nonmucous membrane. The skin of the labia majora is richly supplied with hair follicles and eccrine, apocrine, and sebaceous glands. Lying within the labia majora are the labia minora, two flat folds of skin on either side of the introitus. Like the inner aspect of the labia majora, this skin is also damp and minimally keratinized, but it is not mucous membrane except perhaps near the hymen at the vestibule. Although gynecologic terminology deems mucous membrane to include only secretory epithelium, dermatologic terminology includes nonkeratinizing stratified squamous epithelium as mucous membrane. This encompasses the vagina and oral mucosa. Sebaceous glands that appear as small, yellow-white lobular papules are present.

From the medial aspect of the labia minora to the hymen lies the vulvar vestibule, or introitus. A faint line of texture change called Hart's line is sometimes visible at the medial base of the labia minora and marks the border of the vestibule. The vulvar posterior fourchette divides the posterior aspect of the vulva from the perineum and should not be confused with the vaginal posterior fornix. Anteriorly, the glans of the clitoris is covered by the prepuce, or clitoral hood, and ventrally two flaps of skin, the frenulae, extend posteriorly from the glans. Both the posterior prepuce and frenulae form the anterior origin of the labia minora. Posterior to the glans, but at the anterior portion of the vestibule, is the urethral orifice.

Within the vestibule are the openings of several secretory glands. The ostia of the Bartholin's glands lie posteriorly and laterally in the vestibule and provide lubrication. At the exterior base of the hymen are the openings of the mucus-secreting minor vestibular glands. Skene's ducts lead from paraurethral glands, opening near the urethral meatus, while other paraurethral ducts open into the distal urethra.

Understanding diseases of the female external genitalia also requires familiarity with the vagina, including normal structures and environment. The vagina extends from the hymen to the cervix, and is characterized by extremely extensible folds surrounding a potential space, with anterior and posterior walls in contact. The cervix is located in the anterior, upper vaginal wall, and the pouch behind the cervix is referred to as the vaginal posterior fornix. The lateral fornices are the lateral junctions of the cervix and vagina.

Minor morphologic variations of normal anatomy can produce confusion and may be noticed for the first time when unrelated symptoms occur. The labia minora show wide normal variations in size, shape, and texture, ranging from vestigial remnants of skin to quite large, redundant skin folds. The labia minora may be asymmetrical, and occasionally one or both may be obviously bifid anteriorly. At times the num-

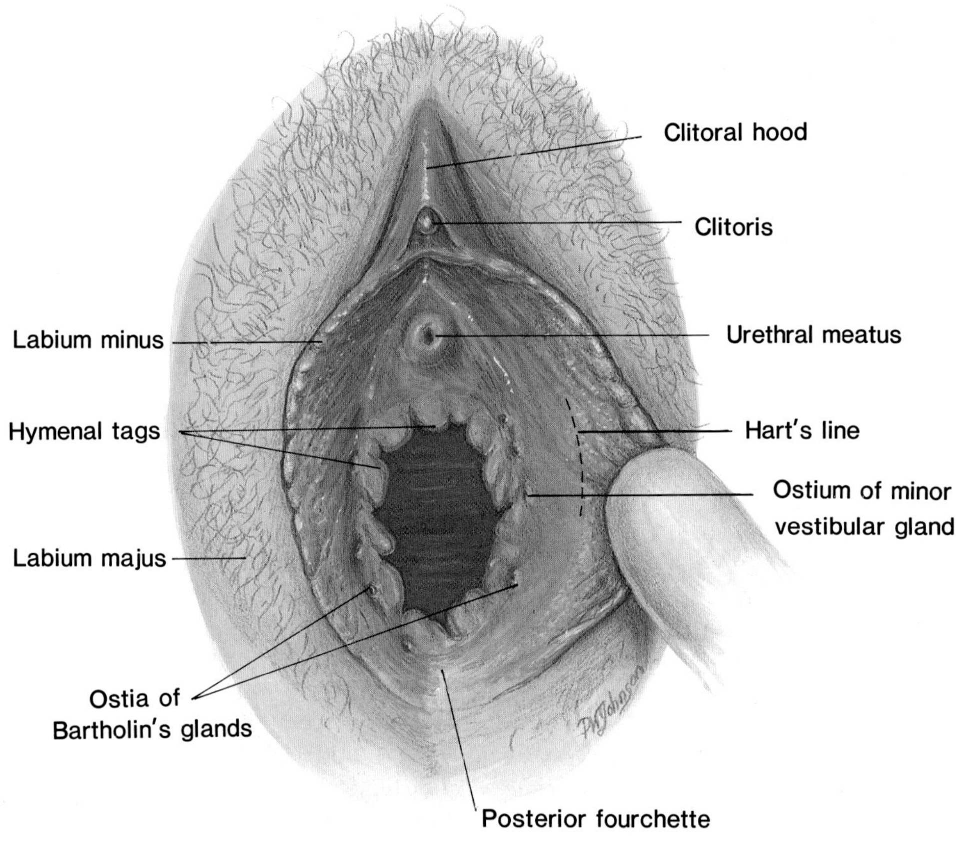

Fig. 1-1. Normal anatomy of the vulva.

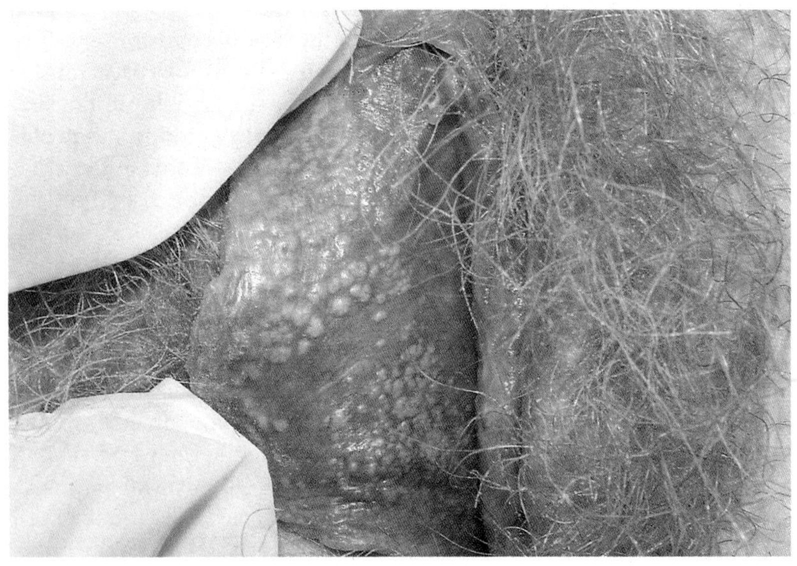

Fig. 1-2. These yellow-white lobules, especially prominent over the inner labia minora, are called Fordyce spots and represent normal, large sebaceous glands.

ber and size of sebaceous glands over the labia minora can be striking (Fig. 1-2). This abundance of large sebaceous glands, called the Fordyce condition, is a normal variant rather than a disease, although some clinicians feel, probably erroneously, that it can be associated with pruritus. There is no medical treatment for this common variant, and surgical removal or destruction is unnecessary.

Vestibular papillae are also normal variants found in up to one half of premenopausal women (Moyal-Barracco M, personal communication, 1993). These small, filiform, tubular projections occurring in the vestibule can be mistaken for condylomata acuminata (see also Ch. 9). Vestibular papillae are more monomorphous than genital warts, taller than they are wide, and have rounded rather than lobular or acuminate tips. They are asymptomatic, and no medical or surgical treatment is needed.

Considerable variation as to the presence and degree of erythema in normal women also exists. This can be especially difficult to evaluate in women with pain or itching who have no other visible abnormalities. Many women report redness, but, because they never had reason to examine their vulva carefully before the onset of symptoms, they do not realize that this degree of erythema may be normal. Similarly, there are substantial differences in the degree of pain normal patients feel to touch and pressure during a routine examination. Many asymptomatic patients may report significant discomfort to pressure in the vestibule with a cotton-tipped applicator.

Male Anatomy

The penis is composed of three major, erectile structures: two dorsal paired bodies, the corpora cavernosa, and the ventral, midline corpus spongiosum, which contains the urethra. The corpora cavernosa are surrounded (and partially separated) by a layer of dense connective tissue known as Buck's fascia (tunica albuginea). The distal end of the corpus spongiosum is enlarged and rounded to form the glans penis, through which the urethra emerges as a vertical slit. The skin of the penis distally is infolded to form the prepuce (foreskin); the prepuce in turn covers the glans unless the prepuce has been removed through circumcision. The prepuce is separated from the glans by a potential space that forms the preputial sac.

The penis is well supplied with arterial blood from the pudendal artery, which branches to form the dorsal artery, the deep cavernous artery, the bulbar artery, and the urethral artery. These vessels can supply the erectile tissue with copious amounts of blood, which fill the endothelially lined maze of vessels that make up the erectile tissue. Venous return occurs through three major vessels, the cavernous vein, the superficial dorsal vein, and the deep dorsal vein. The dorsal nerve of the penis, which is a branch of the pudendal nerve, provides sensory input. The features of the penis pertinent for dermatologic examination are shown in Figure 1-3.

The interior of the scrotum is formed of two sacs separated by a septum. These sacs contain the testicles with the attached vas deferens. The wall of the scrotum, from the outside in, consists of the following layers: the outer skin, the dartos (smooth) muscle, the external spermatic fascia with the cremasteric (skeletal) muscle, the internal spermatic fascia, and the tunica vaginalis.

Several genital anomalies are frequently encountered. At birth the prepuce is adherent to the glans, and it cannot easily be retracted. This condition, known as phimosis, is normal for the first several years of life, but by age 3, separation of the foreskin from the glans has occurred in over 90 percent of boys. If it has not, either surgery or medical treatment with high-potency topical steroids may be necessary.[1] Occasionally, this physiologic phimosis will lead to recurring episodes of balanoposthitis. When this inflammatory process of the glans and foreskin occurs, forcible retraction of the prepuce (after topical steroid therapy) or circumcision or both, are required.

Cysts, which are lined by epidermal cells, sometimes occur on the ventral aspect of the penis along the median raphe.[2] No treatment is necessary for these lesions unless they become symptomatic.

A variety of abnormalities may be encountered as a result of circumcision. These include the formation of partial adhesions between remnants of the foreskin and the glans. Sometimes these adhesions, or "bridges," result in pockets that can be everted, simulating the appearance of wartlike papillomas[3] (Fig. 1-4).

The skin of the penis contains both apocrine and eccrine sweat glands. Hamartomas and tumors of these glands may develop later in life. Pilosebaceous

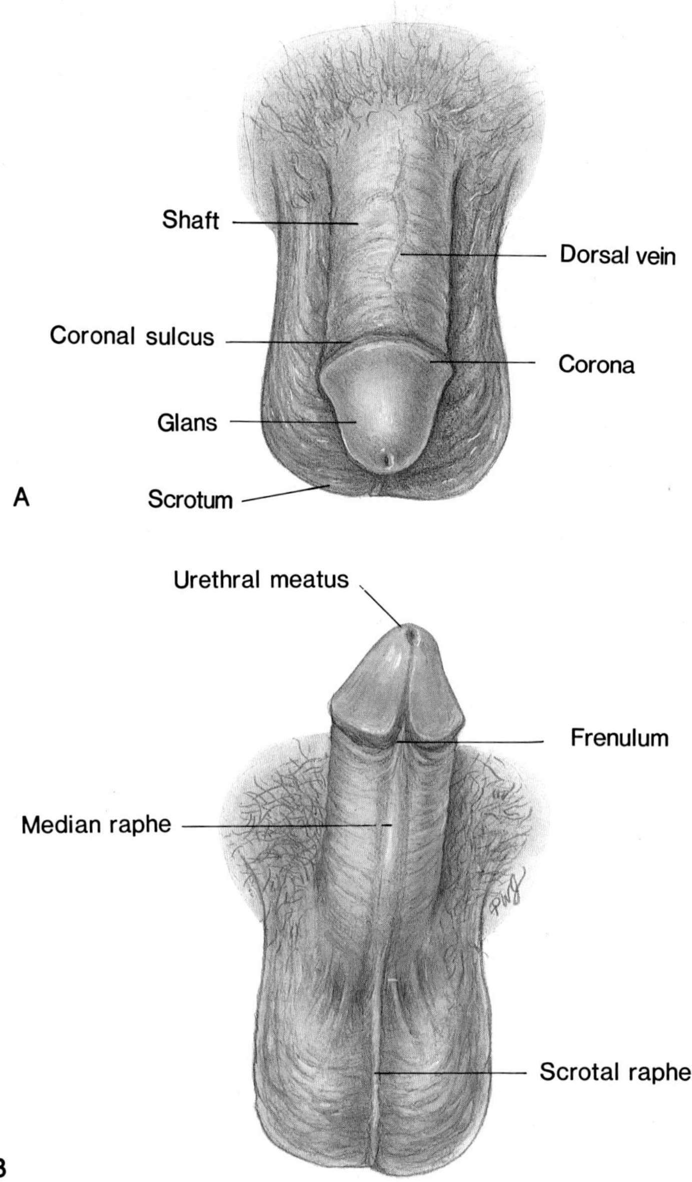

Fig. 1-3. (A & B) Normal anatomy of the penis and scrotum.

units do not normally occur distally beyond the first quarter of the shaft of the penis, but occasionally ectopic pilosebaceous units are found scattered along the entire length of the penile shaft. Free-standing sebaceous glands known as Tyson's glands are found with some frequency on the prepuce.[4] Small soft papules (pearly penile papules) 1 to 2 mm in diameter and 1 to 3 mm in length are found on the corona in 10 to 30 percent of men.[5] These somewhat filiform papillomas often occur in several parallel rows that encircle the corona of the glans. These fibrous papules are often mistakenly diagnosed as genital warts. Additional discussion of these penile papules can be found in Chapter 9.

Fig. 1-4. The appearance of a circumcision fistula **(A)** before and **(B)** after eversion.

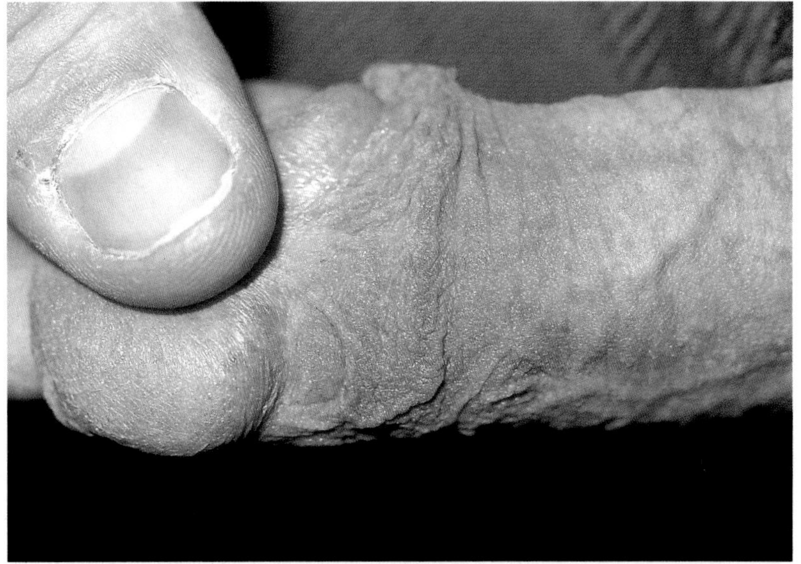

A

B

REFERENCES

1. Jorgensen ET, Svensson A: The treatment of phimosis in boys with a potent topical steroid (clobetasol propionate 0.05%) cream. Acta Derm Venereol (Stockh) 73:55, 1993
2. Sharkey MJ, Grabski WJ, McCollough ML, Berger TG: Postcoital appearance of a median raphe cyst. J Am Acad Dermatol 26:273, 1992
3. Bart BJ, Kempers SS, Rinehart D: A penile-tunnel "pop up wart": an unusual complication of penile adhesions. Arch Dermatol 126:828, 1990
4. Piccino R, Carrel CF, Menni S, Brancaleon W: Preputial ectopic glands mimicking molluscum contagiosum. Acta Derm Venereol (Stockh) 70:344, 1990
5. Magid M, Garden JM: Pearly penile papules: treatment with the carbon dioxide laser. J Dermatol Surg Oncol 15:552, 1989

2 Diagnostic Procedures

SKIN BIOPSY

Skin biopsies are easy, fast and safe procedures that are extremely useful in the diagnosis of some skin diseases and tumors. The punch and the shave biopsies are those most commonly performed; the choice depends on both the disease and the location.

A punch biopsy is preferred for an ulcer or inflammatory skin condition. Because a punch biopsy removes epidermis, dermis, and some fat, the extent of inflammation (which is often a differentiating feature among several similar diseases) can be judged. The tissue is anesthetized using lidocaine 1 percent with epinephrine in a 1-ml syringe with a 30-gauge needle in a single injection at the biopsy site. Although many physicians avoid epinephrine on the penis to prevent vasoconstriction and its resulting ischemia, the volume of anesthetic necessary for a punch biopsy (0.2 to 0.3 ml) is small and is required only in a limited area. This small, correspondingly superficial injection does not pose a threat to the deeper, primary vascular supply. When the procedure is delayed for 10 minutes, epinephrine minimizes bleeding from the biopsy site by inducing vasoconstriction, which is especially useful on the vulva where loose connective tissue can allow impressive hematoma formation. Shaving or vigorous cleansing of the area to be biopsied is unnecessary. The pain produced by the injection of lidocaine can be prevented by the application of topical eutectic mixture of local anesthesia (EMLA) under occlusion with a plastic adhesive cover on the biopsy area. Twenty minutes of contact with mucous membrane or modified mucous membrane and 60 minutes with keratinized skin is sufficient before injecting anesthesia.

A 3-mm punch biopsy is usually adequate for careful microscopic tissue examination without causing a large defect. Occasionally, when complete removal of a specific lesion is desired, a larger punch may be required. The cutting edge of the punch biopsy instrument is applied to the tissue and twisted in a screwing motion until it is buried up to the hub. The biopsy specimen is occasionally retained within the biopsy punch, but more often it remains attached to underlying subcutaneous tissue. Detachment can be accomplished without crushing the specimen by lifting it from the biopsy site with a needle while snipping the base with curved iris scissors. Gentle forceps extraction may be used at the risk of damaging a fragile specimen. One or two sutures can then be placed if desired. Absorbable, soft, 5–0 suture is preferred because these do not require removal from the vulva, and nonabsorbable suture is stiff, potentially pricking the skin. If sutures are not used, a chemical cautery such as ferric chloride, ferric subsulfate (Monsel's solution), or silver nitrate (more caustic and damaging to the skin) may be used to stop bleeding.

A shave biopsy is preferred when the skin lesion is superficial, such as a genital wart or a seborrheic keratosis. It is also useful for the removal of a blister when the rotating motion of the punch might shear off the blister roof. After anesthesia as described above for a punch biopsy, a #15 scalpel blade is used to remove a sample of skin well under the lesion but not through to fat since this causes retraction of the intact skin and results in impressive enlargement of the defect. Sutures are not used to close the defect, and again, Monsel's solution or silver nitrate can be used to stop bleeding. A pedunculated lesion can be removed easily by snipping the base with curved iris scissors.

Although significant adverse reactions are rare, patients should be warned about scarring, infection, soreness, and bleeding or hematoma formation on the vulva.

POTASSIUM HYDROXIDE PREPARATION

The potassium hydroxide (KOH) preparation is extremely useful in diagnosing superficial fungal and yeast infections. Potassium hydroxide dissolves epithelial cells, allowing for better visualization of the fungal organism. However, artifacts are still often confusing, and proper interpretation of a fungal smear requires experience.

If keratinized skin is to be examined, the affected area is swabbed with alcohol both to remove any creams and to allow the damp scale's adherence to a scalpel blade. The scale is scraped from the border of a plaque, or a pustule roof is removed with a #15 scalpel blade. If the vagina is to be studied, a swab of vaginal secretions is used. The specimen is placed on a slide, one drop of 10 or 20 percent potassium hydroxide is applied to the specimen, and a coverslip is affixed. A vaginal swab may be examined immediately, as described below. If keratinized skin is being examined, the slide should be either gently heated over an alcohol flame or it should be set aside for 10 to 15 minutes to allow epithelial cells to dissolve. The coverslip should then be pressed firmly to the slide to flatten and thin the specimen and enhance visibility. The specimen should be examined with the 10× objective under relatively low light. The condenser should be racked down to enhance contrast between the ghost outlines of cells and the darker outlines of organisms. A closer look under the 40× objective can confirm the diagnosis. Superficial fungi exhibit branching hyphae that cross cell borders. *Candida albicans* shows pseudohyphae similar in size and configuration to superficial fungi as well as budding yeasts. Some of the more unusual yeast forms such as *Candida (Torulopsis) glabrata* or *Candida parapsilosis* do not show the fairly easily detected pseudohyphae. Instead, they are subtle, very small, budding yeasts that can only be appreciated with the 40× objective.

Analysis of KOH preparations requires experience and close observation to discern artifacts from actual organisms, but when performed by a skilled and careful clinician, this smear is one of the most valuable tests in the management of genital disease. Yeast forms other than *C. albicans* can be extraordinarily difficult to see, and a culture should be performed when a smear appears negative but the index of suspicion is high. Some yeast forms may require as long as a month of incubation for detection when the inoculum is small.

SALINE WET DROP PREPARATION

A microscopic examination of vaginal secretions diluted with a drop of saline under a coverslip allows for inspection of the morphology of the cells and organisms that constitute a vaginal discharge. Unlike the procedure for the preparation of a fungal smear, the coverslip should not be pressed vigorously to flatten the specimen because this may result in distortion of the cells.

Normal findings include mature epithelial cells and an equal number or fewer white blood cells. Normal secretions show numerous lactobacilli that appear as long rods. Occasionally, lactobacilli may attach to each other end to end to form long filaments previously felt to represent leptothrix bacilli. These can be confused with the hyphae of *C. albicans* except for the much smaller caliber. Anecdotally, these organisms are believed to occur in association with *Trichomonas vaginalis*, but this is not the experience of many clinicians and is disputed by recent investigations. Lactobacilli may produce a symptomatic vaginitis (see Ch. 7) (Horowitz B, personal communication, 1993) or may represent a normal variant.

Occasionally, bacteria adhere to epithelial cells in such numbers that the borders of the cell are obscured and the cytoplasm appears granular. These cells (aptly named "clue cells") are characteristic of bacterial vaginosis. This diagnosis is confirmed by the presence of a high vaginal pH, an absence of lactobacilli, and a positive "whiff test," in which a drop of potassium chloride added to a drop of vaginal secretions produces a fishy odor (see also Ch. 7).

The presence of immature squamous epithelial cells (see Maturation Index below) can be evaluated on a saline wet drop preparation and suggests estrogen deficiency or significant vaginal inflammation.

MATURATION INDEX

Vaginal epithelium is exquisitely sensitive to estrogen. In hormone-deficient states (such as those that follow natural or surgical menopause, oral contraceptive use, or breastfeeding), thinning of the vaginal and vulvar epithelium occurs to varying degrees. The extent of estrogen effect can be estimated by examining vaginal cells for maturity, since estrogen promotes epithelial maturation. A cotton-tipped applicator is gently rolled over the lateral vaginal wall and then rolled onto a glass slide. This slide can then be processed as for a Papanicolaou (Pap) smear for evaluation by a cytologist, or the clinician can examine it in the office with a drop of saline and a coverslip. Well-estrogenized, mature squamous epithelial cells are flattened and large, with abundant cytoplasm and a small nucleus. Intermediate cells are also flattened but show a larger nucleus, while parabasal cells are smaller and round, with a much larger nuclear to cytoplasmic ratio. The more immature the cell, the larger the nucleus and the smaller and more rounded the cell. Although the normal ratios of mature squamous cells to intermediate cells varies with the phase of the menstrual cycle, larger numbers of immature cells are associated with atrophic epithelium from estrogen deficiency or with intense inflammation or erosive disease that has removed the superficial, most mature keratinocytes.

pH DETERMINATION

An examination of vaginal secretions includes a pH determination. Vaginal secretion on a cotton-tipped applicator or residual material on the speculum is applied to pH paper that measures between pH 3 and pH 7. Normal values for premenopausal and postpubertal women vary from 3.5 to 4.5, although asymptomatic women sometimes fall outside this range. The pH is then interpreted in conjunction with microscopic findings. Accurate measurement depends upon the avoidance of lubricating jelly or even water on the speculum, since they can affect the pH. Residual semen from recent intercourse or even small amounts of blood produce falsely alkaline measurements. Lower estrogen states correlate with a higher pH, as do increased numbers of white blood cells. Characteristic pH measurements found in different diseases can be found in Chapter 7.

TZANCK PREPARATION

A Tzanck preparation can be useful for quick confirmation of the diagnosis of herpes simplex or herpes zoster. These viruses cause epithelial cells to coalesce into very large giant cells that can be easily seen on a well-stained scraping of a fresh lesion (Fig. 2-1). The blister roof is removed and a #15 scalpel blade is used to scrape the base of the lesion. The collected material

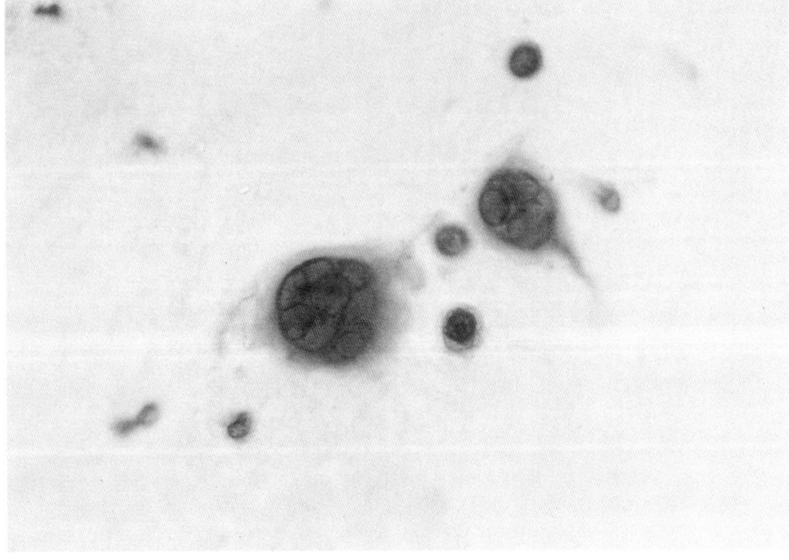

Fig. 2-1. Giant multinucleated keratinocytes that are much larger than surrounding inflammatory cells identify a positive Tzanck preparation, characteristic of herpes simplex virus and varicella zoster virus infections.

is wiped onto a glass slide and then stained with Giemsa's or Wright's stain. When present, these giant cells reliably indicate the presence of one of these viruses. Absence of these cells does not rule out herpesvirus infection, and a viral culture usually provides definitive confirmation of the results of a Tzanck preparation. However, these viruses are relatively fastidious, and a negative culture, while highly suggestive, is also not proof positive of an absence of infection.

CYTOLOGIC PREPARATION FOR SCABIES

Confirmation of a clinical diagnosis of scabies is obtained with direct visualization of the scabies mite, its eggs, or feces. The most difficult aspect of this test is identification of the most appropriate lesion and its removal for examination. A linear edematous papule or vesicle, called a burrow, is most likely to harbor diagnostic material, but intact lesions are difficult to find. Without using anesthesia, the papule is removed by a superficial shave with a #15 scalpel blade, removing the entire top of the lesion but not extending into the dermis, rather than simply scraping off superficial scale. There should be only small bleeding points after the procedure. The removed specimen is then placed on a glass slide with a coverslip and examined under low power. The mite is large and obvious, but the diagnosis can also be verified by the identification of feces or ova. This test frequently produces false-negative results even in the hands of experienced clinicians.

ACETIC ACID APPLICATION AND EXAMINATION FOR HPV INFECTION

Although human papillomavirus (HPV) infection is often visually obvious in the form of genital warts, a subtle variant presents as flat warts or a cobblestoned texture of the skin. The application of 5 percent acetic acid (common white vinegar) to the nonhairbearing portion of the genitalia can be performed by swabbing the area with saturated gauze or cotton. Mucous membranes can be examined immediately; keratinized skin is more impermeable and therefore more efficiently examined after close application of saturated gauze for 10 to 15 minutes. Careful inspection with magnification frequently reveals the whitened lesions of hyperkeratosis that may represent subtle wart infection. Not only is this technique useful in the detection of nearly invisible wart infections, but also it is helpful when differentiating between keratotic wart lesions and, for example, prominent but nonkeratotic sebaceous glands on the penis. Acetic acid application is standard practice when carefully examining the cervix under magnification (colposcopy).

However, any area of hyperkeratosis, thickening of the skin, or inflammation also exhibits aceto-whitening, so this test is not specific and should be confirmed by biopsy. Also, not all warts whiten in response to acetic acid application, and HPV DNA can be present (latent infection) in absolutely normal skin, undetectable by any clinical examination or standard biopsy.

3 Treatment

The basic principles of dermatologic therapy are often somewhat of a mystery to nondermatologists. The material presented in this section is intended to be simple enough, yet sufficiently complete, to allow any clinician to initiate treatment without requiring dermatologic consultation. Additional sources of information regarding these and other therapeutic modalities are listed in the Suggested Readings.

SOAKS

There are two major reasons for using soaks. The first is to gently debride crusted tissue. Debridement is desirable because crust maintains a favorable environment for bacterial overgrowth. The debriding effect occurs as the soaking solution gradually resolubilizes the serum proteins that make up crust.

The second, and more important, reason for using soaks relates to the restoration of a physiologic environment around exposed nerve endings. The sensory nerve endings of the skin, which are responsible for the conveyance of pruritus and pain to the brain, are normally protected from environmental insult by the interposition of the barrier layer present in the outer third of the epidermis. This epidermal barrier may be disrupted, or may be absent, in many types of genital disease. In this setting sensory nerve endings are exposed, with resultant triggering of either itching or discomfort. For the length of time they are used, soaks temporarily bathe the nerve endings with fluid, reducing the noxious environmental stimulation.

The nature of the solution used for soaking is not critical. Tap water is readily available, inexpensive, and easily drawn at a temperature that the patient finds soothing. Normal saline has the advantage of being isotonic, but the nuisance of obtaining (or preparing) saline solutions outweighs this minor advantage. A variety of commercial products for soaks are available; the most commonly used are Burow's solution and colloidal oatmeal (Aveeno). In most circumstances neither has a significant advantage over tap water.

Soaks are administered either as wrapped or immersion preparations. Wrapped soaks involve wetting a gauze bandage, a gauze pad, or cotton toweling, which is then held in place over the area of affected tissue. This approach works well in locations such as the extremities, but (with the exception of penile wraps) this type of soak is not very practical for genital disease. Immersion soaks, in which the patient sits or lies in the soaking fluid, are much more feasible but do require the use of a bathtub or sitz bath chair (rented from medical supply stores). Immersion soaks are carried out for 20 to 30 minutes two or three times a day. Amelioration of symptoms occurs promptly, but exacerbation can be expected within minutes to hours after the soak has been discontinued.

As noted above, the soaking solution restores a physiologic environment to exposed nerve endings. In addition, any remaining epithelial cells take up water, swell, and close off small cracks and fissures. This restoration of a barrier over otherwise exposed nerve endings reduces the symptoms of pain or pruritus. Evaporative loss, with shrinkage of the cells and reopening of the fissures, accounts for the rapidity of symptom return. Application of lubricants (whether or not they contain medication) immediately after the soak retards evaporation and prolongs the soothing effect.

The use of soaks should be viewed as "first aid" for itching or pain. Prolonged use of intermittent soaks can lead to overdrying, and prolonged use of immersion soaks can lead to maceration. If the use of soaks does not lead to marked symptomatic improvement in 2 to 3 days, it is desirable to reexamine the diagnosis or the other portion of the therapeutic plan or both.

LUBRICANTS

Lubricants are generally thought of as therapy for dry skin (e.g., "chapped hands"). Since the anogenital area is not considered a "dry area," one rarely associates the need for lubrication with the treatment of genital disease. This is erroneous, however; lubricants are an essential component of treatment for most genital dermatologic conditions.

Lubricants serve several purposes. First, they retard evaporative loss of water and thus participate in the healing of disrupted epithelium. Second, they replace lipids removed through overly vigorous hygiene, thus preventing the development of certain eczematous diseases. Third, they "smooth" the skin by reducing the roughness associated with scaling diseases. Fourth, they act as the vehicle for almost all topically applied medications. Each of these points is discussed below.

Disruption of epithelium occurs with both eczematous and vesiculobullous disease. This disturbance in epithelial coverage exposes free nerve endings; consequent stimulation of the exposed nerve endings results in pruritus or pain, or both. Lubricants mechanically cover the nerve endings, protecting them from external stimuli. Lubricants also retard the loss of interstitial fluid, thus keeping the nerve endings in a physiologic environment; they also create a moist environment that favors the growth and spread of new epithelial cells. Through these mechanisms lubricants not only reduce the symptoms of pruritus and pain but also play a role in actual repair of the epithelium.

Western civilization is associated with a fetish for cleanliness. This seems to be particularly true regarding the genitalia. Frequent washing of this area, especially if both soap and hot water are used, is associated with removal of the natural lipids produced by epithelial cells. These lipids coat the surface of both skin and mucosae; without them the epithelial surface dries, individual epithelial cells shrink, and microscopic fissures develop. This process is the most common cause of an irritant contact dermatitis, which can occur either as a disease sui generis or superimposed on other dermatologic diseases as patients misguidely try to keep the genital area clean and dry. Restoration of the removed lipids through the use of lubricants is clearly an important therapeutic tool in this setting.

Eczematous and papulosquamous disease is associated with the presence of scale. The scale feels rough and is unattractive in appearance. More importantly, scale provides a focus for picking and scratching. Lubricants smooth over the roughened surface and decrease the apparency of scale. Patients feel better about their disease and are therefore more likely to keep their hands off the diseased skin.

All topically applied medications require a vehicle for their deliverance to the skin and mucosae. Most of the vehicles in use also happen to be lubricants. This dual function provides both the healing effect of lubricants themselves (as detailed in the paragraphs above) and a good delivery system for healing drugs. The role of lubricants as vehicles is, in fact, so important that a section of this chapter is devoted to the subject.

VEHICLES FOR THE DELIVERY OF TOPICAL MEDICATIONS

The most commonly used vehicles for topical medications are ointments, creams, lotions, solutions, and gels. Each will be described in turn.

Ointments

Ointments consist of either pure petrolatum (Vaseline) or water-in-oil emulsions (Polysorb, Aquaphor). They have a slightly opaque, gray appearance and feel quite greasy. For this reason they do not spread as easily as the other types of vehicles. On the other hand, they are excellent lubricants, they provide solubility for a larger number of medical substances, and they require few or no stabilizers and preservatives. The lack of these latter products decreases the likelihood of allergic sensitization, and the absence of alcohol and propylene glycol reduces the likelihood of stinging on application. Ointments are the vehicle of choice for genital application in children (due to the absence of stinging) and can be used effectively in cool dry climates for diseases such as lichen simplex chronicus, in which the need for lubrication is great.

Creams

Creams are considered oil-in-water emulsions; microscopic droplets of oil are distributed in a solid phase of water. They are white in color and feel only slightly greasy. Only a few products (testosterone, for instance) are not soluble in a cream base. They spread easily, are quite cosmetically acceptable, and are satisfactory lubricants. The lubricating quality of creams can be enhanced by the addition of humectants (products that chemically bind water) such as urea, lactic acid, and glycolic acid. However, these humectants, together with the alcohol or propylene glycol (or both) regularly contained in creams, cause stinging when applied to disrupted epithelium. Creams also contain preservatives and stabilizers that represent a possible cause of allergic contact dermatitis. This possibility should not cause avoidance of creams, but it should become a consideration when eczematous disease fails to improve in spite of prolonged use of seemingly appropriate topical medications.

Lotions

Lotions are white, like creams, but are liquid enough to pour from a bottle. They contain little lipid and thus offer only minor benefit in terms of lubrication. While cosmetically very acceptable, the concentrations of alcohol and propylene glycol in lotions are high enough to cause stinging on application in the anogenital area. Lotions are used where easy spreadability, especially in hairy areas, is a prime consideration.

Solutions

Solutions are liquids totally lacking in lipids. They are waterlike in appearance and consistency. Stinging on application prevents their use for genital disease.

Gels

Gels can be considered as "solid solutions." They have a clear appearance but are thick enough to be squeezed out a tube. They have no lubricating property and sting broken skin on application. For this reason they are rarely or never used for genital application.

TOPICAL CORTICOSTEROIDS

Corticosteroids represent the class of compounds most frequently applied to the skin and mucous membranes. Perhaps for this reason, it is not surprising that the number of steroid products is so staggering. Even a small market niche represents very good sales when the market is so large. A reasonably complete list of topical corticosteroid products available in the United States is presented in Table 3-1, but it is worth emphasizing that familiarity with only three or four of these is sufficient to provide excellent topical anti-inflammatory therapy.

Topical steroids are, of course, anti-inflammatory agents, and as such they are useful for all of the eczematous, exudative, and papulosquamous diseases (discussed in Chs. 5 and 6). In addition, other selected diseases (notably lichen sclerosus and several of the blistering and erosive conditions) benefit from the use of topical steroids.

Once a decision has been made to use topically applied steroids, there are several additional considerations: strength, brand, vehicle, size, and frequency of application. Each of these will be considered in turn.

Strength and brand are somewhat interrelated. That is, some steroid products are inherently more powerful than others. This is true regardless of the

Table 3-1. Topical Steroid Products[a]

Maximal potency
Clobetasol propionate 0.05% (Temovate)
Halobetasol propionate 0.05% (Ultravate)
Betamethasone dipropionate 0.05%; optimized vehicle (Diprolene)
Diflorasone diacetate 0.05%; optimized vehicle (Psorcon)
High potency
Halcinonide 0.1% (Halog)
Fluocinonide 0.05% (Lidex)[b]
Amcinonide 0.1% (Cyclocort)
Desoximetasone 0.25% (Topicort)
Midpotency
Flurandrenolide 0.5% (Cordran)
Triamcinolone acetonide 0.1% (Kenalog, Aristocort)[b]
Fluocinolone 0.025% (Synalar)
Betamethasone valerate 0.1% (Valisone)[b]
Betamethasone dipropionate 0.05% (Diprosone)[b]
Mometasone furoate 0.1% (Elocon)
Diflorasone diacetate 0.05% (Florone, Maxiflor)
Low potency
Desonide 0.05% (Tridesilon)
Alclometasone dipropionate 0.05% (Aclovate)
Hydrocortisone valerate 0.2% (Westcort cream)
Hydrocortisone butyrate 0.1% (Locoid)
Dexamethasone 0.1% (Decadron)
Hydrocortisone 1.0% (Hytone, Cort-Dome, and others)[c]

[a] Not all available products are listed. Products within categories are listed in approximate order of decreasing strength. All products are available in creams and ointments and many are available in gels and solutions; percentages given are the highest marketed, and many are available in lower strengths.
[b] Products available generically.
[c] Hydrocortisone 1.0 percent is available without prescription.

actual percentage strength stated on the label. Mild eczematous disease will usually respond to a low-potency product. Hydrocortisone 1.0 percent is a good first choice since it is available generically (and is thus relatively inexpensive) and without prescription. However, the clinician will sometimes want to control tightly the total amount of steroid used. In such instances a low-potency product that requires the use of a prescription, such as desonide 0.05 percent, is preferred.

Midpotency steroid preparations will be necessary for more severe and chronic eczematous disease; they also represent the starting point for therapy of papulosquamous disease involving the genitalia. Triamcinolone 0.1 percent represents a good choice, as it is available generically and thus is quite inexpensive.

High-potency steroid preparations are generally avoided in the genital and perianal area because of the frequency of cutaneous side effects (see below). However, they may be necessary in the treatment of certain diseases such as lichen sclerosus, psoriasis, Darier's disease, and Hailey-Hailey disease. Fluocinonide 0.05 percent is available generically and is fairly inexpensive; Temovate, on the other hand, is more powerful but is also more expensive and troublesome from a standpoint of absorption, cutaneous atrophy, and the induction of striae (Figs. 3-1 and 3-2).

These five products will suffice for nearly all situations, but Table 3-1 lists other equally useful steroids for consideration.

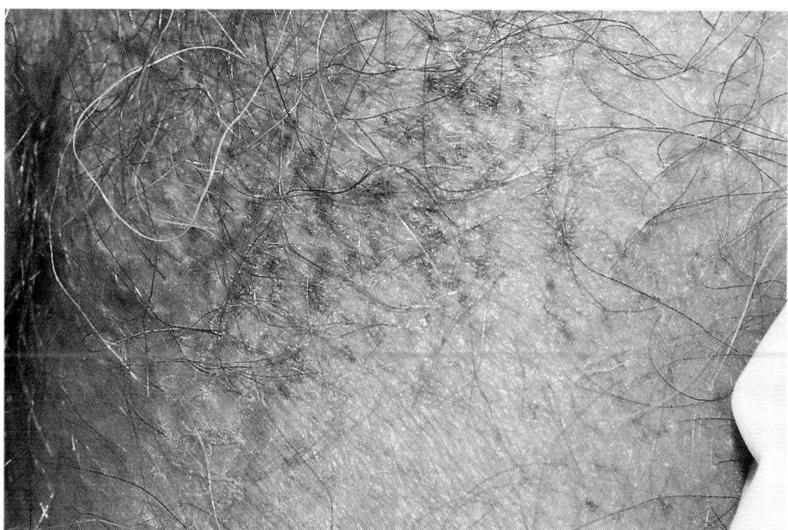

Fig. 3-1. Thinning of the skin from steroid atrophy is evident from telangiectasias and slight shininess of the skin.

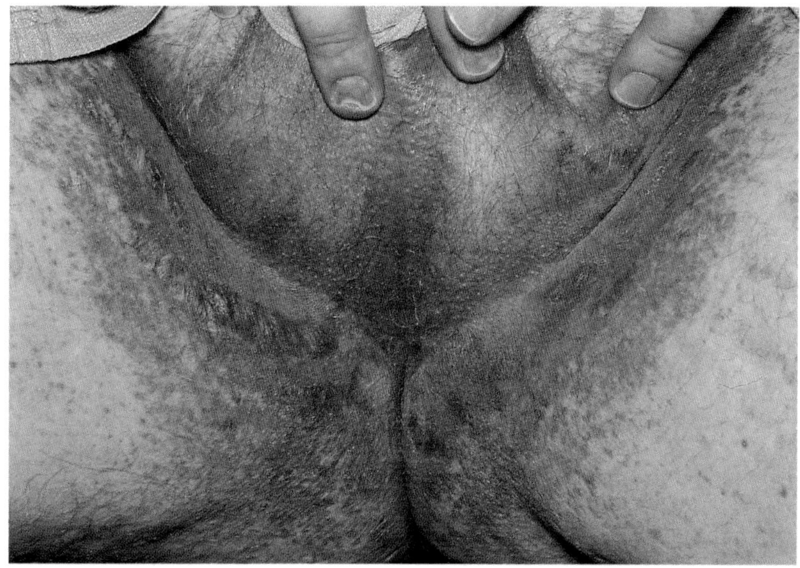

Fig. 3-2. Purple striae of steroid atrophy after using a medium-high potency corticosteroid for 1 month.

In choosing a vehicle it is often helpful, by way of providing samples, to let the patient decide whether a cream or ointment is preferred. Creams are more widely used because they are easy to spread, do not result in the development of maceration, and are cosmetically very acceptable. Their major drawback is that stinging occurs when they are used for inflamed or eroded disease. This is particularly troublesome in infants and children. In such instances the ointment formulations will represent a better choice. Solutions may be preferred for use in the pubic region if pubic hair is thick and matted.

Generally a 30-g tube can be ordered. It provides treatment for about 2 weeks, which is about as long as a steroid product should be used without physician review. Steroid products are best applied twice daily; more frequent use does not result in faster or better response.

TOPICAL ANTIFUNGAL AND ANTICANDIDAL AGENTS

The number of available topical agents in this group has increased dramatically in the last several years (Table 3-2). Fortunately nearly all of the newer agents, regardless of Food and Drug Administration (FDA) labeling, are effective against both *Candida* spp. and dermatophyte fungal infections. This is in contrast to the older products nystatin (effective only against yeasts) and tolnaftate (effective only against dermatophyte fungi). For this reason, and also because of lesser efficacy, these two older agent are no longer often used.

These products are packaged in a variety of ways, but all of them are available as creams, which is the preferred form in which they are applied to the external genitalia and perigenital skin. Twice daily appli-

Table 3-2. Topical Antifungal and Anticandidal Products

Generic Name	*Brand Name*	*Prescription Status*[a]	Labeling[b]
Miconazole 2%	Micatin	OTC	D, C
	Monistat	OTC	D, C
Clotrimazole 1%	Gyne-Lotrimin	OTC	C
	Lotrimin	OTC	D, C
	Mycelex	OTC	D, C
Butoconazole 2%	Femstat	Rx	C
Ciclopirox 1%	Loprox	Rx	D, C
Econazole 1%	Spectazole	Rx	D, C
Haloprogin 1%	Halotex	Rx	D
Ketoconazole 2%	Nizoral	Rx	D, C
Naftifine 1%	Naftin	Rx	D
Sulconazole 1%	Excelderm	Rx	D
Terconazole 0.4%	Terazol	Rx	C
Terbinafine	Lamisil	Rx	D

[a] OTC, over the counter; Rx, prescription.
[b] D, dermatophyte; C, candidal.

cations are sufficient to obtain full effectiveness. A course of treatment is generally 2 to 3 weeks.

TOPICAL ANTIBIOTICS

In a few instances the use of topically applied antibiotics might be considered: bacterial folliculitis, erythrasma, impetigo, and secondarily infected (impetiginized) dermatologic disease.

Neomycin, bacitracin, and polymyxin B (plus various combinations of these agents such as Neosporin, polysporin, and so forth) have a wide spectrum of effectiveness. They are also inexpensive and are available over the counter. Contact allergy has been reported with their use, but at the practical level, especially for short-term application, this is not a contraindication unless a past history of allergic reaction is obtained. Generally these products are packaged as ointments; for this reason they should be applied sparingly two or three times a day, lest maceration (see above) occur under a thick film layer.

Mupirocin (Bactroban) represents the topical antibiotic of choice for persistent or recurring staphylococcal disease. Almost no strains of staphylococcal species are resistant to it, and allergic sensitization does not occur. It is available only by prescription and is quite expensive.

TOPICAL ANTIPRURITIC AGENTS

Pruritus occurs with or without the presence of associated visible disease. Pruritus associated with visible skin disease is most effectively treated with topically applied steroids. These agents, because of their anti-inflammatory effect, reduce the mediators that are responsible for the sensation of itching. Topical steroids are discussed earlier in this chapter.

Pruritus occurring in the absence of visible disease ("idiopathic" or "essential" pruritus) is much harder to control. Several topical agents have been supported by one authority or another, although in our hands they are of limited value. These include pramoxine (Prax), crotamiton (Eurax), antihistamines (Benadryl, Caladryl), and analgesics (Americaine, Xylocaine). Several of these are also formulated in combination with topical steroids, but data to support a synergistic effect are lacking. Many of these products are irritating when applied; safety, however, with the exception of occasional contact sensitivity to benzocaine (Amercaine and other products) and diphenhydramine (Benadryl), is excellent. Thus, questions of efficacy aside, little is lost in a therapeutic trial.

TOPICAL SEX HORMONES

Several forms of estrogen are available for intravaginal use. These include conjugated equine estrogens (Premarin cream), estradiol (Estrace cream, estropipate (Ogen cream), and dienestrol (Ortho Dienestrol) cream. These products are widely and appropriately used for vaginal dryness and atrophy when estrogen replacement is biologically desirable. On the other hand, use of these products for extravaginal conditions is limited to reduction of acquired labial adhesion in infants and children, symptomatic treatment of urethral caruncles, and (possibly) some types of vulvar atrophy. Further discussion of topical estrogen products can be found in standard gynecologic textbooks.

Topically applied progesterone has historically been recommended for the treatment of lichen sclerosus in prepubertal girls and as an alternative to testosterone in treating older women. No commercial product is available for this use, but a 0.5 to 1.0 percent preparation can be formulated by the pharmacist. Limited data are available on both the safety and efficacy of this product; we have not found the product to be useful.

Topically applied testosterone propionate has represented the treatment of choice for adult women with lichen sclerosus, at least until recently. Here, too, no commercial product is available, but a 2 percent preparation can be made up in either Aquaphor or petrolatum. It is usually applied two or three time a day for several months before improvement is noted; thereafter the frequency of application can be reduced to maintain the progress obtained. Testosterone is readily absorbed and serum levels become quite high, but side effects are surprisingly infrequent and mild. Hair growth on the upper lip, increase in libido, deepening of voice, and clitoral enlargement represent the problems most often reported. Women should be warned not to use the product if pregnancy occurs.

TOPICAL CYTOTOXIC AGENTS

Podophyllin Resin

Podophyllin resin is a cytotoxic agent that has been used for many years in the treatment of genital warts. The product has historically been made up as 20 percent podophyllin resin in tincture of benzoin. It is applied, by the clinician, to all visible warts with a cotton-tipped applicator. The product is then washed away by the patient 2 to 8 hours later. Reapplications are generally necessary at 2- to 3-week intervals. Both the efficacy and the degree to which patients develop troublesome, irritant reactions are highly variable.

For this reason Condylox, a product containing 0.5 percent podofilox (the active ingredient in podophyllin resin), was developed. This agent is applied by the patient at home twice daily for 3 consecutive days; after 4 days with no application, the cycle is repeated. Efficacy is at least as good as with the older, crude product; irritant reactions are less troublesome, and, because it is applied at home, patient satisfaction is better. Neither of the podophyllin products should be used in pregnancy because of possible toxicity to the fetus. Care should be taken not to use large amounts of podophylin, especially in the vagina, because of absorption and potential resultant neurotoxicity.

Fluorouracil

Fluorouracil is a cytotoxic agent originally used intravenously for the treatment of certain malignancies. More recently it has been used in the topical treatment of premalignant actinic keratoses and for warts of several types. The product comes in 1 percent (Fluoroplex) or 5 percent (Efudex) creams and solutions. The product most widely used for the treatment of genital warts has been the 5 percent cream. For warts on the external genitalia, it is applied twice daily until an irritant reaction begins to develop (generally 2 to 5 days), at which point the frequency of application is reduced to once daily. For vaginal warts, the cream is placed in a standard vaginal applicator; one half an applicator is inserted in the vagina in various dosing schedules, from nightly to weekly (our preference), to avoid severe irritant effects. To avoid leakage onto the vulva, a tampon can subsequently be inserted.

Treatment with flurouracil is continued for 3 or more weeks. Irritant reactions occur in all patients, and at times they can be quite severe. Data supporting the efficacy of topically applied fluorouracil (used as the sole treatment for genital warts) are very limited. Currently it is most popularly used as adjuvant therapy following laser or electrosurgical destruction of anogenital warts.

INTRALESIONAL TREATMENT

Intralesional treatment, in which medication is introduced by injection directly into the lesion, offers the advantage of a high concentration of medication locally while minimizing systemic side effects.

Intralesional injection bypasses the relatively impervious keratinized surface (barrier layer) of the skin. For this reason intralesional injection is important when disease occurs on nonmucosal surfaces. It is much less often used in the treatment of genital disease both because there is so little barrier to the penetration of creams and ointments but also because the rich nerve supply of genital skin and mucosae makes injection very uncomfortable unless the area has been pretreated with a topical anesthetic such as eutectic mixture of local anesthesia (EMLA) or 2 to 5 percent xylocaine (Lidocaine) ointment.

Intralesional Corticosteroids

In addition to delivering a high concentration of medication to a specific site, intralesional corticosteroids provide very fine control over the area of treatment. Although a higher potency topical corticosteroid cream may be appropriate to use in affected thick skin, creams tend to spread to surrounding thinner genital skin, where they are likely to cause atrophy and other local adverse reactions.

Intralesional corticosteroids serve two purposes in the treatment of skin disease. In a higher concentration a product like triamcinolone acetonide (Kenalog) 10 mg/ml, corticosteroids are useful for thinning lesions (such as hypertrophic scars and limited areas of extreme lichenification) that are too thick to be penetrated easily by topical corticosteroids. In lower concentrations, preparations like triamcinolone acetonide 3 mg/ml are effective anti-inflammatory agents for conditions such as an inflamed cyst or a pruritic trigger point that is too deep for easy penetration by a topical cream. Three tenths of a milliliter of the commercial preparation of triamcinolone acetonide (Kenalog) 10 mg/ml is mixed with 0.7 ml of normal saline in a 1-ml syringe to obtain this anti-inflammatory concentration.

In making the injection, the needle is inserted parallel to the surface of the skin such that the needle point lies just below the surface of the lesion. The technique is similar to that used for tuberculin skin testing. Moderate resistance should be felt as the solution is injected. If there is little resistance, the tip of the needle is too deep, and the material will be ineffectively injected into the subcutaneous tissue.

The primary adverse reactions of intralesional corticosteroids are atrophy and hypopigmentation. These side effects occur most often when higher concentrations or a larger volume of triamcinolone are used and when the injection is very superficial. Hypopigmentation is most obvious and distressful in dark-skinned individuals, and it can be long-lasting.

Intralesional α-Interferon

Intralesional α-interferon is used in the treatment of genital warts and vulvar vestibulitis. The interferons (α, β, and γ) are naturally occurring proteins that normally function as part of the immune system. α-Interferon exhibits antiviral, antiproliferative, and immune-enhancing properties. The three available α-interferon preparations, recombinant α-interferons 2b and 2a (Intron A and Roferon-A) and natural human α-interferon (Alferon N) are probably equal in efficacy, safety, and cost, but direct comparison trials have not been reported. These medications have been studied with different doses, dosing schedules, and injection techniques. However, basic treatment principles and side effects can be generalized to apply to all available forms of interferon, and the details for the treatment of genital warts can be obtained from the package insert. For more information on interferon's use for vulvar pain, see Chapter 21.

The interferon molecule is fragile, so vigorous shaking of the vial should be avoided since it can inactivate the medication. α-Interferon 2b is the only preparation that requires reconstitution, and care should be taken to use only the 10-million-unit vial for intralesional use to avoid a hypertonic solution. A subpotent intralesional medication is produced unless 1 ml of the 2 ml of diluent provided is used. Although any injection is uncomfortable, interferon is not particularly painful when injected, especially when a 30-gauge needle is used. Some patients prefer the use of a topical anesthetic such as lidocaine jelly 2 percent, lidocaine ointment 5 percent, or EMLA applied for 20 to 30 minutes before treatment, while other patients feel that the minimal injection pain, the initial burning from the anesthetic in some, and the limited efficacy of topical lidocaine alone do not warrant the extra time required.

Most patients develop one or more flulike side effects beginning about 4 hours after the first treatment and lasting 4 to 6 hours. These symptoms include fever, headache, myalgias, chills, malaise, nausea, and fatigue. The usual flulike side effects are minimized with acetaminophen administered at the time of the injection and every 4 hours during the next 12 hours. The first injection should be given late in the day so that symptoms occur at night. Symptoms will disappear by the next morning, and significant side effects are unusual after the first treatment unless there is a lapse of 1 week or more between injections. Although a decrease in white blood cell counts occurs in about 15 percent of patients, this is never clinically significant, and even patients with the acquired immunodeficiency syndrome are treated routinely with interferon.

The exact dose and dosing schedule of α-interferon depends upon the disease to be treated and which preparation is used. When genital warts are treated, the doses and schedules in *Physicians' Desk Reference* are appropriate, and details of therapy for vulvar vestibulitis are found in Chapter 21.

Intralesional Alcohol Injections

Some clinicians use alcohol injections to destroy nerves in areas of well-localized, persistent pruritus refractory to topical therapies. Alcohol injections are not beneficial for pain syndromes and may even exacerbate them.

The disadvantages of this therapy include the necessity of general anesthesia to prevent extreme pain with injection, the occasional sloughing of skin and subcutaneous tissue, and the recurrence of symptoms secondary to the regeneration of nerves. Because of these drawbacks, alcohol injections should be used only rarely and then as a last resort with careful patient education and understanding of the limitations and adverse reactions of the procedure.

ORAL AND INTRAMUSCULAR CORTICOSTEROIDS

Corticosteroids may be administered systemically if an adequate response cannot be obtained with topical or intralesional steroid treatment. This is most likely to happen in patients with chronic itching and scratching (lichen simplex chronicus), but systemic steroids are warranted in most patients with immunobullous disease and in some with lichen planus.

Systemic steroids are used on a short-term basis ("burst therapy") in the treatment of lichen simplex chronicus. Generally prednisone is given in a dose of 40 mg orally each day for 7 to 10 days. The entire dose is taken in the early morning to reduce the suppressive effect on the pituitary-adrenal axis. If prednisone is given for less than 14 days, no tapering of the dose is necessary. Some clinicians taper the dose anyway, believing that this approach reduces rebound of disease activity. Many generalists use Medrol Dosepaks for steroid burst therapy, but dermatologists usually find that this 5-day, tapered dose is insufficient and unnecessarily expensive.

Alternatively, corticosteroids can be administered intramuscularly. Triamcinolone in the form of Kenalog-40 is most often used because of the depot effect provided by this preparation. The usual dose is 60 to 80 mg given deep into the upper outer quadrant of the buttock. Maximum effect is reached in about 3 to 4 days, with some effect still present for an additional 2 weeks. In terms of therapeutic equivalence, 80 mg of triamcinolone IM is about the same as 20 to 30 mg PO of prednisone administered for 1 week. Intramuscular administration of triamcinolone allows for better physician control over usage and is probably associated with fewer side effects.

Side effects are rarely encountered when steroids are given in short-term therapy as described above. Increases in blood pressure and glucose levels may occur in patients with preexisting hypertension and diabetes, respectively. An increase in appetite and some tendency to retain water are occasionally noted. Mild euphoria and agitation may also be experienced. Women may develop menorrhagia, especially after intramuscular triamcinolone.

Long-term systemic steroid therapy is occasionally required for immunobullous disease and vulvovaginal lichen planus; the use of steroids in these two situations will be discussed separately in each disease section.

ORAL ANTIBACTERIAL AGENTS

The most commonly encountered bacterial infections of the genitalia and perigenital skin are folliculitis, furunculosis, cellulitis, impetigo, and impetiginized eczematous disease. These are almost always staphylococcal in origin and will respond to standard therapy directed toward *Staphylococcus aureus* organisms. Dermatologists generally prefer to use dicloxacillin or erythromycin for these infections, but the incidence of erythromycin-resistant staphylococcal organisms seems to be increasing. Others find that Keflex, ampicillin, amoxicillin or Augmentin also work well. All of these agents are used in similar dosage: 250 mg taken four times a day. Therapy for minor infections can be discontinued in 5 to 7 days; more serious infections should be treated for 10 to 14 days.

Side effects are rarely a problem with these agents. The use of erythromycin is sometimes associated with gastrointestinal problems, but even this is usually not severe enough to require disruption of therapy. Care should, of course, be taken not to use any of the penicillin derivatives when a past history of allergic reaction is present. In this situation, Keflex or erythromycin can be used. For more serious infections, it may be necessary to consider ciprofloxacin (Cipro) in a dose of 500 mg twice daily or the new erythromycin-like drugs, clarithromycin (Biaxin) or azithromycin (Zithromax).

Streptococcal infections are less often encountered and will respond to the same agents discussed above. Therapy for the bacterial sexually transmitted diseases will be discussed in the chapter sections dealing with each condition.

Dermatologists use antibiotics as nonsteroidal anti-inflammatory drugs. Tetracycline and erythromycin (both at 500 mg twice a day) are very effectively for acne and other sterile pustular diseases. Doxycycline (Vibramycin) and minocycline (Minocin), in a dose of 100 mg twice daily, work as well, or better, for this purpose. Sunlight sensitivity (in the case of doxycycline) and high cost (in the case of minocycline) limit the frequency with which these agents are used.

ORAL ANTICANDIDAL AND ANTIFUNGAL AGENTS

Griseofulvin

Griseofulvin was the first of the antifungal agents, and it remains in widespread use today. It has a fairly narrow spectrum of activity and is only effective against dermatophyte fungal infections. It represents the treatment of choice for dermatophyte fungal folliculitis and for those cases of tinea cruris unresponsive to topical antifungal therapy.

Two types of griseofulvin are available. The older preparation is termed "microsized" because the particle size was smaller than the original product. It can be ordered generically. The newer preparation has an even smaller particle size (ultramicrosized), and it is solubilized in polyethylene glycol (Gris-PEG, Fulvicin P/G). The dosage for the former is 500 mg twice daily; that for the solubilized form is 250 or 330 mg twice daily. Both forms should be taken with meals. Treatment for fungal folliculitis and tinea cruris requires about 3 weeks of medication.

Mild gastrointestinal upset and headaches occur fairly often; urticaria and photosensitivity reactions develop in less than 1 percent of patients taking the drug. Griseofulvin is contraindicated in patients with porphyria and should be used with caution in patients with liver problems. It also interacts with warfarin-type anticoagulants. Laboratory testing is not necessary for patients taking the drug for only a few weeks.

Ketoconazole

Ketoconazole (Nizoral) is effective against both yeast and dermatophyte fungi. Interestingly, it also has some antiandrogen and corticosteroid-like effects in doses higher than those used for its antimicrobial effect. Ketoconazole may be used for fungal infections resistant to griseofulvin and may be necessary in some cases of chronic or chronically recurring vulvovaginal yeast infections.

Ketoconazole comes as a 200-mg tablet; the usual dose is 200 mg each morning. The length of treatment for yeast infections may be as short as a few days to as long as few months (see discussions of candidiasis in Chs. 5 and 7). When used for fungal infections, treatment duration is about 3 weeks.

Side effects are few, with two exceptions. First, very rare, severe idiosyncratic hepatotoxic reactions have been reported, and for this reason long-term therapy with this agent is discouraged; if used for more than 3 weeks, liver function studies should be obtained on a regular basis. Second, a number of drug interactions occur. Specifically, erythromycin and the nonsedating antihistamines terfenadine and astemizole should not be used concomitantly with ketoconazole.

Fluconazole

Fluconazole is a triazole antifungal agent somewhat related to ketoconazole. Currently it is not labeled in the United States for use in mucocutaneous yeast or fungal infections, but nevertheless, it is used rather widely for nonsystemic infection.

Fluconazole has a long serum half-life. This allows for intermittent dosing (a good thing, considering its very high cost) but has also led to great variability in recommended dosage schedules. Thus as little as a single dose of 150 mg has been used in uncomplicated candidal vulvovaginitis, whereas 50 mg a day or 100 mg every other day have been suggested for chronic yeast and dermatophyte infections.

Side effects occur infrequently. Hepatotoxicity, such as is seen with ketoconazole, is not a problem. It is not clear whether the drug can be used in patients taking erythromycin or nonsedating antihistamines, but because of its chemical similarity it is probably wise to avoid its use when these other drugs are being taken. Other drug interactions do occur, and appropriate precautions in this regard should be taken before prescribing the drug.

Itraconazole

Itraconazole is a new azole that has been labeled in the United States only for histoplasmosis and blastomycosis. Nevertheless, studies in other countries indicate that it is quite effective in candidal and dermatophyte infections. It is similar to ketoconazole in terms of drug interactions, but no significant hepatotoxicity has been reported. Its role in treating various diseases discussed in this textbook has not yet been determined.

ORAL ANTIVIRAL AGENTS

Acyclovir (Zovirax) is an antiviral agent specifically effective in the treatment of infections due to herpes simplex virus (HSV) and varicella zoster virus (VZV). It can truly be said that its availability has revolutionized the treatment of recurring genital herpes.

Good results in the treatment of genital herpes require that acyclovir be started within 24 to 36 hours after symptoms have first occurred. Unfortunately, patients often do not seek medical attention that quickly and thus for practical purposes the drug has had little impact on the treatment of primary cases of HSV infection. However, when taken prophylactically, the drug is extremely effective in preventing recurring outbreaks of genital disease.

The dose of acyclovir used for primary herpes simplex infection is one 200-mg capsule PO five times a day. Generally, treatment is carried out for about 10 days. This regimen decreases both discomfort and the time to healing if it can be started sufficiently soon after symptoms have first developed.

The dosage used to prevent recurrences of genital herpes is 400 mg two times a day. This dose can sometimes be reduced further after efficacy at the higher dose has been documented. Suppressive therapy for recurring disease has demonstrated to be effective for at least 5 years.

The use of acyclovir on a prophylactic basis presumably reduces the quantity of virus shed asymptomatically, but it probably does not eliminate it. For this reason, patients should take appropriate precautions to prevent unexpected transmission of the disease even in the absence of clinical symptoms and signs.

A larger dose of acyclovir is necessary for the treatment of VZV infections. Specifically, adequate treatment of herpes zoster (shingles) requires 800 mg five times a day for ten to 14 days. An 800-mg capsule has recently become available. Unfortunately, treatment with acyclovir does not appear to decrease significantly the incidence or severity of post-herpetic neuralgia.

The use of oral acyclovir in the doses discussed above is, for practical purposes, unassociated with significant side effects. Resistance of herpesviruses to the drug rarely, if ever, occurs in immunocompetent patients.

ORAL ANTIPRURITIC, ANALGESIC, AND PSYCHOTROPIC AGENTS

Antihistamines

Antihistamines are the most widely used oral antipruritic agents. They achieve their effect through two different mechanisms.

First, antihistamines have an effect at the mucocutaneous level. Histamine is released during the course of some inflammatory conditions. Antagonists of histamines block this effect at the site of inflammation. The importance of this local effect is most notable in urticaria and angioedema. Second, antihistamines have a central mode of action. The exact mechanism through which these drugs alleviate pruritus at the central nervous system (CNS) level is unknown, but only those antihistamines that have a sedating effect seem to be useful. Possibly the receptors for itch are similar in type to those for sedation.

Diphenhydramine (Benadryl) is the antihistamine most widely used in the treatment of pruritus. The conventional dose is 25 mg PO taken four times a day, but better effect, with less daytime sedation, can be obtained if the medication is given primarily at suppertime or in the early evening. Thus the entire dose (from as little as 25 mg to as much as 200 mg) can be given at a single point in time. Specifically, the sounder sleep induced with this medication schedule significantly reduces nighttime scratching and helps interrupt the "itch-scratch" cycle (see atopic/neurodermatitis in Ch. 5).

Other antihistamines work equally well. Dermatologists especially favor hydroxyzine (Atarax, Vistaril) given in the same dose and schedule as described for diphenhydramine above. Chlorpheniramine (Chlor-Trimeton) and cyproheptadine (Periactin) may also be used. The dosage for both is 4 to 24 mg taken in the evening as indicated above. As noted previously, the nonsedating antihistamines terfenadine (Seldane), astemizole (Hismanal), and claritidine (Claritin), while effective for the pruritus associated with urticaria, have little or no effect on other types of itching.

Analgesics

Analgesics, as used for standard types of pain, will not be covered here, but note the beneficial effect of the tricyclic antidepressants (see below) in chronic pain unresponsive to classical analgesics. These agents are particularly valuable in treating postherpetic neuralgia, vulvodynia, and other genital pain syndromes.

Psychotropic Medications

Psychotropic medications are remarkably helpful in treating several of the diseases discussed in this mongraph. First, they can have a powerful effect on pruritus, and second, they may be the only medications helpful in treating chronic mucocutaneous pain.

Tricyclic Antidepressants

The tricyclic antidepressants such as amitriptyline (Elavil) and doxepin (Adapin, Sinequan) happen to also be excellent antihistamines. This may account for some of their effectiveness in the treatment of itching. However, because they also have sedative side effects, a CNS effect on pruritus is probably more important (see Antihistamines above). Since depression occurs in patients with chronic disease of all types, these agents might also work directly through a mechanism of mood elevation. Interestingly, however, they tend to work more quickly and at lower doses than is necessary for the treatment of depression. Side effects, in addition to sedation, include dryness (mouth and eyes), constipation and nighttime problems with balance in the elderly. A significant minority of patients experience weight gain due to an increased appetite. These drugs are not habituating.

Amitriptyline and doxepin are given in identical dosages. The starting dose is 10 to 25 mg given in the early evening. This is gradually increased until pruritus is relieved or side effects prohibit further increase, or until a total dose of 150 mg is reached. Most patients require only 25 to 75 mg. These tricyclic agents also have a good effect on certain types of pain unrelieved by classic analgesics. For this reason, they are widely used (in the same dose as for pruritus) in the treatment of postherpetic neuralgia, vulvodynia, and other genital pain syndromes.

Anxiolytic Agents

Patients with recalcitrant pruritus often have high levels of anxiety. In such situations anxiolytic agents can be quite helpful. Classically, benzodiazepines have been used for this purpose. Diazepam (Valium) can be given orally in doses of 5 to 10 mg twice daily or in a total dose of 10 mg in the early evening if daytime drowsiness presents a problem. More recently, the shorter acting product alprazolam (Xanax) has become quite widely used in an oral dosage of 0.25 mg two or three times a day. These agents should not be used for more than about 3 consecutive weeks because of the risk of habituation; side effects are not otherwise very troublesome.

Buspirone (Buspar) is an antianxiety agent unrelated to the benzodiazepines. In addition, it has a low incidence of drowsiness and it does not appear to be habituating. Some patients experience mild dizziness or agitation when they start therapy, but this decreases after several days of medication. The starting dose is 10 mg a day increased to 10 mg two to three times a day over a period of about 2 weeks. Buspirone is probably less effective than the benzodiazepines, but its safety makes it a very attractive alternative.

ORAL RETINOIDS

The audience to whom this book is directed will not have much reason to use these agents, but a short discussion is warranted because of their increasing use for dermatologic diseases (psoriasis, lichen planus, and so forth) that may effect the genitalia and perigenital skin. Retinoids are derivatives of vitamin A and have a remarkable array of effects on keratinization, cell differentiation, inflammation, and the immune system. In addition, they have some antioncogenic effect.

Unfortunately, side effects occur frequently and may be quite severe. These include cheilitis, dryness of the eyes, skin chapping, hair loss, myalgia, arthralgia, and photosensitivity. In addition, retinoids are mildly hepatotoxic and tend to elevate serum cholesterol and triglyceride levels. Most importantly, they are the most potent teratogens used in clinical medicine today. They must never be used unless there is absolute assurance that pregancy is not present and will not occur during treatment.

Isotretinoin (Accutane) is used primarily for the treatment of acne, but because of its short half-life it is also used in place of etretinate when retinoids are warranted in women of child-bearing age. The usual dose is 40 mg taken orally twice daily; higher doses are sometimes indicated. Etretinate (Tegison) is the agent most often used for psoriasis and lichen planus. The usual dose is 25 mg taken two or three times a day. Etretinate remains stored in body fat for years; this means that any toxicity encountered lasts for a long time after the drug is discontinued. Additional material on the use of these drugs will be found in individual disease sections.

ORAL IMMUNOSUPRESSIVE AND CYTOTOXIC AGENTS

Corticosteroids administered systemically are among the most potent immunosupressive drugs used. Discussion of corticosteroids can be found earlier in this chapter. Methotrexate is the cytotoxic agent most often used in the treatment of mucocutaneous disease; additional discussion of this agent will be found in Chapter 6, Psoriasis. The systemic use of other agents such as cyclosporine and azathioprine, although important in the care of some of the diseases discussed in this book, is not covered in this chapter.

SUGGESTED READINGS

Lubricants

Lazar AP, Lazar P: Dry skin, water, and lubrication. Dermatol Clin 9:45, 1991

This review article covers the entire subject of skin lubrication but there is little information on specific products.

Topical Corticosteroids

Maibach HI: Bioequivalence of topical corticosteroids. Int J Dermatol 31:1, 1992 suppl 1.

This whole supplement is devoted to the subject of topical steroids. There is more technical detail than a clinician will need but there is good discussion about relative steroids strengths.

Topical Antifungal and Anticandidal Agents

Lesher JL, Smith JG Jr: Antifungal agents in dermatology. J Am Acad Dermatol 17:383, 1987

Although a bit outdated, this article contains good material on some of the older topical agents.

Topical Antibiotics

Hirschmann JV: Topical antibiotics in dermatology. Arch Dermatol 124:1691, 1988

This review article covers the various agents available (including Mupirocin) and the indications for their use.

Topical Sex Hormones

Bracco GL, Carli P, Sonni L, et al: Clinical and histologic effects of topical treatments of vulval lichen sclerosus. A critical evaluation. J Reproduct Med 38:37, 1993

This article discusses topical testosterone and progesterone. A comparison is made in a randomized study between these topical sex hormones and high potency corticosteroids.

Serrano G, Millan F, Fortea JM et al: Topical progesterone as treatment of choice in genital lichen sclerosis (sic) et atrophicus in children. Pediatr Dermatol 10:201, 1993

Topical Cytotoxic Agents

Marcus J, Camisa C: Podophyllin therapy for condyloma acuminatum. Internat J Dermatol 29:693, 1990

This review article covers the various types and methods of use of podophyllin.

Intralesional Treatment

Friedrich EG Jr: p. 71. Vulvar Disease. 2nd Ed. WB Saunders, Philadelphia, 1983

This book section describes the practical specifics of alcohol injections of the vulva.

Stadler R, Mayer-da-Silva A, Bratzke B et al: Interferons in dermatology. J Am Acad Dermatol 20:650, 1989

This article briefly reviews background information and the mechanisms of action of interferon, and then summarizes the literature regarding effectiveness of α-interferon in skin diseases, primarily condylomata acuminata.

Oral and Intramuscular Corticosteroids

Arnold Jr HL: Oral prednisone-an illogical therapy. Int J Dermatol 26:286, 1987

Dr. Arnold was the foremost proponent of the use of intramuscular depot steroids. He outlines his arguments regarding efficacy and safety of this approach in this older article.

Gallant C, Kenny P: Oral glucocorticoids and their complications. J Am Acad Dermatol 14:161, 1986

Although the article was published almost 10 years ago, most of the material in it is up-to-date and usable today.

Oral Antibacterial Agents

Wilkowske CJ: General principles of antimicrobial therapy Mayo Clin Proc 66:931, 1991

This article is the first of a series of review articles on antimicrobial therapy published over several months in Mayo Clinic Proceedings. This opening manuscript provides a good overview of the various agents available together with the most common indications for their use.

Oral Anticandidal and Antifungal Agents

Jacobs PH, Nall L: Systemic antifungals. Cutis 52:165, 1993

Additional material on agents useful in yeast infections can be found in this reference.

Stiller MJ, Sangueza OP, Shupak JL: Systemic drugs in the treatment of dermatophytoses. Int J Dermatol 32:16, 1993

This article reviews those agents useful in the treatment of dermatophyte infections but there is an appreciable overlap in the usefulness of these agents for the treatment of candidiasis as well.

Oral Antiviral Agents

Whitely RJ, Gnann JW Jr: Acyclovir: a decade later. N Engl J Med 327:782, 1992

This review covers all aspects of the use of acyclovir.

Oral Antipruritic, Analgesic, and Psychotropic agents

Floweres FP, Araujo OE, Nieves CH: Antihistamines. Int J Dermatol 25:224, 1986

This review article covers the older antihistamines to include their use as antipruritic agents.

Goldsmith P, Dowd PM: The new H_1 antihistamines. Dermatol clinics 11:87, 1993.

This article reviews the new nonsedating antihistamines that unfortunately, are not effective in the relief of pruritus except in situations where the pruritus arises as a result of an urticarial reaction.

Koo JYM: The use of psychotropic medications in clinical dermatology. Dermatol Clin 10:641, 1992

This article represents a thorough review of agents used for anxiety and depression.

Oral Retinoids

Shalita AR: Introduction-retinoids: present and future. J Am Acad Dermatol 27:S1, 1992

This is the first article in a series of nine, all contained in this supplement, that deal with various aspects of retinoid therapy.

4 Principles of Problem-Oriented Diagnosis

PRINCIPLES OF MORPHOLOGIC DIAGNOSIS

Most textbooks organize the diseases covered on the basis of etiology or pathogenesis, or both. Thus, for example, infectious diseases are considered in one chapter and malignancies in another. This is an intellectually satisfying way of classifying disease, but any book using this system can only be used as a reference source *if you already know the diagnosis.* For this reason we have elected to use a morphologic, problem-oriented approach.

The diseases in Chapters 5 through 21 are classified on the basis of morphology. That is, diseases that look alike are grouped together. This approach allows a clinician, on the basis of physical examination, to turn to the section of the book covering the specific diseases that share the patient's disease morphology. Then, after a quick perusal of the photographs and the paragraphs describing the clinical features, one can establish either a single best diagnosis or a short list of differential diagnoses. In most instances it is even possible to arrive at a correct diagnosis when the disease in question has never been encountered previously.

An overview of this organizational structure is contained in Table 4-1. The major sections are separated on the basis of color and lesional type; within these sections there are 17 groups of disease. These 17 groups are arranged in chapters; the diseases contained within each of these groups are listed at the start of each chapter. Some of the morphologic terms used in this schema may be unfamiliar to nondermatologists; for this reason they are defined below. Additional material on the philosophy and use of problem-oriented dermatologic diagnosis may be found in *Dermatology for the House Officer* and *Principles and Practice of Dermatology.*

DEFINITIONS

The world of dermatologic terminology is a foreign one to most physicians. However, as is true for all foreign languages, a very small number of words will allow for surprisingly good communication. The following list of words, modified from a similar list in *Principles and Practice of Dermatology,* will enable any clinician to have a clear understanding of the basic dermatologic terms used in the description of mucocutaneous disease. (For a more complete listing, see Glossary.)

A **macule** represents a small area of color change. As such, a macule is not palpable. Generally macules are less than 1.5 cm in diameter. The surface of a macule is usually smooth, but sometimes a small amount of fine scale is present.

A **patch** is an extension of a macule in length and width. Thus a patch is a nonpalpable area of color change 1.5 cm or larger in diameter. Again, the surface is usually smooth but fine scale is sometimes recognizable.

A **papule** is a small palpable lesion less than 1.5 cm in diameter. Some dermatologists require that a lesion be elevated in order to be termed a papule, but we and others believe that there are intracutaneous papules that are palpable even though not elevated.

Table 4-1. Problem-Oriented Diagnosis of Anogenital Disease

Red plaques, papules, and nodules
Red plaques with eczematous features
Red plaques with papulosquamous features
Vulvovaginitis and balanitis
Red papules and nodules
Skin-colored and white lesions
Skin-colored papules
Skin-colored nodules
White patches and plaques
Brown, blue, and black lesions
Dark-colored papules and nodules
Pigmented patches and generalized pigmentation
Pustules, vesicles, bullae, and erosions
Pustules and pseudopustules
Vesicular disease
Bullous disease
Ulcers
Infectious primary ulcers
Noninfectious primary ulcers
Ulcerated nodules and plaques
Pruritis and Pain
Anogenital pruritus
Anogenital pain

The surface of papules may be smooth (nonscaling) or rough (scaling).

A **plaque,** by analogy to a patch, is an enlargement of a papule in two dimensions: length and width. That is, a plaque represents a planar extension of a papule. Most plaques are elevated, but as noted for papules, some are intracutaneous and palpable but not elevated. Plaques may be smooth (nonscaling) or rough (scaling).

A **vesicle** is a small blister less than 1 cm in diameter. Conceptually it can be considered as a fluid-filled papule in which the fluid is loculated. (A fluid-filled papule with nonloculated fluid is a wheal or hive.) If a vesicle is incised, fluid runs out and the compartment collapses. When the roof of a vesicle has been removed or has disintegrated, an underlying erosion remains visible.

A **pustule** is a vesicle that is packed with neutrophils. The fluid in a pustule (pus) is white or yellow-white. Vesicles may accumulate a few neutrophils with the passage of time and thus appear cloudy. These cloudy vesicles are not pustules; a pustule by definition must be opaquely white both presently and from the time of its inception.

A **bulla** is a large vesicle that is 1 cm or more in diameter. The fluid in a bulla is usually contained in a single compartment, but occasionally clustered vesicles and bullae coalesce to form *multiloculated* bullae.

An **erosion** is a shallow defect in the skin; it occurs when the overlying epithelium is destroyed or removed. Primary erosions arise as a result of trauma —usually scratching. These erosions are linear or angular in shape and lack the collarlike remnants ("collarette") of a blister roof at the periphery. Secondary erosions arise when a blister roof breaks down or is removed. These erosions are round and regularly have a collarette of scale encircling the defect. The surface of an erosion may be "clean" and red or may be covered with crust. A *fissure* is a special type of an erosion that forms as a thin crack between adjacent islands of intact epithelial cells. Fissures form when clusters of epithelial cells shrink due to dryness. They may be viewed as analogous to the cracking seen at the bottom of a dried lake bed.

An **ulcer** also represents a defect in the skin, but the defect is deeper than that occurring in an erosion. Dermal connective tissue and blood vessels are destroyed, leaving fibrin and old blood pigment (heme) at the base. For this reason the crusts formed within an ulcer are dark and adherent.

Scale represents a buildup of the flattened, dead, superficial keratinizing cells—the stratum corneum. Since mucosal epithelium does not keratinize, scale is normally not found on mucosal lesions. Scale is palpable as roughness on the surface of lesions and sometimes is visible as small white flakes. Scale is obscured when the surface of the lesion is wet (as so often happens in genital and perigenital locations) or when greasy medications or lubricants have been applied.

Crust occurs when plasma exudes through a missing or damaged epithelial surface. It represents the dried serum proteins that remain when plasma water has evaporated. Crust feels rough on palpation. Crust differs in appearance from scale because crust is amorphous (rather than disclike) and is yellow, or because of brown, blue, or black heme pigment.

SUGGESTED READINGS

Lynch PJ: Problem-oriented algorithm. In: Dermatology for the House Officer. 3rd Ed. Williams & Wilkins, Baltimore, 1994.

Lynch PJ: Problem-oriented diagnosis. p. 27. In Sams Wm Jr, Lynch PJ (eds): Principles and Practice of Dermatology. Churchill Livingstone, New York, 1990.

II Red Plaques, Papules, and Nodules

5 Red Plaques with Eczematous Features

The diseases considered in this chapter are characterized morphologically by the presence of red plaques with superimposed features of epithelial disruption. That is, because of damage to, or partial loss of, the epithelial barrier layer, the clinical appearance of the erythematous plaques will include some evidence of weeping, crust formation, or yellow scale. Margination of the lesions (the transition between diseased and nondiseased skin) tends to be less sharp than is true for the papulosquamous diseases discussed in the next chapter.

In the context of this chapter, the terms *eczema* and *dermatitis* are used as synonyms; thus atopic dermatitis can just as appropriately be called atopic eczema. Additional material describing the morphologic aspects of eczematous disease can be found in Chapter 4. Note that two of the conditions included in this chapter (Darier's disease and Hailey-Hailey disease) are considered in most general dermatology textbooks as papulosquamous diseases. However, probably because of the effects of maceration, the anogenital lesions in both diseases lose their papulosquamous features and take on an eczematous morphology.

ATOPIC DERMATITIS, NEURODERMATITIS, AND SQUAMOUS CELL HYPERPLASIA

A cluster of closely related diseases can be considered in this section. The degree to which they are separable and the terminology to be used depends on the physician's age, the specialty practiced, the location of specialty training, and the degree to which the physician is, philosophically, a "lumper" or a "splitter." A capsule description of each of these conditions follows, but thereafter they will be considered as a single entity using the term *atopic/neurodermatitis.*

Atopic dermatitis implies that there is a genetic predisposition to acquire certain "atopic" diseases such as hay fever, asthma, and atopic eczema. Certain cutaneous sites (especially the antecubital and popliteal fossae) are characteristically involved. The pathogenesis of atopic dermatitis is thought to depend on immunologic mechanisms including lymphocytic attack on the epidermis, heightened IgE responsiveness, and a tendency for peripheral eosinophilia.

Neurodermatitis suggests that the induction of pruritus is mediated by psychological factors and that the eruption following is directly and physicially caused by the trauma of scratching. Individuals with this condition are thought to be highly "nervous" individuals with many "type A" personality features. An atopic personal or family history is not required.

Lichen simplex chronicus is a term, beloved by dermatologists, that emphasizes the chronic nature of the condition, the morphologic feature of lichenification, and the role that habitual scratching or rubbing, or both, plays in its continuation.

Infantile eczema or *childhood eczema* are terms most often used by pediatricians. These rather general terms were used because the patients were generally too young to have developed the atopic features of hay fever or asthma. Moreover, there was no unanimity regarding psychological factors as a cause of the disease.

Hyperplastic dystrophy was the name preferred, in the setting of vulvar involvement, by the International Society for the Study of Vulvovaginal Disease (ISSVD), as published in a 1976 classification of vulvar dystrophies.[1] Uneasiness on the part of some ISSVD members with the meaning of the word *dystrophy* led to substitution of a new term *(squamous cell hyperplasia)* in a 1989 revised classification of vulvar non-neoplastic epithelial disorders.[2]

We believe that all of these eczematous conditions have three elements in common. First, itching precedes both the scratching and the subsequent appearance of inflammatory disease. This phenomenon has led to the tongue-in-cheek description of the process as the "itch that rashes." Second, when chronic disease is present, biopsy reveals a readily recognized, characteristic histologic pattern demonstrating marked epidermal acanthosis and hyperkeratosis occurring in a setting of mild to moderate lymphocytic inflammation. Third, an "itch-scratch cycle" is invariably present. Initial itching leads to a little scratching; the scratching, which many patients find pleasurable, intensifies the itching. The intensified itching leads to even more vigorous scratching. This, in turn, recreates and reinforces the cycle. Eventually a habit develops in which scratching occurs subconciously. This subconcious scratching is particularly characterized by the presence of nighttime scratching even while asleep. This itch-scratch habit becomes so ingrained that patients cannot break it by the force of willpower alone.

These important and consistently present unifying features lead to our belief that all the eczematous patterns described above can be considered as a single entity. The term we have somewhat arbitrarily chosen to use is *atopic/neurodermatitis.*

Clinical Presentation

Patients present with the complaint of intractable itching that has been present for weeks to months. Generally the process starts insidiously, although in some cases a specific trigger such as a vaginal yeast infection can be recalled as the initial event. The itching is described as worse at night; patients state that during the day they can usually avoid scratching. Identification of the itch-scratch cycle is a key point in making the diagnosis. This is done by asking the patient (or sometimes a spouse) whether or not scratching occurs without the patient being aware of it. More specifically, one can ask if scratching occurs during sleep or during sleepless intervals throughout the night. A positive answer is nearly pathognomonic in terms of diagnosis.

Patients may, on questioning, identify a personal or family history of hay fever, asthma, or childhood eczematous disease. This information is helpful if present but is not required in order to make the diagnosis.

In men, the most common areas of involvement are the anterior and posterior wall of the scrotum and the proximal, ventral aspect of the penis. In women the labia majora, labia minora, and portions of the vestibule are most often involved. The perianal area may be involved alone or in conjunction with disease elsewhere in both sexes.

The appearance on physical examination is quite variable. Patients who scratch lightly and intermittently may have no visible disease. Patients with a moderate degree of severity have at least slight inflammation (redness), and on careful examination there will be evidence of lichenification (Figs. 5-1 and 5-2) (see below). Patients with more severe disease have readily recognizable angular and linear erosions (excoriations) as a result of vigorous scratching (Fig. 5-3). In all instances, the margination of the involved patches and plaques tends to be indistinct; this is in contrast to the sharp margination of lesions found in the papulosquamous diseases (see Ch. 6).

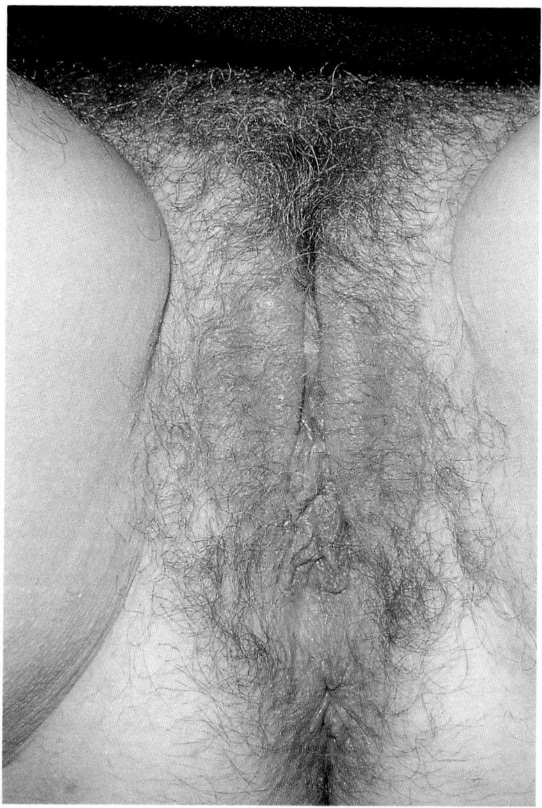

Fig. 5-1. Poorly demarcated, red, lichenified plaque with excoriation of neurodermatitis.

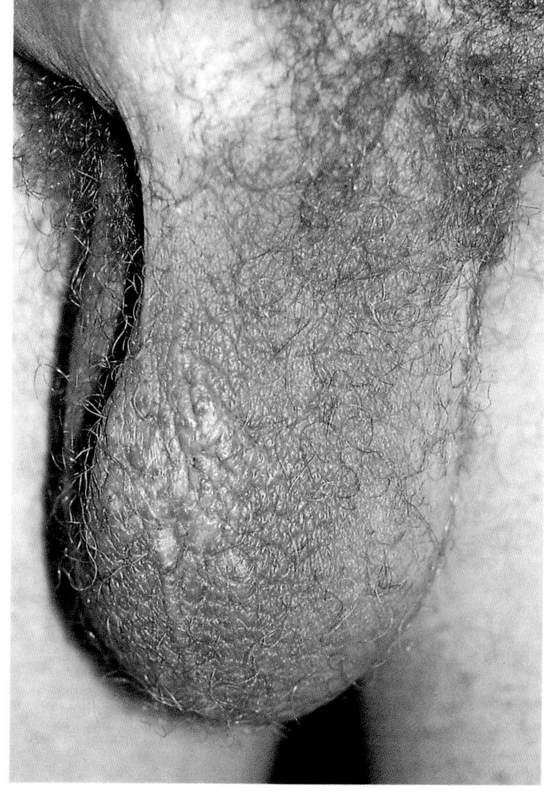

Fig. 5-2. Neurodermatitis of the scrotum showing typical erythematous, thickened skin with hyperpigmentation and excoriations.

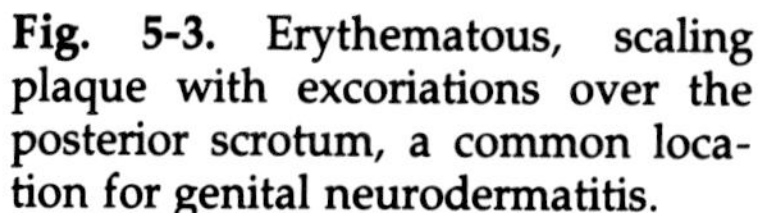

Fig. 5-3. Erythematous, scaling plaque with excoriations over the posterior scrotum, a common location for genital neurodermatitis.

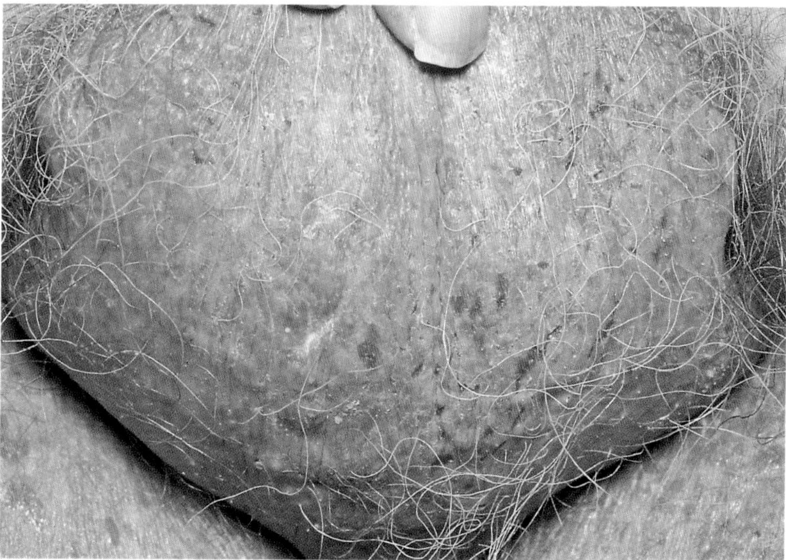

The appearance in dark-skinned blacks and Hispanics is somewhat different (Fig. 5-4). The redness is masked by the dark skin color, leading examiners to underestimate the severity of the inflammatory process. Lichenification is often exaggerated. Postinflammatory hyperpigmentation is always present, and it often surrounds areas of postinflammatory hypopigmentation (Fig. 5-5). The increased pigmentation develops because chronic inflammation stimulates melanocytes, while hypopigmentation occurs because melanocytes are traumatically destroyed by scratching. These pigmentary responses are very slow to resolve and may be present for a year or more after treatment has resolved the underlying eczematous disease.

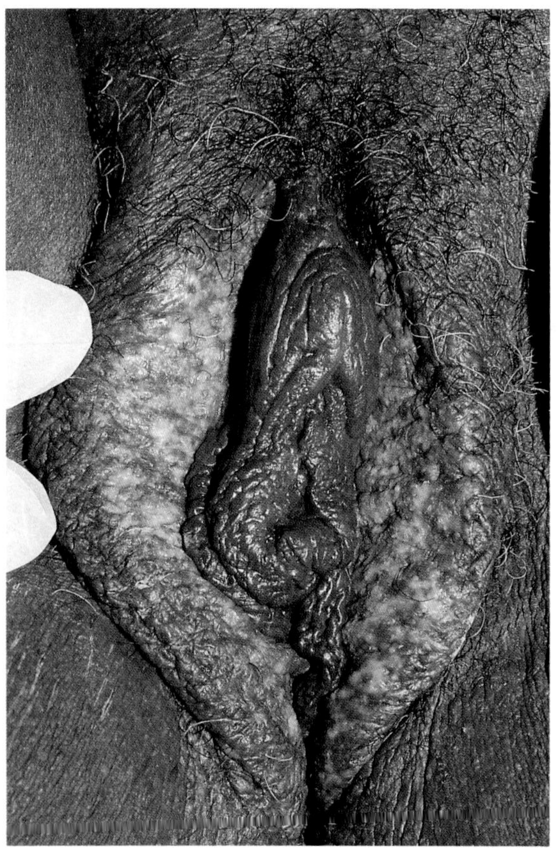

Fig. 5-4. Lichenification, excoriations, and postinflammatory hypopigmentation of vulvar neurodermatitis. Although significant inflammation is present, obvious erythema is not visible in this black patient.

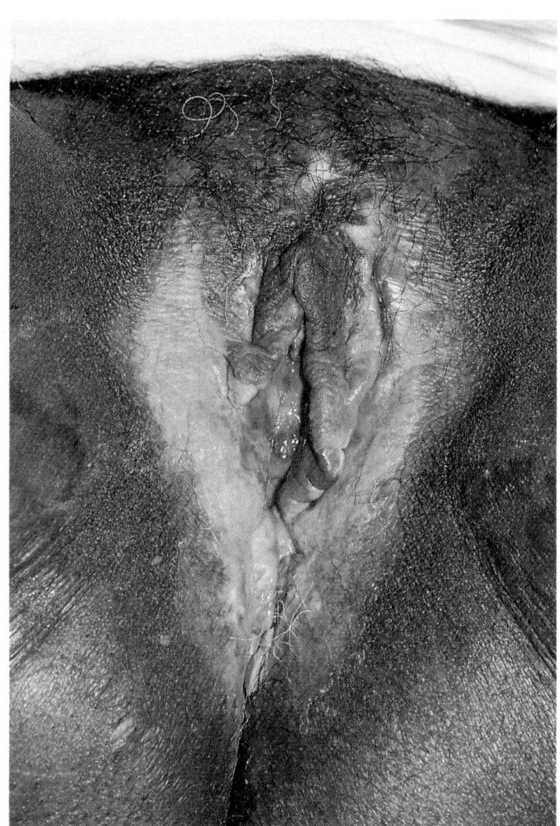

Fig. 5-5. Marked lichenification, linear fissures, and hypopigmentation characterize neurodermatitis in this patient.

Lichenification is a key feature of atopic/neurodermatitis (Figs. 5-6 and 5-7). It represents the skin's protective, thickening reaction when subjected to chronic rubbing or scratching trauma. In some ways lichenification can be viewed as analogous to the formation of callus on tramatized portions of the palms and soles. Lichenification is recognized clinically as palpable thickness of the involved tissue accompanied by visual accentuation of the normally present, but usually unnoticed, crosshatch-type skin markings. Also, in nonmucosal areas of involvement, lichenification is accompanied by a small amount of scale that may be visible as such or may only be appreciated as a slight surface roughness on palpation.

Lichenified areas appear white when the involved surface is moist (Figs. 5-7 and 5-8). This white color represents hydration of a thickened stratum corneum

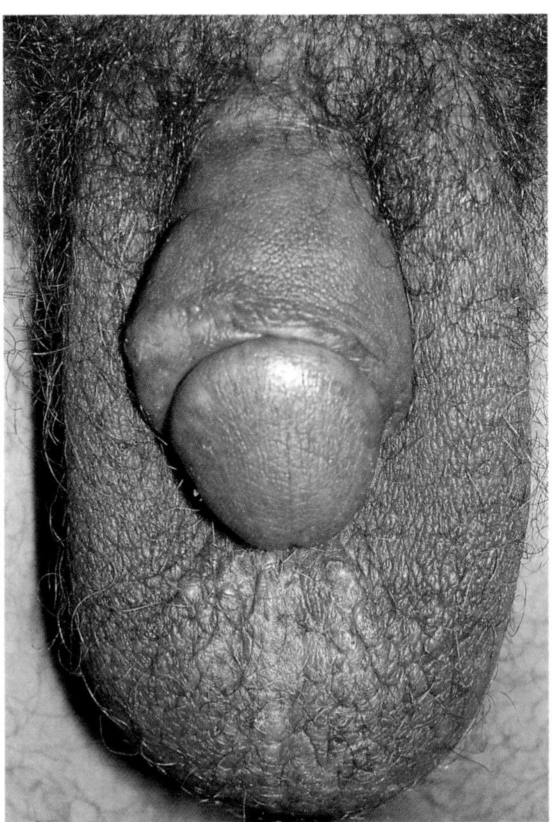

Fig. 5-6. Both superficial lichenification and deeper fibrosis of the penis from chronic edema as well as midline scrotal thickening and excoriations are seen in this patient with lichen simplex chronicus.

and is entirely similar to the whitening of the fingertips after prolonged water immersion. Examination immediately after patients have removed their underwear usually reveals some whiteness of the lichenified areas, but the white color disappears minutes later as evaporation leads to drying of the tissue.

Diagnosis

A diagnosis of atopic/neurodermatitis can usually be made if two key features are present: (1) historical documentation that the itch-scratch cycle has become established and (2) the presence of lichenification, with or without accompanying excoriation, on physical examination.

Course and Prognosis

Atopic/neurodermatitis is a chronic disease punctuated by episodes of exacerbations and remissions.[3] Environmental triggers such as sweat retention, binding from tight clothing, and irritation from yeast infections commonly set off a new episode. Likewise, patients whose disease is related to psychological factors are likely to worsen when stress levels increase or depression recurs.

As indicated above, the presence of chronic disease is accompanied by changes in pigmentation. Postinflammatory hyperpigmentation occurs at sites where the inflammation is mild or moderate in intensity, whereas postinflammatory hypopigmentation

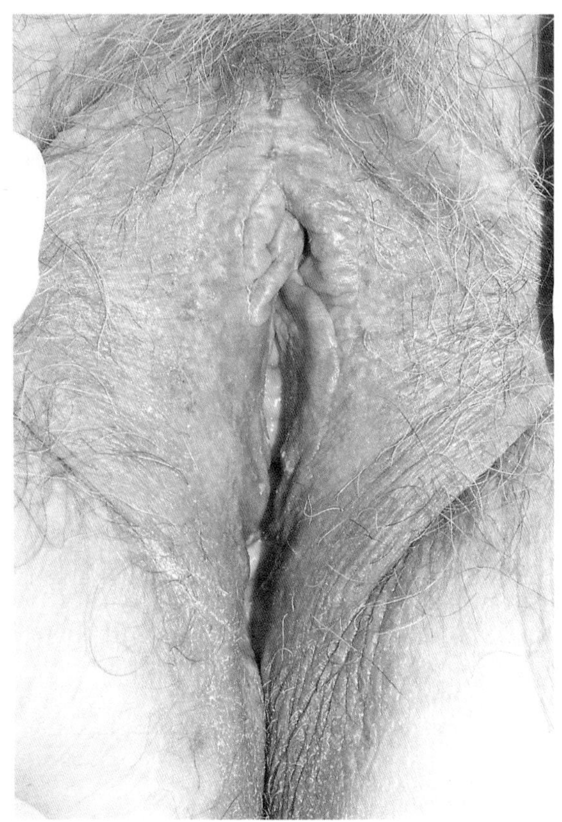

Fig. 5-7. Lichenification easily detectable from the accentuation of skin markings over the posterior vulva as well as erythema and white color from hydration of the hyperkeratotic epithelium are typical of neurodermatitis. Linear fissures within skin folds are present anteriorly.

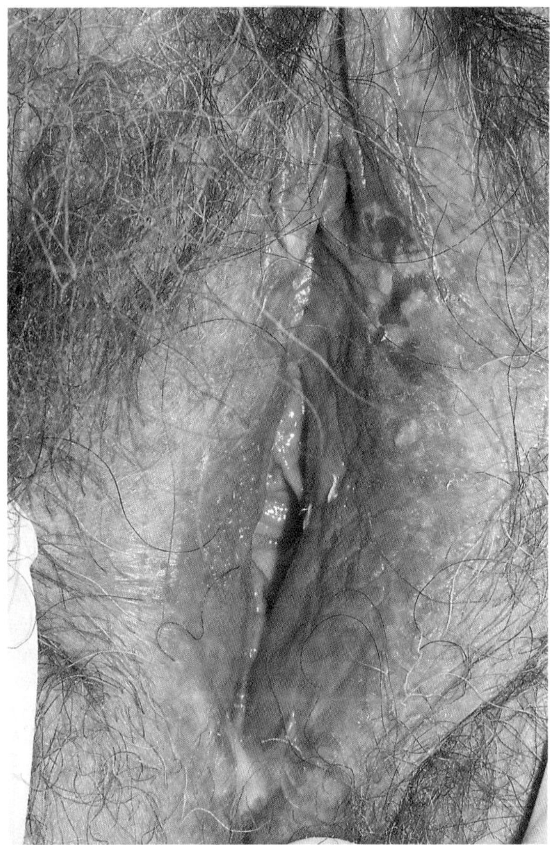

Fig. 5-8. Erythema and excoriations within white, hyperkeratotic skin of neurodermatitis. The differentiation from erosive lichen planus can be made by the better response to therapy or by biopsy.

occurs where the inflammation is severe or where scratching (through removal of bits of epidermis) has mechanically led to loss of melanocytes. These pigmentary changes may remain for a year or more; in some instances they are permanent.

True connective tissue scar formation is usually not seen, but on rare occasions the degree of damage done by deep, repetitive gouging is sufficient to result in permanent scars.

Pathogenesis

A large proportion of those who develop atopic/neurodermatitis are genetically predisposed to do so.[4] These predisposed individuals have inherited, usually in an autosomal dominant pattern, the "atopic diathesis" that in turn puts them at risk for the development of hay fever, asthma, and atopic dermatitis. These atopic individuals also develop one or more phenotypic characteristics such as a double lower eyelid fold (Dennie-Morgan fold), xerosis of the skin, keratosis pilaris, and pityriasis alba.[5]

Certain hematologic and immunologic abnormalities may also be present. These include idiopathic peripheral eosinophilia, elevated IgE levels to specific antigens, and a slight decrease in cell-mediated immune response. This latter abnormality is reflected by increased susceptibility to cutaneous viral and fungal infections.

Approximately 20 percent of the population inherits the atopic diathesis. About one quarter of them develop atopic dermatitis.[4] Of those with atopic dermatitis, 10 to 20 percent (0.5 to 1.0 percent of the total population) experience lesions in the anogenital region. Conversely, of all the patients with anogenital atopic/neurodermatitis, about 60 to 70 percent can be identified as atopic. Thus, while the inherited presence of the atopic diathesis favors development of the disease, atopy would not appear to be absolutely required for such development.

If atopy plays such an important role, it might be expected that specific etiologic antigens could be identified, as is possible for patients with hay fever and asthma. Unfortunately, this is not true for atopic/neurodermatitis even though high levels of IgE antibodies to antigens such as staphylococcal and house mite proteins are often found. Nevertheless, certain environmental substances (such as sweat, wool fibers, and candidal proteins) do seem to serve as precipitating factors by acting as irritants rather than as antigens.[6]

One of the most characteristic features of atopic/neurodermatitis is the type and duration of reaction to the precipitating factors such as those described above. Individuals who develop atopic/neurodermatitis seem to have a heightened awareness of, and a more vigorous response to, anything that causes itching. First, these individuals describe the itching as being much more severe than do "normal" people when exposed to the same precipitating factors. Second, nonaffected individuals scratch only as long as the trigger is present, whereas affected individuals quickly develop a habit of scratching that persists long after the trigger has disappeared. This habit of scratching is defined as the itch-scratch cycle and is described phenotypically under Clinical Presentation (see above).

Psychological factors play an important role in the development of atopic/neurodermatitis. Many affected individuals possess readily recognized obsessive-compulsive features that can be summarized by describing the patients as having type A personalities. It is tempting to relate the continued scratching and subsequent development of the itch-scratch cycle directly to the compulsive behavior, but doing so almost certainly is an oversimplification of a much more complex mechanism. Anxiety, depression, or both together are frequently found in patients with atopic/neurodermatitis. Some would say that these features develop because of the chronic and troubling nature of the disease. This may be true, but others, including ourselves, believe that psychological disability also plays an important etiologic role, which must be addressed in the course of therapy.

Treatment

Scratching must be stopped. This is the cardinal rule for care of patients with atopic/neurodermatitis. There is no hope of long-term improvement unless the itch-scratch cycle is interrupted. The following paragraphs describe the steps through which this goal may be attained.

The first therapeutic step involves a search for "trigger factors" in the form of preceding or concomitant disease. This is particularly important for women in whom chronic candidiasis, lichen sclerosus, or even squamous cell carcinoma may be playing an important role in perpetuating the cycle. If there is uncertainty about the presence of an underlying disease, one or more biopsies should be obtained.

Modification in routine skin care is helpful. First, fingernails should be cut very short once every 3 days and should be filed so that no sharp edges remain. Second, patients often believe that their eczematous disease is occurring because of inadequate hygiene. In an ill-considered attempt to remedy the problem, they increase the frequency of bathing, the amount of soap used, and also the vigorousness of scrubbing. This only worsens the situation because of the drying effect that ensues. Bathing should be done no more than once a day. Warm (*not* steaming hot) water is usually all that is necessary; the use of soap should be discouraged. Third, since heat and sweat are often provoking factors, clothing should be chosen to maximize coolness and air movement. Fourth, all topical products currently being used by the patient should be discontinued. Some of these agents may be acting as irritants, and a few may even be responsible for the induction of allergic contact dermatitis.

Historically, soaks (see Ch. 3) have represented the first line of treatment for all types of pruritic, eczematous disease. While less in favor today, soaks can still be used as an excellent "first-aid" approach for patients with intractable itching. Soaks restore a fluid, physiologic-like environment around nerve endings that have been exposed through broken or absent epithelium. This restoration of a fluid environment reduces nerve stimulation with consequent reduction in perceived pruritus. Unfortunately, within minutes after the soaks have been discontinued, the tissues dry out and nerve endings are reexposed to environmental stimulation. The good effects of soaks can, however, be prolonged if lubricants (which retard evaporative loss of moisture) are applied immediately after each soak. Moisturizing products such as hand creams, rather than lotions, should be used, inasmuch as the thicker products enhance the emollient effect and reduce the risk of stinging on application. Lubricants are discussed in greater detail in Chapter 3.

Topically applied steroids (see Ch. 3) are indispensible in the treatment of atopic/neurodermatitis. These agents reduce inflammation (and thus itching), and they also provide a protective layer of lubrication. Theoretically a nonfluorinated product such as 1 percent hydrocortisone cream would be appropriate, but often a stronger, fluorinated steroid such as triamcinalone 0.1 percent cream is necessary. A high-potency steroid such as 0.05 percent fluocinonide is rarely required. The cream vehicle is nongreasy and is easier to use, but if stinging occurs, if lichenification is prominent, or if additional lubrication is desirable, the ointment form can be substituted.

Patients with mild disease require the use of topical steroids for about 3 weeks. Patients with moderate disease or significant lichenification may require longer use, but these patients should be alerted to the possible development of tissue atrophy and striae development.

Patients with severe, extensive, or very chronic disease may require short-term use of systemic steroids (see Ch. 3). Orally administered prednisone in a dose of 40 mg each morning for 7 to 10 days leads to dramatic improvement, but rapid exacerbation occurs unless the patient also carries out an excellent topical program. Alternatively, 80 mg of triamcinalone acetonide (Kenalog-40) can be given intramuscularly.

Systemically administered antihistamines, given in the early evening, are almost always necessary to control nighttime scratching.[7] Hydroxyzine (Atarax, Vistaril) works well for this purpose, although patients frequently object to the morning "hangover" effect. This morning drowsiness can be reduced by giving the antihistamine earlier in the evening; often suppertime dosing works best. The correct dose of hydroxyzine (or other antihistamines) can be arrived at only by trial and error. Generally 25 mg provides a good starting point, but a rare patient will only tolerate 10 mg. Thereafter the dose is increased by 25-mg increments until all nighttime scratching stops or until the side effects prevent a further increase. Generally the most appropriate dose lies between 25 and 75 mg. The sedative-type tricyclic antidepressants (see Ch. 3) are probably even more effective than conventional antihistamines. Either doxipen or amitriptyline can be used; the dosing is exactly the same as is used for hydroxyzine.

For some patients psychological factors may have an impact on the disease process. As indicated above, anxiety occurring because of work- or home-related stress is often present. Sometimes this can be handled simply by bringing this possibility to the patient's attention, but more often life-style changes are desirable. Unfortunately, it is often impossible to change the life-style factors that are causing the stress. In this situation, it is more helpful to recommend either stress-reduction techniques (relaxation tapes, biofeedback, hypnosis, and so forth) or short-term tranquilization.

In the elderly, genital and anal itching is more often associated with depression than with anxiety. When depression is recognized, the use of tricyclic antidepressants can be very helpful. In most instances the sedating tricyclic products, as described above, are most effective. When these agents are used for their antidepressant effect, is is usually necessary to administer doses in the range of 100 to 150 mg a day. At this dosage level there is an increased risk of nighttime falls. For this reason it is sometimes preferable to use nonsedating antidepressants such as Prozac or Zoloft. Additional information regarding the use of psychotropic agents can be found in Chapter 3.

CONTACT DERMATITIS

Contact dermatitis is inflammation of the skin caused by contact with irritating or allergenic substances. *Allergic* contact dermatitis is a specific immunologic response to a sensitizing agent that has touched the skin. *Irritant* contact dermatitis is a nonimmunologic cutaneous reaction resulting from direct damage to the outer skin layers caused by occasional exposure to a harsh irritant, or frequent or chronic exposure to a less caustic agent. Both forms of contact dermatitis produce inflammation, scaling, and (when severe) blistering and exudation. Patients describe sensations of irritation, rawness, or stinging, as well as itching and swelling. Distinguishing between irritant contact dermatitis and allergic contact dermatitis can be difficult, and identifying the offending agents is often a challenge.

ALLERGIC CONTACT DERMATITIS

Allergic contact dermatitis is an immunologically mediated cutaneous inflammatory response to an allergen that comes in contact with the skin of a sensitized person. The clinical differentiation of an allergic contact dermatitis from an irritant contact dermatitis can be extremely difficult, and patients often have a combination of factors contributing to their dermatitis.

Clinical Presentation

Patients with an allergic contact dermatitis complain of pruritus and, especially when acute in the genital area, burning and stinging. Symptoms usually begin within 1 or 2 days of exposure, although sometimes after a longer interval. If symptoms occur immediately after exposure, irritant contact dermatitis or contact urticaria should be considered. The clinical appearance of an allergic contact dermatitis varies with the severity of the allergic response and the chronicity of the reaction. An acute allergic contact dermatitis due to a strong allergen such as poison ivy is vesicular, pink, and often displays sharply demar-

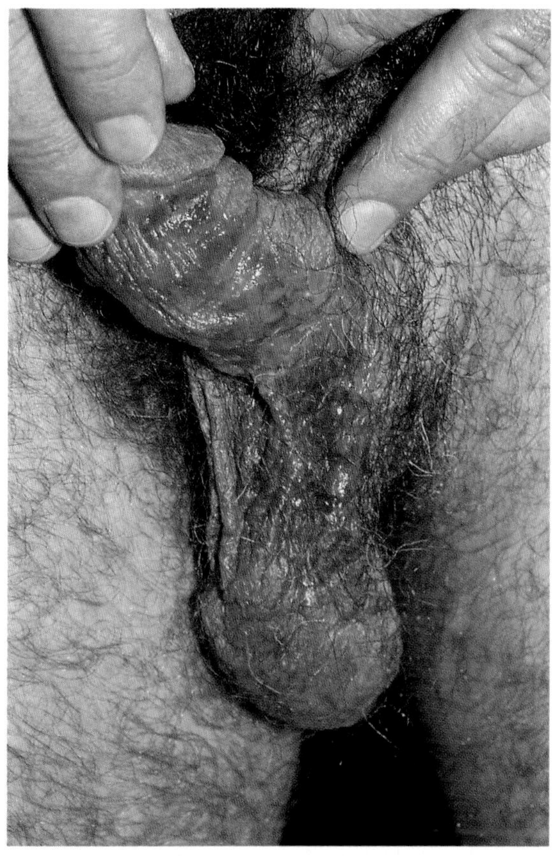

Fig. 5-9. Intense erythema and exudation from an acute allergic contact dermatitis to topical Mycolog, which contained several allergens.

cated, irregular, linear papules and plaques where the contactant has touched or been wiped across the skin. In the genital area, dampness and friction may spread the contactant so that the pattern and linearity may be less obvious than on other skin surfaces. Also, the fragility of the skin in this area and friction from clothes or between skin folds result in early rupture of blisters so that exudative, denuded skin like that of a severe irritant dermatitis may predominate (Fig. 5-9). Non-hair-bearing areas of genital skin, such as the labia minora, may show marked edema rather than identifiable vesiculation. In instances of acute allergic contact dermatitis, patients are often able to identify the likely causative agent.

The findings in a chronic allergic contact dermatitis are less specific, showing erythema, scale, and sometimes lichenification in the general area where the agent touches the skin; also plaques have less distinct borders. In the damp genital area, scale is often less visible, and skin changes may be limited to shininess, thickening from edema or lichenification, or fissuring of the skin (Fig. 5-10). Black patients often show hyperpigmentation rather than erythema, and lichenification is frequently marked. The vagina is usually spared by allergic contact dermatitis, but agents used in the vagina, such as douches and vaginal creams, flow onto the vulva, producing vulvar and medial thigh signs and symptoms.

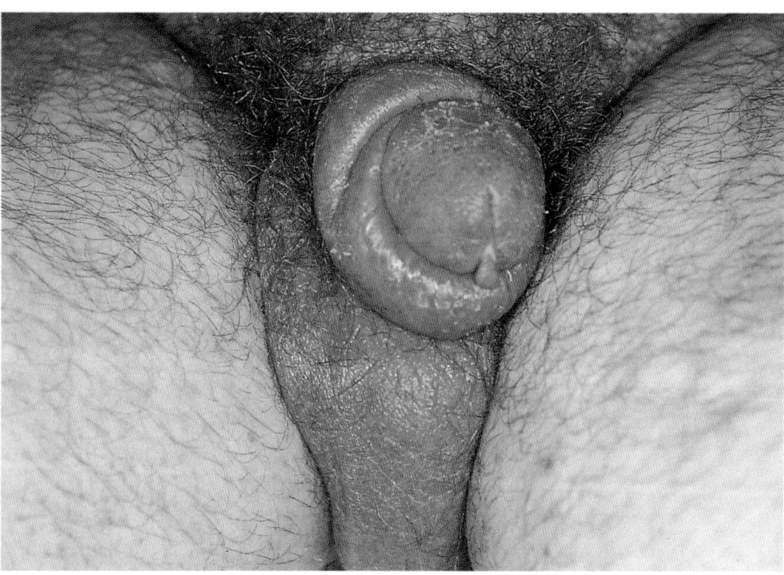

Fig. 5-10. Erythema and marked edema with crusting due to an allergic contact dermatitis.

Diagnosis

The differential diagnosis of an acute allergic contact dermatitis includes an irritant dermatitis; atopic/neurodermatitis; a *Candida* or bacterial skin infection; seborrheic dermatitis; psoriasis; and, less often, extensive Paget's disease or Bowen's disease. A biopsy can be helpful in ruling out some of these diseases in unclear cases, but it cannot separate irritant from allergic dermatitis.

Often the diagnosis of an allergic contact dermatitis is based on the history, while clinical examination is secondary since it is not specific. Occasionally patients will have already identified the offending agent, and at other times careful questioning regarding habits suggests possible causes. As with irritant contact dermatitis, patients often need to be questioned carefully. Asking what is applied to the area generally does not yield all contactants. It is generally necessary to ask specifics: What do you use for cleaning the area? Do you use a deodorant in this area? What medications have doctors (pharmacists, friends) given you to try? Many patients deny application of any substance unless they are reminded of its existence with pointed questions. Because an allergic contact dermatitis can occur from materials inadvertently spread to the genital area, questions about and an examination of other cutaneous surfaces may reveal dermatitis in another area as well, providing clues to both the diagnosis and responsible agent. For example, allergens in nail polish classically cause eyelid dermatitis when eyes are touched before nail polish is completely dry, and vulvar dermatitis can result in similar fashion. It may be helpful to ask about the habits of sexual partners. For example, a rubber diaphragm, feminine hygiene spray, or vaginal lubricant used by a woman may cause dermatitis in her partner.

If the clinical findings suggest an allergic contact dermatitis and if the history is not obviously helpful, patch testing can be useful in some patients. Standard patch testing consists of the application of known concentrations of common allergens under occlusion to the back for 2 days. The area is evaluated on the day of removal and 24 to 48 hours later to observe resulting changes in the skin. The differentiation between irritant and allergic patch test reactions in the skin can be difficult, and patch testing should be performed by an experienced clinician. It is recommended that the patch tests be done only with standardized allergens, or with appropriate preparations (dilutions and so forth) of a patient's own products to avoid uninterpretable results. In addition, the skin of the back is less sensitive than the vulva, scrotum, and penis, making false-negative results of a standard patch test more likely. If questioning has produced a possible offender, a "use" patch test can be performed. The suspected substance is applied to uninvolved skin above the antecubital fossa or medial upper arm twice a day for a week as a crude method of evaluating its effect on the skin.

A recent study examined the frequency and relevance of careful patch testing in patients with vulvar disease using both a standard patch test tray and agents expected to be likely offenders in that area.[8] Twenty-nine percent of women with persistent and resistant vulvar symptoms had relevant positive patch tests, but the vast majority had allergic contact dermatitis as a secondary event occurring in the setting of another disease. The majority of positive reactions were to medications.

Course and Prognosis

Patients who are allergic to one substance are at risk of developing other sensitivities, and cross-reactivity among some allergens can occur. Patients who develop an acute allergic contact dermatitis to an obvious agent usually do quite well with avoidance of the causative substance along with short-term local and anti-inflammatory care. Those patients with chronic symptoms, no obvious single etiology, and multiple positive patch tests often continue to have ongoing local manifestations.

Pathogenesis

Allergic contact dermatitis represents a type IV delayed hypersensitivity to an allergen that comes in contact with the skin of a sensitized person. Initially, local antigen-presenting cells in the skin (Langerhans cells) recognize and process the antigen, initiating the sequence of events that results in sensitivity in some patients. Then, with subsequent exposures, Langerhans cells present the allergen to helper T cells with specific receptors for that allergen. Lymphokines are recruited, and the inflammatory reaction is set into motion.

Of the many allergens that produce allergic contact dermatitis, some are more common in the genital area (Table 5-1). Most genital allergic dermatitis results from the use of topical cosmetic products and medications. As with stasis dermatitis, patients with preexisting vulvitis are at high risk for sensitization and the subsequent development of allergic contact dermatitis. Active medical ingredients that may produce an allergic contact dermatitis include topical antibiotics, especially sulfonamides, neomycin, and nitrofurantoin. Topical penicillin is available in several countries outside the United States and is a potent sensitizer. Anticandidal medications can occasionally produce an allergic contact dermatitis, and cross-sensitization is common, especially between miconazole and econazole. The common sensitizers benzocaine (Anbesol, Dermoplast, Hurricaine) and diphenhydramine (Benadryl) are ingredients in widely used over-the-counter topical preparations for relief of pain and itching. Surprisingly, even corticosteroids have been found to produce allergic contact dermatitis in some individuals, although more often the reaction is due to an additive. Preservatives in these and other medications that may produce contact dermatitis include quaternium 15, imidazolidinyl ureas, parabens, and formaldehyde. Fragrances and preservatives are incorporated in soaps, douches, vaginal lubricants, and deodorants as well. Spermicides may be directly allergenic or produce disease as a result of preservatives.

Other causes of allergic contact dermatitis include the latex in condoms and diaphragms. The dermatitis from rubber condoms can affect not only the penis, but also the scrotal, inguinal, and suprapubic areas, as well as the vulva and inner thighs of the partner. Rarely, semen and saliva can be allergenic. Snaps and buckles can produce dermatitis in nickel-sensitive individuals, and formaldehyde in clothing can result in contact dermatitis; these reactions are not usually restricted to the genital area.

Treatment

The treatment of an allergic contact dermatitis is initially the same as described below for irritant contact dermatitis. The offending agent should be identified and removed. In severe disease or when the offending substance has not been identified, all contactants other than water and prescribed treatment

Table 5-1. Allergens in Genital Allergic Contact Dermatitis

Type of Substance	*Offending Agents*
Medications	
Anesthetics	Benzocaine, crotamiton, diphenhydramine, tetracaine, xylocaine
Antibiotics	Sulfonamides, neomycin, gentamicin, polymyxin, nitrofurantoin, penicillin
Anticandidal agents	Miconazole, econazole, isoconazole, tioconazole, clotrimazole, clioquinol, chlordantoin
Antiseptics	Thimerosal (Merthiolate), merbromin (Mercurochrome), iodine, povidine-iodine, quaternary ammonium salts (disinfectant)
Corticosteroids	Almost any
Spermicides	Phenylmercuric acetate, oxyquinolone sulfate, quinine hydrochloride, hexylresorcinol, phenoxypolyetoxy ethanol
Additives to personal hygiene products, cosmetics, medications	
Preservatives	Parabens, formaldehyde, quaternium 15, stearyl alcohol, imidazolindinyl urea, diazolidinyl urea
Fragrances	Balsam of Peru, cinnamic alcohol, cinnamic aldehyde, hydroxycitronellal, isoeugenol and eugenol, musk ambrette, benzyl alcohol
Emollients	Lanolin, propylene glycol, isopropyl myristate
Materials	
Panty liners, sanitary napkins	Formaldehyde, cu (II)-acetyl acetonate, acetyl acetone, fragrances
Condoms, diaphragms, examination gloves	Rubber, spermicides
Body fluids	Semen, saliva
Snaps, buckles, pins	Nickel
Clothing	Formaldehyde, dyes, synthetic resins
Nail polish	Toluene sulfonamide, formaldehyde resin
Poison ivy, oak, and sumac	Urushiols

should be discontinued. Unfortunately, not all patients improve significantly with withdrawal of the apparent causative agent(s), because of irritant and other factors that may also be contributing to their local disease. A topical corticosteroid hastens healing and minimizes itching in milder disease, but the clinician should be certain that the cause is not an ingredient in this or any other medication to be used. The physician should also be aware that many patients are sensitized to multiple allergens. If the skin is mildly inflamed, a low-potency medication such as hydrocortisone 1 percent in a cream or ointment base may be sufficient. With greater inflammation, short-term use of a midpotency agent such as triamcinolone 0.1 percent can be more beneficial, and an ointment base is less painful on broken or very inflamed skin. A very acute, vesicular, or exudative dermatitis is soothed by cool compresses, and oral corticosteroid therapy is usually preferred over topical. Oral prednisone at a dose of 40 mg each morning for 7 to 14 days is a standard regimen, sometimes requiring a taper to minimize rebound of the disease. In all patients who have pruritus or pain, nighttime sedation is extremely useful. This can be accomplished with an antihistamine in soporific doses, tricyclic medications, or even benzodiazepines.

Long-term therapy includes the avoidance of known allergens in the same and unsuspected forms.

IRRITANT CONTACT DERMATITIS

Many patients with genital symptoms have an irritant contact dermatitis. This may be a primary disease or the result of vigorous cleaning, an irritating vaginal discharge, or the application of irritating substances for preexisting symptoms.

Clinical Presentation

Patients complain of burning, soreness, rawness, or irritation and frequently report that any medications applied to the area sting and worsen the problem overall. In atopic patients, pruritus sometimes occurs as a major symptom, and the resulting scratching initiates atopic/neurodermatitis (see above).

On physical examination, a mild irritant contact dermatitis may be manifested only by slight erythema, with or without subtle edema and scale. Because the scrotum and vulva are naturally and variably pink or dusky, the recognition of mild erythema can be difficult and its clinical significance unclear. Black patients may show only slight hyperpigmentation. Edema can also be hard to discern because of the natural thickness of the labia majora and rugae of the scrotum. Finally, the moist nature of genital skin may mask scale. Accordingly, a patient who has symptoms of an irritant contact dermatitis should be examined carefully for subtle signs of disease. The possibility of contact dermatitis should be considered in symptomatic patients even in the absence of observable pathology, and even if "nothing" has been applied to the skin.

More severe (acute to subacute) irritant contact dermatitis is manifested by definite erythema (or, in dark skin, hyperpigmentation), edema, scale, and

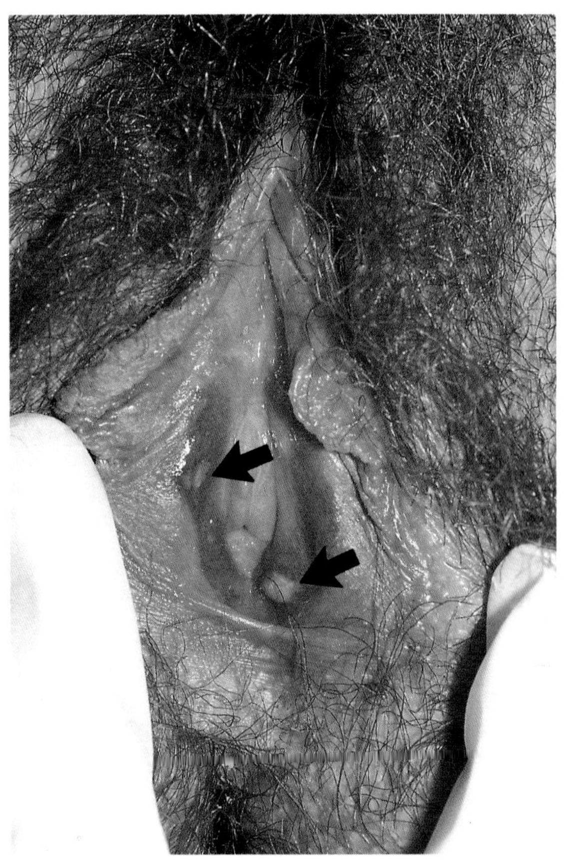

Fig. 5-11. Erosion and superficial ulceration *(arrows)* from an acute irritant contact dermatitis to fluorouracil inserted into the vagina for the treatment of genital warts.

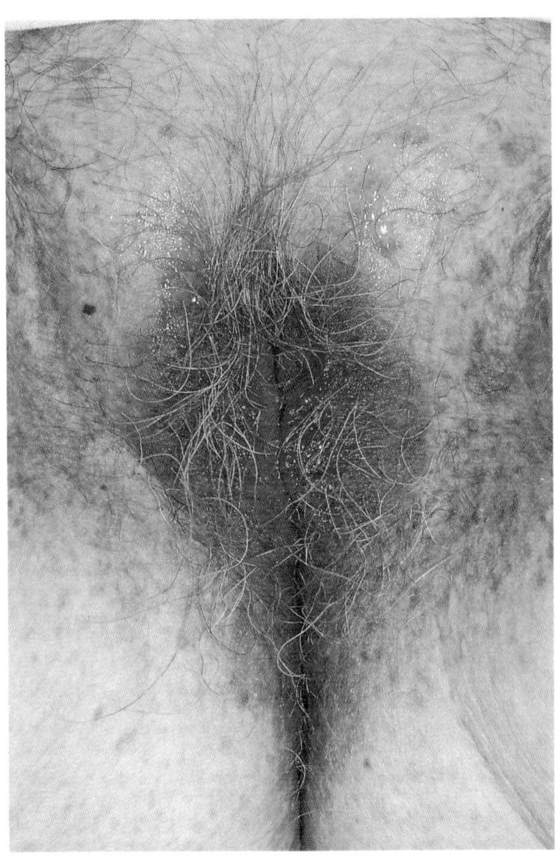

Fig. 5-12. Deep erythema, vesiculation, and exudation in an elderly woman using multiple products for hygiene and washing her vulva 5 to 10 times each day.

even exudative or erosive skin (Figs. 5-11 through 5-13). Although these skin findings occur in the general area of contact, dampness and friction between skin surfaces tend to spread substances to other areas. For example, an irritating substance inserted into the vagina may cause symptoms and redness in the vestibule, and medication applied to the scrotum often spreads to the ventral shaft of the penis and proximal inner thighs. Unless the irritant is directly applied to skin folds, these areas may be spared because of the natural topographic protection afforded by the intertriginous areas. Chronic irritant contact dermatitis (symptoms present more than 3 to 4 weeks) may have hyperkeratosis, and perhaps mild lichenification. Black patients often show marked lichenification.

Histology

A skin biopsy of irritant dermatitis is nonspecific and generally not helpful except to rule out other processes. The histology is similar to that of allergic dermatitis, atopic dermatitis, and its variants. Acutely, spongiosis and ballooning are prominent, and with severe disease intraepidermal vesicles occur. A lymphocytic infiltrate is present both in the epidermis and in the upper dermis. More chronic disease is characterized by acanthosis, hyperkeratosis, and spongiosis. A lymphocytic inflammatory infiltrate is again seen in the upper dermis, especially around vessels.

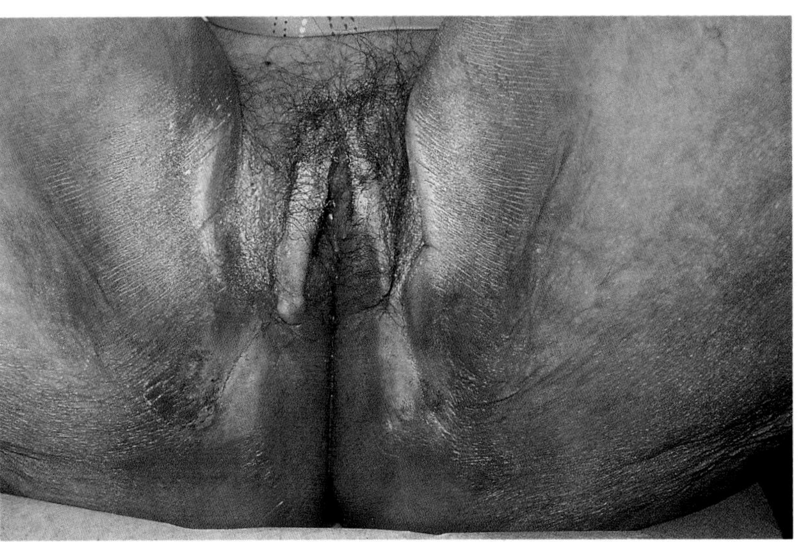

Fig. 5-13. Erythema, edema, superficial necrosis, and erosion are prominent in this incontinent patient with an irritant contact dermatitis from urine and feces. (From Edwards,[42] with permission. Courtesy from Ronald C. Hansen, MD)

Diagnosis

A thorough history is needed to confirm the diagnosis and identify the offending agent or agents. Although some patients will have recognized a relationship between a contactant and their disorder, others may not connect their symptoms with even the most obvious substance. Careful and detailed questioning is often required.

It is not sufficient to ask what substances have been applied to the area. Rather, the patient should be questioned with various and specific questions. For example, what cleansing agents, lubricants, deodorants, powders, and medications are used? What have doctors prescribed? What have pharmacists recommended? What over-the-counter medications have been used? What medications have been used locally for itching, pain, or discharge? Have any other family member's or friend's medications or remedies been tried? What has made the problem better? What has made it worse?

Sometimes, after exhaustive nonproductive questioning, the patient is counseled to use nothing on the area but once-a-day tepid water; she may then ask if it is permissible to continue some heretofore unmentioned soap or medication. Energetic, recent, or frequent sexual activity or unusual sexual practices may result in edema and erythema, or even in human bites or other injury, especially of the penis. Questions about sexual activity may therefore be useful.

Course and Prognosis

Once the integrity of the skin is damaged, irritation from the friction between skin folds, vigorous use of a washcloth or towel, or scratching exacerbates the problem. Until the skin has healed and until inflammation and hyperreactivity have disappeared, which may take many weeks, even the mildest irritation may drive the disease.

Pathogenesis

The cause of an irritant contact dermatitis may be obvious, such as acid treatment (for warts) or use of other destructive materials. Sometimes the cause is subtle, such as the frequent use of soap and water (or water alone), or another usually innocuous material. An irritant generally causes disease by producing overdrying (xerosis), overwetting (maceration), or inflammation from an acid or alkaline pH or heat (Table 5-2). Strong irritants most often result in chemical or thermal burns. They usually produce immediate stringing or burning, so the patient can often identify the cause. However, even some harsh irritants such as fluorouracil can cause delayed pain and erosions, and patients may not notice the association. Surprisingly destructive substances are sometimes intentionally applied to the genital area but not revealed in the history. For example, a patient who feels physically or morally dirty as a result of a sexual encounter may use extraordinarily caustic agents for "cleansing."

Weak irritants are more frequent and insidious offenders. Genital skin is damp, thin, warm, and naturally occluded, so that substances penetrate more easily, and normally nonirritating materials may cause inflammation. Dermatitis produced by mild irritants is often multifactorial. Often too, the causative agents are normally harmless substances such as a mild soap and water. The patient may not realize

Table 5-2. Causes of Irritant Dermatitis of the Genital Area

Strong irritants
Destructive therapies for genital warts (tri- or bichloroacetic acid, liquid nitrogen, 5-fluorouracil, podopyllum resin)
Heat, extreme
Quaternary ammonium compounds (high-concentration disinfectants, algicides)
Sodium hypochlorite (Chlorox)
Solvents
Weak irritants
Alcohol (in topical medications)
Astringents
Deodorants
Fluorinated hydrocarbons (feminine sprays)
Hair-dryers
Heat
Methyl benzethonium
Povidone-iodine
Powders
Propylene glycol (in topical medications)
Perfumes
Semen
Soap
Sweat
Urine, feces
Vaginal secretions/discharge
Water

that, when used many times daily, even clear water alone dries and irritates the skin by evaporation and removal of naturally occurring lipids. Symptoms resulting from overly conscientious cleaning of the genitals are extremely common. Patients may apply deodorants, moisturizers, wipes, perfumes, astringents, and antiseptics (which are then forgotten during the history), or, because symptoms may predate the use of some of these materials, patients are likely to exclude them as a cause of present problems and neglect to mention them. Alternatively, patients may feel that a product they have used for years cannot be causing problems now even though the frequency of use or the product formulation may have been changed.

Other contactants include urine, feces, and sweat, especially when these substances are held against the skin by a diaper, skin folds, or clothing. Occasionally, an irritant contact dermatitis may precipitate psoriasis or flares of atopic dermatitis. If withdrawal of the offending substances and appropriate treatment of the skin do not produce healing, these diseases as well as secondary dermatophyte, *Candida,* or bacterial infections should be considered. Caution should be used in the selection of any topical therapy, however, because some ingredients (see Table 5-2) can further irritate the inflamed skin. Unfortunately, some patients are psychologically unable to discontinue their home therapies and washing routines. Both their skin disease and their emotional disorder must be addressed.

Treatment

The first order of treatment of an irritant contact dermatitis is removal of the offending agents. A low- or midpotency topical corticosteroid such as hydrocortisone 1.0 percent or triamcinolone 0.1 percent can hasten healing and rapidly improve symptoms. Creams are used for mild disease with intact skin; ointments are used for inflamed or fissured skin. In exudative disease, cool compresses may provide amelioration of pain and itching. Because topical corticosteroids are less effective for and promote maceration on weeping skin, patients with severe disease often benefit more from a short burst of oral prednisone at 40 mg each morning for 7 to 10 days. Uncircumcised men with significant erosions or exudative disease of the glans and foreskin require careful attention to this area to prevent strictures and phimosis that could require circumcision. Patients with significant disease should abstain from intercourse because friction, semen, vaginal secretions, artificial lubricants, and spermicides are all irritants and may prevent or prolong healing. In those patients with pruritus or pain, nighttime sedation is extremely useful. This can be accomplished with an antihistamine in soporific doses, tricyclic medications, or even benzodiazepines.

SEBORRHEIC DERMATITIS

Seborrheic dermatitis is a common red, scaling eruption of the scalp, ears, and central face, sometimes referred to as "inflammatory dandruff." When severe, it can affect the central chest and back, axillae, genitalia, and (rarely) the entire skin surface.

Clinical Presentation

Seborrheic dermatitis is more common in men and is notoriously more common and worse in patients with the acquired immunodeficiency syndrome or those debilitated with neurologic disease such as Parkinson's disease or stroke. It occurs primarily in adults and during early infancy when sex hormones from the mother are still circulating. The skin lesions are erythematous, poorly marginated plaques that exhibit a characteristic yellowish scale with a somewhat greasy texture. Evidence of excoriation and crusting is usually absent or subtle. Lesions begin in the scalp, particularly at the anterior hairline and behind the ears, but with worsening disease, erythema and scale progress to involve the entire scalp and the central face, especially in the eyebrows and in the nasolabial fold. Individual lesions outside the scalp area are sometimes more sharply circumscribed or annular, and facial lesions on black skin may be hypopigmented and sharply demarcated. The eruption occasionally involves the trunk, predominately affecting the midline and intertriginous areas, including the axillae and groin. Some feel that seborrheic dermatitis of the vulva is characterized by fissures along the skin lines in the interlabial cleft, but this finding also occurs in other forms of dermatitis and superficial infection.

Histology

A skin biopsy is characteristic but not specific. Mild or moderate psoriasiform hyperplasia of the epidermis is present, usually with some spongiosis and exostosis of neutrophils. Focal parakeratosis, sometimes with neutrophils, occurs.

Diagnosis

The diagnosis can usually be made on the clinical appearance and distribution of the eruption. Other diseases to be considered in the differential diagnosis include atopic dermatitis, psoriasis, lupus erythematosus, fungal infection, and contact dermatitis. An examination of other skin surfaces for signs of seborrheic dermatitis or other diseases in the differential diagnosis is usually very helpful. When the diagnosis is not clear, such as severe disease presenting as nonspecific, widespread erythema and scale, a skin biopsy is often suggestive of seborrheic dermatitis and is sometimes useful in ruling out some other diseases.

Course and Prognosis

Seborrheic dermatitis is a chronic disorder, but ongoing treatment can usually control it. Reaccumulation of scale or repopulation with the pityrosporum organism, or both, result in rapid reappearance of the disease.

Pathogenesis

The etiology is debated. Because seborrheic dermatitis of the scalp is sometimes associated with decreased frequency and vigor of hairwashing, one theory is that retained scale anchored by hair results in the trapping of sweat and sebum next to the skin, producing inflammation that in turn produces an irritant contact dermatitis manifested by increased cell turnover and scale production. This irritant dermatitis in the skin folds and hairy areas of the groin may be caused by heat and moisture retention. Terminology is confusing, since some clinicians refer to this phenomenon as an intertrigo dermatitis, reserving the name seborrheic dermatitis for those with scalp involvement and the characteristic yellow, greasy scale. Another theory as to the cause of seborrheic dermatitis is the presence of *Malassezia furfur* (also known as *Pityrosporum ovale, P. orbiculare*), the causative agent of tinea versicolor, either as a direct infection or by producing hypersensitivity in some hosts.[9] This organism has been found in skin affected with seborrheic dermatitis, but the involved skin improves whether treated with either an appropriate antifungal agent or corticosteroids.[10] In either case, chronic treatment is necessary.

Treatment

Treatment is first directed at vigorous mechanical removal of scale from hairy areas with medicated shampoos. Treatment of the scalp generally improves affected skin in other areas. Medicated shampoos promote scale removal with keratolytic agents such as salicylic acid and decrease scale production with antiproliferative substances such as tar that reduce cell turnover. These should be scrubbed vigorously into the scalp and left for 5 minutes before rinsing so that the medications have adequate contact with the skin. More cosmetically pleasing shampoos or cream rinses can be used afterward to remove any objectionable odor and improve texture of the hair.

Disease sufficiently advanced to produce genital lesions will also require the use of corticosteroids. Low-potency topical corticosteroids such as hydrocortisone 1 percent are usually adequate in mild to moderate disease in the genital area, although occasionally midpotency steroids may be necessary periodically or initially. In the hair-bearing skin of the genitalia, creams tend to stick to hair and are often unacceptably greasy, while a lotion vehicle is more cosmetically acceptable. However, the alcohol base of a lotion may be irritating to significantly inflamed skin. Patients with widespread or extremely inflamed skin benefit from a short course of oral prednisone at a dose of 40 mg each morning for 5 to 10 days. The topical measures discussed above remain important in maintaining the benefit obtained by this course of systemic therapy. More recently, topical antifungal agents effective against the pityrosporum organism, especially ketoconazole 2 percent cream applied twice a day or the 2 percent shampoo used twice a week, have been found useful. This medication is effective when applied twice a day, but is more expensive than antiseborrheic shampoos and low-potency corticosteroids.

Careful attention should be paid to local measures in the genital area. The possible presence of a coincident dermatophyte or *Candida* infection should be addressed. Patients with crural maceration should be careful to keep the area as dry as possible by separation of skin folds using dry, soft cotton fabric or gauze.

DARIER'S DISEASE

Darier's disease (Darier-White disease, keratosis follicularis) is an uncommon disease of keratinization that is inherited in an autosomal dominant fashion with variable phenotypic expression. Patients with this disease exhibit keratotic, crusted papules and plaques that usually develop at adolescence but can present later.

Clinical Presentation

The skin lesions of Darier's disease consist of skin-colored papules that quickly develop hyperkeratosis and scale-crust. These yellowish papules coalesce into poorly demarcated, warty, yellow or brown, rough plaques. On casual examination, skin lesions show a predilection for the same areas affected by seborrheic dermatitis, including the scalp, ears, central face, central trunk, and skin folds, but other areas are also classically involved. The lower legs are likely to show thickened, hyperkeratotic plaques. Intertriginous areas including the groin sometimes develop irregular, verrucous plaques. Papules on the dorsal hands and feet tend to remain discrete, and palms and soles may exhibit papules with or without central pits. Nails show longitudinal erythematous and white lines as well as ridges with fragility and splitting of the distal nail plate, leaving irregular notches; subungual hyperkeratosis is common. The face may be affected, and disfigurement can be considerable. Mucous membrane lesions, especially of the mouth but also of the vulva, can occur and show coalescent papules in a cobblestoned texture. The hyperkeratotic, inelastic plaques on the most involved skin surfaces crack and break, creating fissures and crusts. Bacterial colonization and superinfection are common; they not only produce discomfort but also worsen the odor of retained keratotic debris. Odor can also be particularly marked in the genital area because hyperkeratotic skin is moist and maceration is likely.

Histology

A biopsy of Darier's disease shows hyperkeratosis, acanthosis, and papillomatosis. Dyskeratosis results in keratinocytes (called "corps ronds") with small, homogeneous, basophilic nuclei surrounded by a clear halo. Suprabasalar acantholysis results in clefts, and papillae covered with a single layer of basal cells project upwards within these clefts.

Diagnosis

Although the clinical appearance, time of onset, and family history are usually distinctive, other diseases should sometimes be considered in the differential diagnosis of Darier's disease of the genital area. These include Hailey-Hailey disease, pemphigus vulgaris and vegetans, warts, acanthosis nigricans, and impetigo. A biopsy is usually diagnostic.

Course and Prognosis

Patients exhibit a wide range of expression of this chronic disease. Some have minimal genital signs, while others have thickened, hyperkeratotic, and malodorous genital plaques poorly managed by conservative methods. Severe disease is often controlled relatively well with oral retinoids or surgical intervention.

Pathogenesis

The etiology of Darier's disease is unknown, although some studies have shown decreased attachment between epidermal cells because of defective desmosomes and tonofilaments, with resulting microscopic blisters and disordered keratinization.[11] Whether these are primary or secondary changes is unknown.

Treatment

The treatment of Darier's disease consists of minimizing aggravating factors, such as heat, maceration, yeast, and bacterial overgrowth. Keratolytic medications, especially oral retinoids, and local supportive care are mainstays of treatment. Topical retinoids and keratolytic lotions and creams such as salicylic and lactic acids can remove keratinous debris and crust, but their usefulness is limited by irritant effects, especially when the skin is fissured and crusted or inflamed by infection. These agents are of no benefit in the genital area where the natural occlusion of skin folds enhances penetration and irritant effects. The only therapy with remarkable benefit is chronic oral retinoid therapy, either isotretinoin, 40 mg bid, or especially etretinate, 25 mg bid.[12,13] Although these medications produce benefit overall, hypertrophic flexural disease in the genital area often does not respond well.[14] Other major drawbacks to this treatment are the risk of teratogenesis and, because of the chronicity of treatment, the development of hyperostoses. The multiple other adverse reactions that occur with systemic retinoids (such as hypertriglyeridemia, extreme dryness, bone and joint pain, and headaches) mandate that the clinician be familiar with these medications before prescribing them. Also, these medications and the necessary close monitoring are expensive.

Local care of the genitalia includes aggressive treatment of superinfections and encouraging measures to promote dryness. Irritating cleansers and medications should be avoided. Gauze pads inserted between skin folds may minimize dampness and maceration, as may loose-fitting cotton clothes. Topical antibiotics are useful in decreasing bacterial superinfection and controlling the odor resulting from bacterial overgrowth. Topical antiperspirants can be useful when the skin is in good condition, but they burn if applied to broken skin. Careful observation for yeast and fungal infection is also important, and empiric topical or oral antifungal and anticandidal treatment should be used early. For significant disease recalcitrant to other treatments, surgical excision or ablation of genital skin with grafting,[15] dermabrasion,[16,17] or CO_2 laser ablation[18] can be beneficial.

Because of the disfigurement and odor that can be caused by this disease, patients with Darier's disease often have difficulty coping with their disorder. Suicidal depression is not uncommon, and the physician should be alert to the sometimes serious adjustment problems of their patients. Genuine sympathy, psychoactive medications, and professional counseling may be required in those with severe disease.

HAILEY HAILEY DISEASE

Hailey-Hailey disease (benign familial pemphigus) is a familial superficial blistering disease that preferentially affects the intertriginous areas of the axillae and groin.

Clinical Presentation

The blistering nature of this disease is often difficult to appreciate clinically. The blister occurs within the epidermis so that the very thin and fragile blister roof quickly ruptures, leaving crusted and scaling plaques or erosions (Figs. 5-14 and 5-15). A high index of suspicion is needed to recognize the vesicular nature of the eruption after the flaccid vesicles have disappeared. Plaques extend peripherally with central healing or damp vegetations.

The distribution is characteristic. Lesions are most common in the axillae, genital area, and lateral neck, but may also occur over the trunk, skin folds of the abdomen, scalp, and extremities. True mucosal lesions are rare but do occur, as do lesions of the modified mucous membranes of the vulva. This disease is

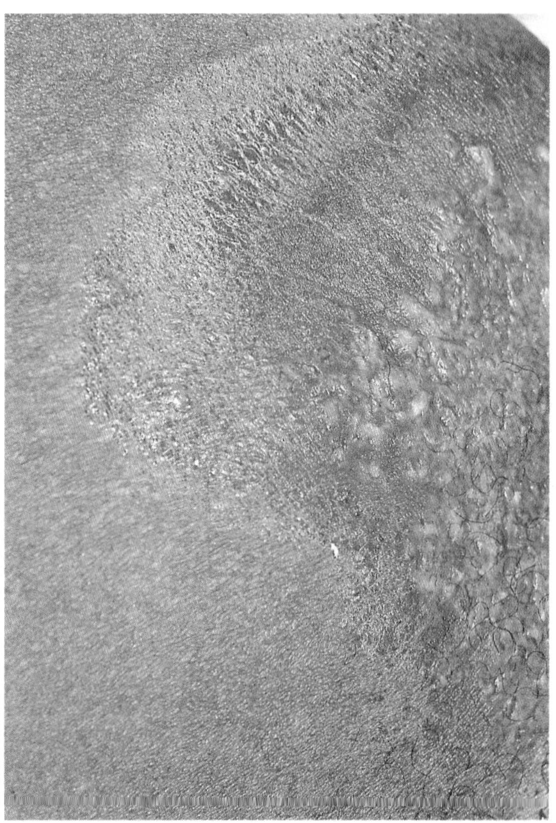

Fig. 15-14. Erosions in the intertriginous folds of the groin are typical of Hailey-Hailey disease. The linear nature of the erosions is particularly characteristic of this blistering disorder.

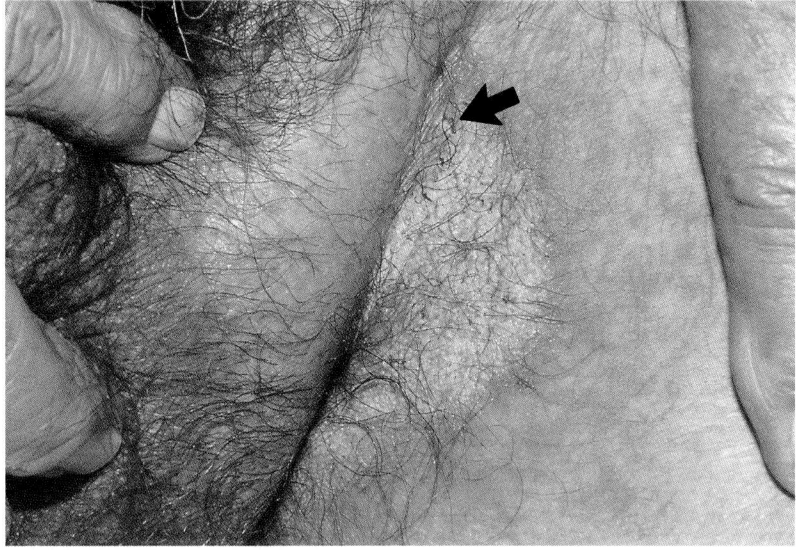

Fig. 5-15. Some patients with Hailey-Hailey disease develop hyperkeratosis and maceration that appear white from hydration, although erosions are still visible *(arrow).*

generally worse in summer, when dampness and heat are greatest and bacterial overgrowth is most likely.

In the genital area, erosions and crusts may extend from the scrotum or vulva to the upper, inner thighs (Fig. 5-16). Bacterial superinfection or colonization is common and may worsen the odor that occurs in some patients. Yeast and dermatophyte infections may occur as well. Genital warts and herpes simplex virus infections spread locally more easily when epithelial disruption allows easy access of viruses to the surrounding skin.

Histology

On skin biopsy, Hailey-Hailey disease is an acantholytic disorder, showing primarily suprabasilar acantholysis that generates clefts containing

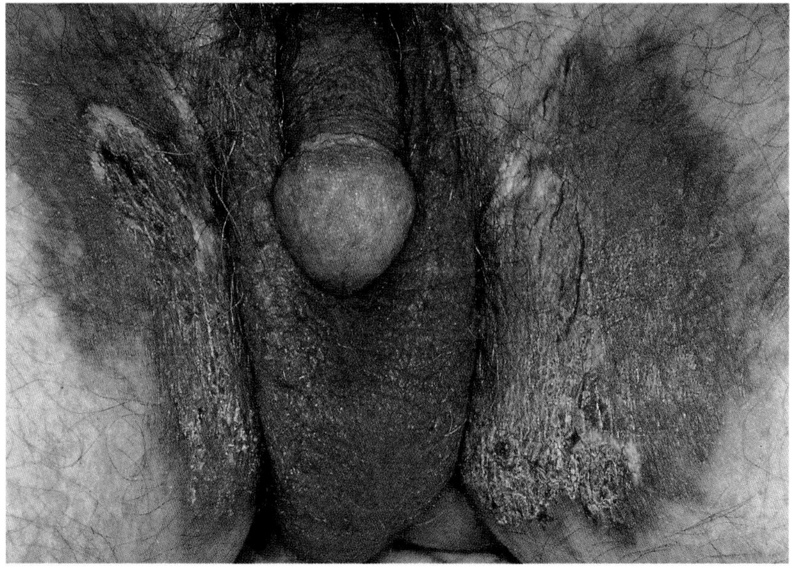

Fig. 5-16. Extreme hyperkeratosis with fissuring and cracking, often accompanied by malodor, occurs in some with Hailey-Hailey disease.

acantholytic cells. Some of these cells show premature keratinization, but not the extent seen in Darier's disease. Dermal papillae covered with one layer of basal cells produce villi that protrude upward into epidermal clefts.

Diagnosis

The differential diagnosis includes other intertriginous erosive or crusting diseases, including Darier's disease, impetigo, herpes simplex virus infection of eczematized skin, and pemphigus vulgaris or vegetans.

Course and Prognosis

This disease is variably expressed and ranges from mild to severe. It is characterized by flares and amelioration that depend at least partially upon warmth and secondary bacterial and yeast colonization and infection. The debilitation, odor, and discomfort of Hailey-Hailey can be minimized by aggressive local care. Some do well with more aggressive surgical intervention.

Pathogenesis

Hailey-Hailey disease is inherited in an autosomal dominant fashion, so that a positive family history can usually but not always be elicited. Keratinocytes lose cohesiveness, and clefts within the epidermis occur, resulting in the characteristic small, fragile blisters and ensuing crusting. Even minor friction produces these vesicles, and fragility is worsened by dampness, warmth, and any superimposed inflammation such as that caused by colonizing or infecting bacteria or *Candida.*

Treatment

The treatment of Hailey-Hailey disease is aimed primarily at control of the local environment and superinfections. Avoidance of overheating should be recommended. Weight loss to minimize skin-fold area, heat, and sweating is useful in those who are overweight. Gauze pads may be placed between damp skin folds in obese patients to decrease moisture and friction. The application of powder to skin folds can also decrease friction, but care should be taken to avoid the buildup of powder (caking) that can occur when excess sweat or exudate mix with powder. Although a topical antiperspirant is extremely irritating and painful when applied to broken or eroded skin, its use after the skin disease is controlled helps to manage dampness of the area. Frank bacterial infection or probable colonization of exudative or crusted skin should be treated using an oral antibiotic with antistaphylococcal coverage such as erythromycin, cephalexin, or dicloxacillin. Some patients do best when treated with chronic oral antibiotics, but when the skin is intact, bacterial overgrowth often can be controlled with a topical antibiotic. Cultures with sensitivities may be useful with recalcitrant flares. Secondary yeast infections are also common both because of the local maceration and moisture and because of antibiotic use. Topical or oral anticandidal agents should be used for infections; in some patients with frequent recurrences, they can be used chronically.

Topical corticosteroids are sometimes beneficial for patients with Hailey-Hailey disease even though this is not a primary disease of inflammation. In patients with a severe flare that prevents the use of topical medications, oral prednisone at 40 mg each morning for 7 to 10 days allows for some healing and the subsequent use of topical agents. Cyclosporine oral solution applied topically to affected intertriginous areas has been reported to be useful.[19] Grenz ray therapy has been useful in some patients,[20] and excision with grafting can produce long-term healing in recalcitrant patients.[21] This disease has also been successfully treated by dermabrasion and CO_2 laser ablation.[22,23]

CANDIDIASIS AND RELATED YEAST INFECTIONS

Mucocutaneous disease as a result of yeast infection is extremely common. Nearly all of the yeasts involved are *Candida* spp., but controversy exists as to whether *Torulopsis glabrata* is a member of the *Candida* genus, and some authorities believe that *Saccharomyces cerevisiae* can be a pathogen in the anogenital region. Nevertheless, for simplicity's sake, all these yeast organisms will be referred to collectively as *Candida* spp. in the remainder of this section.

The yeast organisms responsible for anogenital infections are almost universally found (though usually in small numbers) in the gastrointestinal tracts of both men and women. From there, because of the warmth and moisture of the anogenital region, spread to the vagina is almost inevitable. The prevalence of *Candida* spp. in the vagina is about 10 to 20 percent, but it rises to as high as 30 percent in women who are pregnant or who are using contraceptives of various types.[24,25] The lifetime incidence of vaginal colonization with these organisms is almost 100 percent. For these reasons about 75 percent of women will have candidal vulvovaginitis at some time during their lives. Men are also affected but at a lower rate. Balanitis in the uncircumcised male occurs with appreciable frequency, and "jock itch" due to candidal infection is not uncommon.

Clinical Presentation

Men and Women

Perianal candidiasis occurs in both sexes. It is most often seen in patients taking antibiotics and in those who have diarrhea due to any cause. On examination, bright red erythema is seen on the perianal skin. Small red papules and pustules may be surmounted on a background of flat redness, or they may exist as discrete "satellite" papules and pustules peripheral to the more central patch of flat erythema. Itching is usually present.

Babies

Most diapered babies will experience one or more episodes of candidiasis. In fact, candidiasis is the second most common cause of "diaper rash" (see also Diaper Dermatitis in Ch. 22). The initial lesions are similar to those described for the perianal area in the paragraph above, but, because of the warmth and moisture under the diaper, there is rapid spread of papules, pustules, and patches of flat redness to the nonintertriginous skin covered by the diaper. Distinction from irritant contact dermatitis due to constant wetness is usually possible on clinical examination, inasmuch as irritant contact dermatitis has a duskier red color, a shiny surface, lacks pustules, and tends to spare the intertriginous skin folds.

Women

Vaginitis due to candidal infection is described in the following section. Vulvitis most often occurs in the setting of an accompanying vaginitis but can be an independent process. Candidal vulvitis usually presents with moderate to severe itching or burning. On examination, inflammation is present within the vestibule, in the interlabial crease, and over the labia minora and majora (Fig. 5-17). In mild infections the inflammation is light red in color and is unaccompanied by a papular or pustular component.

In more severe infections the inflammation is also found in the crural fold and on the upper, inner aspect of the thigh (Figs. 5-18 and 5-19). In this location the lesions are similar in appearance to those found in men (see below).

Erosions, usually in skin folds, are encountered only in the most severe instances of candidiasis and for this reason are especially likely to occur in patients who have diabetes mellitus, human immunodeficiency virus (HIV) infection, or malignancy and in those who are receiving chemotherapy or corticosteroids. Smaller erosions in the form of scratch marks

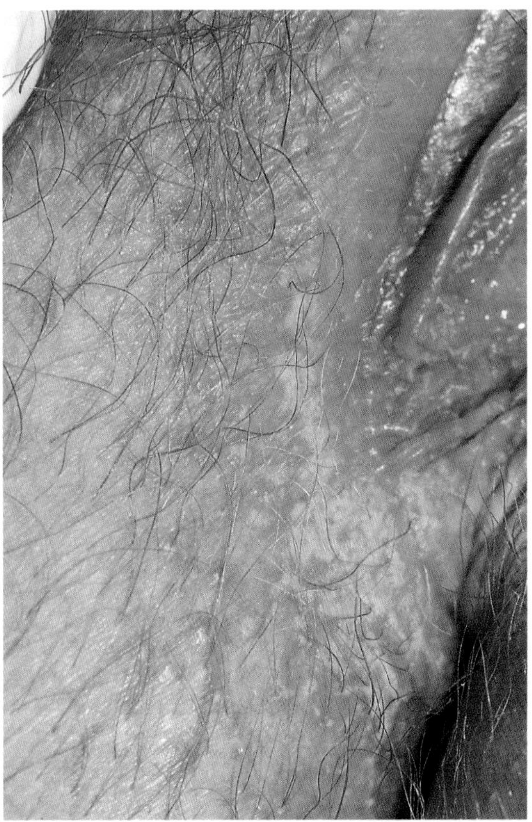

Fig. 5-17. Poorly marginated, pink plaque of a candidal infection with white material that shows budding yeast forms on a KOH preparation.

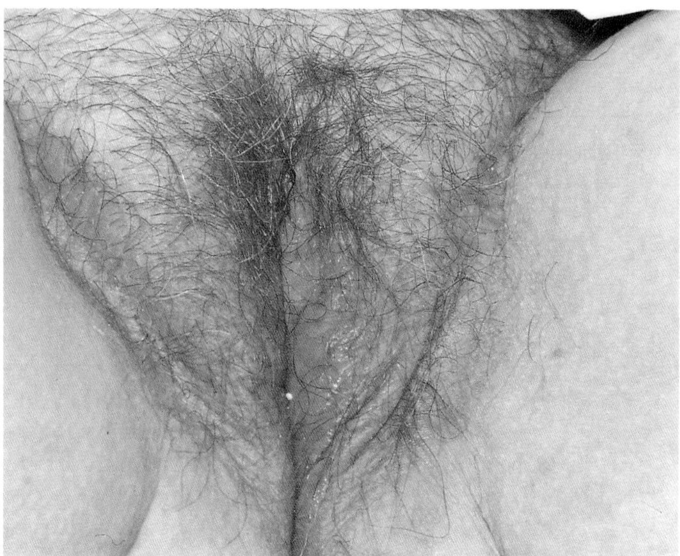

Fig. 5-18. Patchy erythema of a vulvovaginal candidal infection without obvious scale or pustules. This morphology can be easily confused with a contact dermatitis or neurodermatitis.

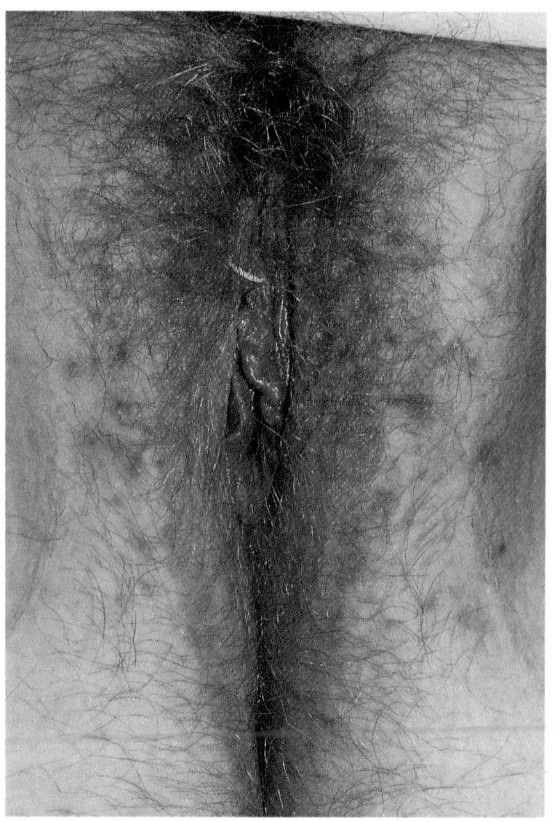

Fig. 5-19. Erythematous vulvar plaque of candidiasis with superficial KOH-positive white material and satellite papules and pustules.

(excoriations) may be seen in any patient experiencing intractable itching.

Men

The inguinal-scrotal fold (crural crease) is the initial site of candidiasis in men. The fold becomes bright red, often with a linear fissure at the apex of the fold (Fig. 5-20). The surface of the involved area is often white due to excess hydration of the mild scaling that accompanies the disease. As the disease progresses, there is spread to the scrotum and the upper, inner thigh, first with flat erythema, and subsequently with the appearance of small (1 to 3 mm) papules and pustules (Fig. 5-21). The papules and pustules may overlie the flat erythema or may occur as discrete satellite lesions peripheral to the central confluent patch of erythema. Itching is usually present and can be severe.

Uncircumcised men often develop balanitis as a result of candidal infection. The clinical appearance and treatment of this infection is described below in the section on balanitis.

Differential Diagnoses

Intertrigo (irritation due to moisture retention) appears as flat red patches perianally and in folded areas; no papules or pustules are present. Seborrheic dermatitis occurs as flat red patches with slight over-

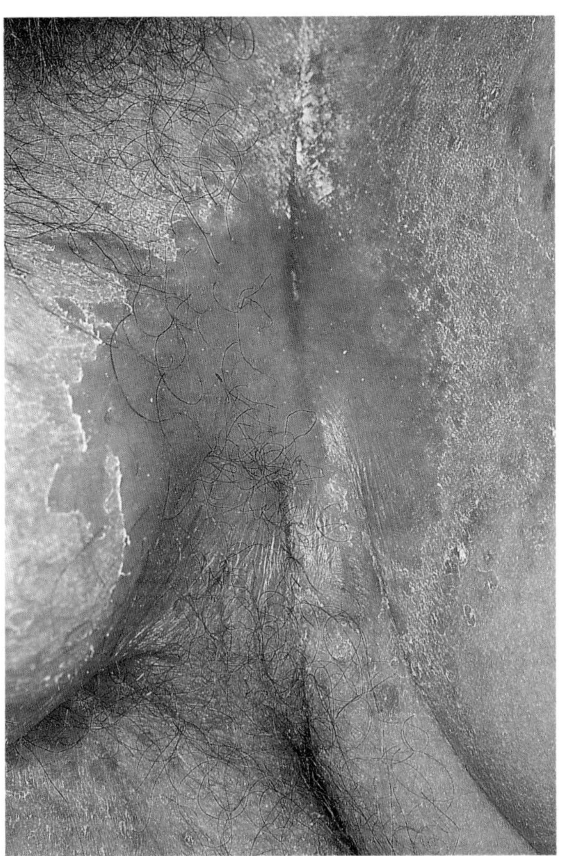

Fig. 5-20. Crural crease with an inflamed, moist, superficially eroded plaque typical of a candidal infection, and a characteristic fissure within the crease.

lying yellow scale; no papules or pustules are present. Secondary colonization of seborrheic dermatitis with *Candida* spp. frequently occurs. In these cases differentiation between the two conditions may not be possible or necessary. Darier's disease and Hailey-Hailey disease often present with the clinical appearance of candidiasis; in fact, the two conditions frequently coexist.

Course and Prognosis

In some instances candidal infections will clear spontaneously, but in most cases treatment will be necessary. Recurrences following treatment are frequent, especially for babies with diaper dermatitis and for women with vulvovaginitis. The high frequently of recurrences is due to the fact that *Candida* spp. are normal inhabitants of the gastrointestinal tract and, to a lesser degree, the vagina. Thus total and permanent eradication of the organisms from these two locations is probably not possible; reinfection occurs whenever predisposing factors (see below) favor overgrowth of the organisms.

Pathogenesis

Candida spp. are a family of commensal yeasts that can live symbiotically in human hosts. *C. albicans* is the species most commonly encountered and accounts for approximately 90 percent of the infections described above. *T. glabrata,* (also known as *C. glabrata*), *C. tropicalis,* and *C. parapsilosis* account for most of the rest of the infections.

Yeasts such as *Candida* spp. were originally identified as such because it was believed that they repro-

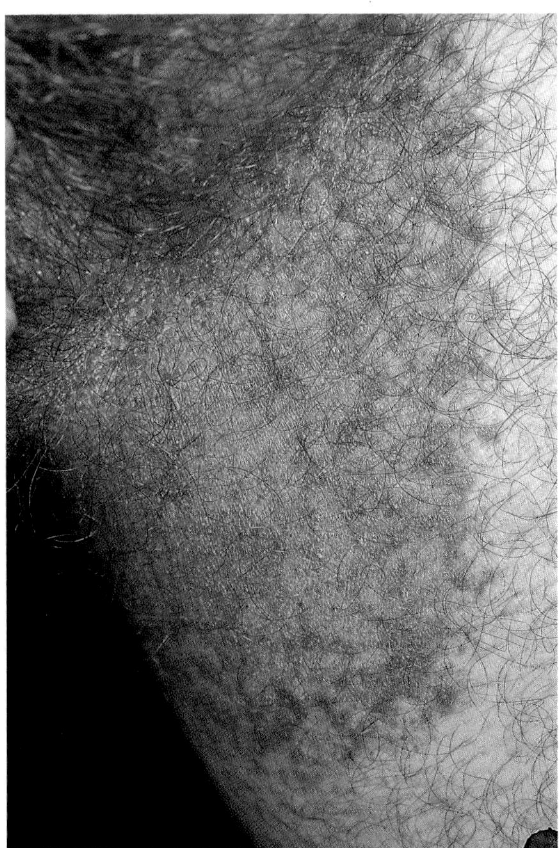

Fig. 5-21. Red papules coalescing into a scaling plaque of candidiasis with irregular borders and satellite papules and pustules.

duced only by cell budding. Later studies showed, however, that some yeasts may form pseudohyphae or even true hyphae, and thus separation from the other fungi is not completely clear-cut. In any event, in the nonpathogenic state, yeasts exist in the small, rounded spore form. In most instances the mycelial forms are present when *Candida* spp. cause mucocutaneous disease. *T. glabrata* and other *Candida* spp. provide an exception to this rule and thus one cannot automatically assume that the absence of hyphae on potassium hydroxide (KOH) examination excludes the possibility of candidal infection.

On the other hand, the presence of mycelia together with spores on KOH examination provides essentially certain evidence that the process is a fungal infection. Unfortunately, most clinicians do not have sufficient skills to separate dependably *Candida* spp. from dermatophytes microscopically. Thus a diagnosis of candidiasis, in the presence of a positive KOH, requires a compatible clinical presentation and/or a positive culture.

C. albicans grows well on all conventional fungal media such as Sabouraud's agar, but a few strains of other species will not grow in the presence of the usually included cyclohexamide. In critical instances, then, laboratory media designed specifically for the support of *Candida* spp. are necessary. When cultures are positive, laboratories generally report only the presence of *Candida* spp. without further identification of the different species. In most instances more specific identification is not necessary, but occasionally, in the face of apparent therapeutic resistance (see below), further information will be necessary.

A positive culture is not certain proof that the organisms recovered are causing the symptoms and signs.[25] As indicated above, *Candida* spp. can be normal inhabitants of the vagina and (somewhat less often) the skin.[26] Moreover, *Candida* spp. can colonize mucocutaneous disease of other types. For this reason, the failure of anogenital disease to respond to anticandidal therapy should suggest a possible need for biopsy.

Many (although somewhat arguable) factors play a role in allowing *Candida* spp. to switch from a commensal role to that of a pathogen.[27] Of these, environmental conditions favoring warmth and moisture retention are among the most important. Diabetes mellitus seems to facilitate the development of candidiasis for reasons that are not completely clear. Usually any diabetes associated with candidiasis is rather severe and is poorly controlled; thus routine screening of patients with candidiasis for latent diabetes is not cost-effective. Trauma, whether frictional such as during coitus or from maceration due to sweat retention, also creates a favorable environment for the development of candidiasis.

Immune suppression due to congenital factors, HIV infection, or advanced malignancy also favors the development of candidiasis, as does chemotherapy and the use of antibiotics and corticosteroids. Previously, the use of oral contraceptives was thought to be problematic. This is less clear now because of the use of products with lower doses of estrogen. In fact, it appears as though the use of intrauterine devices, spermicides, and diaphrams may be more troublesome than birth control pills.[24,28] Pregnancy, possibly because of its effect on the immune system, also serves as a predisposing factor.

For the vagina at least, pH seems to be important. *Candida* spp. grow best in the slightly acid pH found in the vaginas of women between puberty and menopause. This observation probably accounts for the infrequency of candidal vulvovaginitis in children and the elderly. Finally, it is possible that "allergic" reactions to *Candida* spp. occur and that these allergies, rather than true infection, may play a role in vaginitis.[29]

Much discussion has occurred as to whether or not candidiasis should be considered a sexually transmitted disease.[30] The only setting in which this seems to be an important factor is that of balanitis, in which there is a high likelihood that the patient's sexual partner has either clinical candidal vaginitis or at least large numbers of culturable organisms. In all other instances it is probably better to assume that the disease occurred because of overgrowth of the patient's own organisms.

Treatment

Removal or improvement of predisposing factors represents the first step in the treatment of candidiasis. Clothing should be nonocclusive (cotton and cotton blends) and should be loose enough to allow for air movement. Reduced environmental temperature (air conditioning if available) is valuable for the home, office, and car. In some cases it may be desirable to reduce or discontinue medications such as contraceptives, antibiotics, and steroids.

Drugs, both topical and systemic, used for the treatment of candidiasis are discussed in Chapter 3. In most settings, topical therapy twice daily with any one of the azole agents for 7 to 10 days is sufficient. As better and safer oral agents have become available, there is an increasing tendency to use agents such as fluconazole (Diflucan) and itraconazole (Sporanox) in spite of the high cost.[31] Sometimes a combination of both topical and systemic therapy provides the most advantagous approach.

The agents discussed in the paragraph above serve quite well when *C. albicans* is the etiologic agent. Unfortunately, the less frequently encountered infections due to *T. glabrata* and other *Candida* spp. respond somewhat less well to azole derivatives and may require higher doses, longer periods of treatment, or use of alternative remedies such as genetian violet. This product can be made up as a 0.25 or 0.5 percent aqueous solution for use once daily at home or may be applied in the physician's office as a 1.0 percent solution applied once weekly. Patients should be warned that this product will permanently stain most types of clothing a brilliant purple. Some patients experience significant irritation from this treatment.

Infection due to *Candida* spp. causes appreciable inflammation, which in turn favors growth of the yeasts. For this reason, some patients require concomitant anti-inflammatory therapy in the form of topically applied, low-potency corticosteroids. The cream form of these agents is generally preferred because of easy spreadability, but if stinging occurs on application an ointment can be substituted. Most dermatologists prefer hydrocortisone (1 to 2.5 percent) or desonide 0.05 percent for this purpose. Combination products such as Mycolog and Lotrisone are available, but a relatively ineffective anticandidal agent (nystatin) in Mycolog and concerns about the high potency of the steroid (betamethasone dipropionate) in Lotrisone limit their usefulness. Topically applied steroids may also be useful when the presence of itching has led to the development of an itch-scratch cycle and accompanying symptoms and signs of lichen simplex chronicus. The problem of chronic pruritus is discussed in Chapters 5 and 20.

Additional discussion of therapy as it relates specifically to candidiasis of the vagina and penis can be found in the sections on vaginitis and balanitis below.

CANDIDAL VULVOVAGINITIS

Additional material on the more general aspects of candidiasis can be found in the preceding section.

Clinical Presentation

Vulvovaginitis due to *Candida* spp. begins with itching and sometimes burning; these symptoms are accompanied by a varying amount of vaginal discharge. If the discharge is copious, the patient notes that it is thick in consistency, white in color, and odorless. Vulvar itching or burning may be present before the discharge starts or may appear shortly thereafter. Sometimes these symptoms can be remarkably severe even when there is little in the way of visible disease, but usually within 2 or 3 days, notable vulvar inflammation occurs. Later, the redness can spread to the labial folds and upper, inner thighs. Vulvar itching becomes increasingly severe and, because of the vestibular inflammation, burning on urination is frequently present. Dyspareunia is present, and the sexual partner may notice inflammatory changes on the shaft and glans of the penis several hours after intercourse. The clinical appearance of the vulva and surrounding affected skin is further described in the section on candidiasis above.

Speculum examination of the vagina reveals little erythema in mild cases. When the process is severe, inflammatory changes are more pronounced. Sometimes pathognomonic white, loosely adherent plaques are noted on the vaginal wall. These white lesions are identical to the patches of thrush sometimes seen in the mouths of infants. Microscopic examination of material from these patches reveals dense mats of intertwined mycelia. A strip of pH paper applied to the discharge shows a normal, slightly acid pH of less than 5.0.

Diagnosis

Physiologic desquamation of epithelial cells from the vagina can result in a thick white "discharge" that mimics the discharge of candidiasis. Similar desquamation occurs as white patches ("smegma") in the labial folds of women and under the prepuce in men. Some authorities believe that a similar appearing vaginitis occurs in the presence of massive human papillomavirus infection of the vagina. Microscopic examination of the material in any of these situations reveals only sheets of epithelial cells; no mycelia are found.

Course and Prognosis

Almost all women will experience an episode of *Candida* vulvovaginitis at one time or another. For most of these individuals the process responds rapidly to treatment; symptoms and signs disappear completely within 24 hours of treatment. For a few, probably those who are genetically atopic, itching persists and develops into a chronic itch-scratch cycle, which then persists long after the infection has resolved. The itch-scratch cycle must be treated separately from the candidiasis (see Chs. 5 and 20).

In 2 to 5 percent of women, recurrent vulvovaginal candidiasis becomes a major problem. There is little or no evidence that the yeast organisms become biologically resistant to the anticandidal therapy. In most instances either predisposing factors are present (see the earlier section on candidiasis) or the infection is with a yeast other than *C. albicans* that is inherently less susceptible to conventional treatment.

Pathogenesis

Most women, and men for that matter, have small numbers of *Candida* spp. in the gastrointestinal tract. It is likely that this represents the source of organisms that periodically and asymptomatically colonize the vagina.[32] In certain situations (see predisposing factors above) the number of organisms present in the vagina increases to a point at which symptoms and signs of vulvovaginitis occur. Treatment then reduces the number of organisms below this "critical mass," and the problem resolves. Note that it is not necessary, or even possible, to eradicate *Candida* spp. totally from the vagina.

Controversy exists regarding the role of sexual transmission of yeasts. Historically, contagiousness between sexual partners has been downplayed, but some evidence exists suggesting that this is possible and that it may even be an important route of infection.[30] In our experience, sexual transfer seems to occur infrequently except when the male consort is uncircumcised. In any event, it does not appear that treating the male consorts of women with vaginal candidiasis influences either the cure rate or the likelihood of recurrence.[33]

Treatment

First, the correct diagnosis must be made. This statement may seem unnecessary, but amazingly often the diagnosis is established over the telephone or in the absence of a KOH examination or culture, or both. Incorrect diagnosis is the most common cause of therapeutic failure. Second, predisposing factors (see the general section on candidiasis) should be identified and remedied where possible.

Any one of the azoles designed for vaginal use represent the first line of treatment. Either the cream form or vaginal suppositories can be used; women generally prefer the latter because they are less messy, but regardless of which preparation is chosen, an anticandidal cream (sometimes automatically included with the vaginal inserts) should be used for concomitant treatment of the vulva. Most physicians prefer that treatment be continued for 5 to 7 days even though symptoms and signs usually improve significantly within the first day or two. In most instances the brand used is not terribly important. Clotrimizole (Gyne-Lotrimin) and miconazole (Monistat) are available over the counter. Butoconazole (Femstat) may be more effective for short-term use,[34] and terconazole (Terazol) and tioconazole (Vagistat) may be more effective in the small percentage of cases in which the infection is due to *Candida* spp. other than *C. albicans.*

Most of the older topical vaginal products marketed for the treatment of vulvovaginal candidiasis have been supplanted by the azoles. Treatment with gentian violet is covered in the previous section. Since the number of normally present lactobacilli are decreased during candidal vaginitis, some have suggested that therapy would be more effective if these organisms could be reinstated. However, controversy exists regarding the value of yogurt, administered either orally or intravaginally, when used for this purpose.[35]

Many women prefer to use an oral rather than vaginal product. Oral therapy may be employed for these individuals and should be used for women whose infections fail to respond to topical therapy, for those who have frequent recurrences, or for those who experience burning with topical agents. Ketoconazole has been the most widely used product, usually in a dose of 200 mg for several days in a row,[36] but concerns about hepatotoxicity and drug interactions have limited its popularity. Currently there is enthusiasm for use of the newer azoles such as fluconazole (Diflucan) and itraconazole (Sporonox).[36,37] Safety and efficacy appear to be excellent, but high cost represents a significant drawback. No consensus is available regarding the dosage to be used, although 150 mg of fluconazole[36] taken as single dose and itraconazole 200 mg/day for 3 days[38] seem to work quite well. Oral nystatin, since it is not absorbed, can not be used in the systemic treatment of candidiasis.

A small number of women have unusually troublesome recurrences. A variety of approaches have been suggested, ranging from prophylactic vaginal treatment for several days each month[39] to long-term, continuous oral therapy with nystatin or imidazoles.[40,41] Long-term orally administered nystatin has been used historically in an attempt to minimize the number of yeasts in the gastrointestinal tract, but evidence that this is really helpful is lacking. A certain amount of trial and error is often necessary in instances of chronically recurring disease.

CANDIDAL BALANITIS

Balanitis (inflammation of the glans), or balanoposthitis (inflammation of the glans and prepuce), is most often caused by infection with *Candida* spp. Two sources of infection are possible: autoinoculation and sexual transfer. As indicated previously, small numbers of *Candida* spp. are present in the gastrointestinal tract. Given the warmth and moisture found throughout the anogenital region, and especially under the foreskin, it is not surprising that yeasts may spread to those locations. Likewise, intercourse with a woman whose vagina is heavily colonized may lead to deposition of organisms under the foreskin or even on the shaft of the penis. Minimal growth causes no symptoms, but in the setting of poor hygiene, local trauma, and other predisposing factors (see above), clinical evidence of candidiasis can develop.

Candidal balanitis begins as flat erythema on the inner aspect of the foreskin and over whatever portion of the glans penis is covered by the foreskin. Closely set, extremely minute (less than 1 mm) yellowish pustules will be found in profusion when the infection is severe. These pustules then break down, leaving a moist, bright red, eroded surface (Fig. 5-22). Phimosis because of foreskin inflammation and swelling is possible. Occasionally, satellite papules and pustules are found on the shaft of the penis as well. Dysuria may be present, and intercourse becomes quite painful.

The presence of pustules in this setting is, for practical purposes, diagnostic of candidal balanitis, but laboratory confirmation can be obtained by way of KOH preparations taken from the roofs of intact pustules. Recovery of *Candida* spp. on culture provides helpful, but not certain, evidence of etiology, since candidal colonization on other types of balanitis may occur.

Mild cases of balanitis and balanoposthitis can be treated with topical therapy. Any of the azole creams described in the general section on candidiasis can be applied two or three times per day.

If the inflammation is severe, wrapped tap water soaks (see Ch. 3) can be used. Low-potency topical steroids (usually in the cream form) such as hydrocortisone 1 percent or desonide 0.05 percent can be applied concomitantly with the anticandidal therapy. Phimosis to the point that the foreskin cannot be retracted is sometimes encountered. This will require

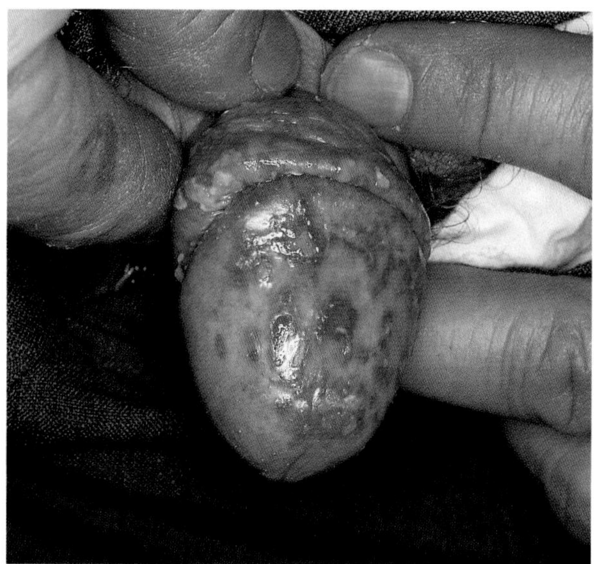

Fig. 5-22. Red papules and erosions over the glans and inner prepuce are typical of candidal infection over the uncircumcised penis.

treatment with an oral azole (see under Vaginitis and in the general section on candidiasis) along with topical steroids. Once the edema has lessened, conventional topical therapy can be initiated.

Recurring disease is best treated by scrupulous attention to hygiene with daily retraction of the foreskin for purposes of soap and water washing. Weekly prophylactic use of topical anticandidal agents and application after intercourse may also be helpful. Rarely, circumcision is necessary to achieve a permanent cure.

REFERENCES

Atopic Dermatitis, Neurodermatitis, and Squamous Cell Hyperplasia

1. Friedrich EG Jr: International Society for the Study of Vulvar Disease. New nomenclature for vulvar disease: report of the committee on terminology. Obstet Gynecol 47:122, 1976
2. Ridley CM, Frankman O, Jones ISC et al: ISSVD: New nomenclature for vulvar disease. Am J Obstet Gynecol 160:769, 1989
3. Lammintausta K, Kalimo K, Raitala R, Forsten Y: Prognosis of atopic dermatitis. A prospective study in early adulthood. Int J Dermatol 30:563, 1991
4. Diepgen TL, Fartasch M: Recent epidemiological and genetic studies in atopic dermatitis. Acta Derm Venereol (Stockh), suppl. 176:13, 1992
5. Kang K, Tian R: Atopic dermatitis. An evaluation of clinical and laboratory findings. Int J Dermatol 26:27, 1987
6. Rajka G: Atopic dermatitis. Correlation of environmental factors with frequency. Int J Dermatol 25:301, 1986
7. Healsmith M, Berth-Jones J, Graham-Brown RAC: Histamine, antihistamines and atopic dermatitis. J Dermatol Treat 1:325, 1991

Contact Dermatitis

8. Marren P, Wojnarowska, Powell S: Allergic contact dermatitis and vulvar dermatoses. Br J Dermatol 126:52, 1992

Seborrheic Dermatitis

9. Heng MCY, Henderson CL, Barker DC et al: Correlation of Pityrosporum ovale density with clinical severity of seborrheic dermatitis as assessed by a simplified technique. J Am Acad Dermatol 23:82, 1990
10. Stratigos JD, Antoniou C, Katsambas A et al: Ketoconazole 2% cream versus hydrocortisone 1% cream in the treatment of seborrheic dermatitis: a double-blind comparative study. J Am Acad Dermatol 19:850, 1988

Darier's Disease

11. el-Gothamy Z et al: Ultrastructural observations in Darier's disease. Am J Dermatopathol 8:306, 1988
12. Dicken CH, Bauer EA, Hazen PG et al: Isotretinoin treatment of Darier's disease. J Am Acad Dermatol suppl. 6:721, 1982
13. Orfanos CE, Kurka M, Strunk V: Oral treatment of keratosis follicularis with a new aromatic retinoid. Arch Dermatol 114:1211, 1978
14. Burge SM, Wilkinson JD: Darier-White disease: a review of the clinical features in 163 patients. J Am Acad Dermatol 27:40, 1992
15. Dellon AL, Chretien PB, Peck GL: Successful treatment of Darier's disease by partial-thickness removal of skin. Plast Reconstr Surg 59:823, 1977
16. Zachariae H: Dermabrasion in Darier's disease. Acta Derm Venereol (Stockh) 59:184, 1979
17. Zachariae H: Dermabrasion of Hailey-Hailey disease and Darier's disease (letter). J Am Acad Dermatol 27:136, 1992
18. McElroy JA, Mehregan DA, Roenigk RK: Carbon dioxide laser vaporization of recalcitrant symptomatic plaques of Hailey-Hailey disease and Darier's disease. J Am Acad Dermatol 23:893, 1990

Hailey-Hailey Disease

19. Jitsukawa K, Ring J, Weyer U, Kimmig W, Radloff H: Topical cyclosporine in chronic benign familial pemphigus (Hailey-Hailey disease) J Am Acad Dermatol 27:625, 1992
20. Sarkany I: Grenz-ray treatment of familial benign chronic pemphigus (Hailey-Hailey disease). Br J Dermatol 71:247, 1959
21. Shelly WB, Randall: Surgical eradication of familial benign chronic pemphigus from the axilla. Report of a case. Arch Dermatol 100:275, 1969
22. Kirtschig G, Gieler U, Happle R: Treatment of Hailey-Hailey disease by dermabrasion. J Am Acad Dermatol 784, 1993
23. Kartamaa M, Reitamo S: Familial benign chronic pemphigus (Hailey-Hailey disease). Treatment with carbon dioxide laser vaporization. Arch Dermatol 128:646, 1992

Candidiasis and Related Yeast Infections

24. Martinez de Oliveira J, Cruz AS, Fonseca AF et al: Prevalence of Candida albicans in vaginal fluid of asymptomatic Portuguese women. J Reprod Med 38:41, 1993
25. Odds FC, Webster CE, Riley VC et al: Epidemiology of vaginal Candida infection: significance of numbers of vaginal yeasts and their biotypes. Eur J Obstet Gynecol Reprod Biol 25:53, 1987
26. Elsner P, Maibach HI: Micrbiology of specialized skin: the vulva. Semin Dermatol 9:300, 1990
27. Reed BD: Risk factors for candidia vulvovaginitis. Obstet Gynecol Surv 47:55, 1992
28. Hooten TM, Hillier S, Johnson C et al: Escherichia coli bacteriuria and contraceptive method. JAMA 265:64, 1991
29. Witkin SS, Jeremias J, Ledger WJ: A localized vaginal allergic response in women with recurrent vaginitis. J Allergy Clin Immunol 81:412, 1988
30. Horowitz BJ, Edelstein SW, Lippman L: Sexual transmission of Candida. Obstet Gynecol 69:883, 1987
31. Coldiron BM, Manders SM: Persistent Candida intertrigo treated with fluconazole. Arch Dermatol 127:165, 1991

Candidal Vulvovaginitis

32. Poirier, 1990
33. Bisschop MPJM, Merkus JMWM: Co-treatment of the male partner in vaginal candidosis: a double blind randomized control study. Br J Obstet Gynecol 93:79, 1986

34. Kaufman RH, Henzl MR, Brown D et al: Comparison of a three-day butaconazole treatment with a seven-day miconazole treatment for vulvovaginal candidiasis. J Reprod Med 1988
35. Drutz, 1992
36. Kutzer E, Oittner R, Leodolter S, Brammer KW: A comparison of fluconazole and ketoconazole in the oral treatment of vaginal candidiasis: report of a multicentre trial. Eur J Obstet Gynecol Reprod Biol 29:305, 1988
37. Alcantra R, Garibay JM: Itraconazole therapy in dermatomycosis and vaginal candidiasis: efficacy and adverse effects profile in a large multicentre study. Adv Ther 5:326, 1988
38. Stein GE, Mummaw N: Placebo-controlled trial of itraconazole for treatment of acute vaginal candidiasis. Antimicrob Agents Chemother 37:89, 1993
39. Roth AC, Milsom I, Forssman L, Wahlen P: Intermittent prophylactic treatment of recurrent vaginal candidiasis by postmenstrual application of a 500 mg clotrimazole vaginal tablet. Genitourin Med 66:357, 1990
40. Nystatin Multicenter Study Group: Therapy of vaginal candidiasis: the effect of eliminating intestinal Candida. Am J Obstet Gynecol 155:651, 1986
41. Sobel JD: Recurrent vulvovaginal candidiasis. N Engl J Med 315:1455, 1986
42. Edwards L: Desquamative vulvitis. Dermatol Clin 10:334, 1992

SUGGESTED READINGS

Contact Dermatitis

Fisher AA: Contact Dermatitis. pp. 61–169, 88–91, 346–348, 633–634. Lea & Febiger, Philadelphia, 1986

This book provides comprehensive information on all aspects of allergic and irritant contact dermatitis with specific discussions on causes of genital contact dermatitis.

Marren P, Wojnarowska, Powell S. Allergic contact dermatitis and vulvar dermatoses. Br. J Dermatol 126:52, 1992

The authors report 135 patients with unusually refractory or diagnostically difficult vulvar dermatoses for patch testing. Twenty-nine percent showed relevant positive tests. The offenders are listed, and readers are warned that patients with preexisting dermatoses are at high risk for the development of allergic contact dematitis.

Darier's Disease

Burge SM, Wilkinson JD: Darier-White disease: a review of the clinical features in 163 patients. J Am Acad Dermatol 27:40, 1992

This article reviews the clinical manifestations, therapeutic results, and the course of this disease in 163 patients.

Hailey-Hailey Disease

Burge SM: Hailey-Hailey disease; the clinical features, response to treatment and prognosis. Br J Dermatol 126:275, 1992

This article reviews the clinical findings, complications, therapy, and course of Hailey-Hailey disease in 58 patients.

Candidal Vulvovaginitis

Sobel JD: Vulvovaginitis. Dermatol Clin 10:339, 1992

The entire spectrum of types of vulvovaginitis is covered; the section on candidiasis is complete and up to date.

Candidal Balanitis

Odds FC: Genital candidosis. Clin Exp Dermatol 7:345, 1982

This is a good review of all forms of genital candidiasis including candidal balanitis.

6 Red Plaques with Papulosquamous Features

PSORIASIS

Psoriasis is a skin disease characterized by erythema and scale; it is sometimes associated with arthritis. Inflammation and epidermal proliferation usually result in characteristic skin lesions in a distinctive distribution.

Clinical Presentation

The skin lesions of typical, untreated psoriasis are red, sharply demarcated, thickened plaques covered with dense, silvery scale. Lesions occur preferentially on the scalp, over the elbows and knees, and in the gluteal cleft and umbilicus. Psoriatic plaques occurring on the face and genitalia are often less well demarcated and show substantially less scale. Lesions in these areas and on intertriginous skin are much thinner than those on exposed skin. Some patients exhibit Köbner's phenomenon, in which lesions tend to occur at the exact site of injury or irritation. This probably accounts in part for the common distribution pattern of psoriasis over the elbows and knees. Köbnerization may also play a role in localization of the disease in the genital area, where continual heat, sweat, and friction often produce ongoing mild irritation.

Whereas typical psoriasis (psoriasis vulgaris) is usually easily diagnosed from the appearance and distribution of skin lesions, several distinct variants can present a more difficult diagnostic challenge. Among the more common variants is pustular psoriasis, often showing yellowish, serum-stained scale early in its evolution, and red plaques with pustules and crust in more developed disease. This form may be generalized, or it may remain localized, especially on the hands and feet. Inverse psoriasis preferentially affects skin folds, including the groin and axillae. Finally, erythrodermic psoriasis occurs when the disease becomes generalized, affecting all areas of the body. Inflammation is more marked and the scale loses its characteristic silvery, thick appearance. Because of the generalized distribution, plaques become confluent and less well demarcated. Erythrodermic and pustular psoriasis are most likely to occur in association with arthritis. At times, one variant of psoriasis may evolve into another, or two variants may overlap.

Psoriasis of the hairy, well-keratinized, and relatively nonoccluded skin of the genitalia such as the

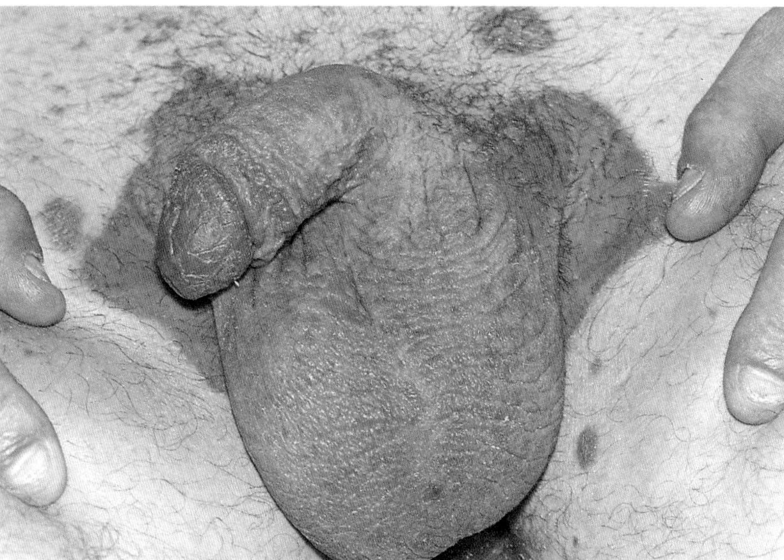

Fig. 6-1. Sharply marginated, scaling, red plaque of genital psoriasis.

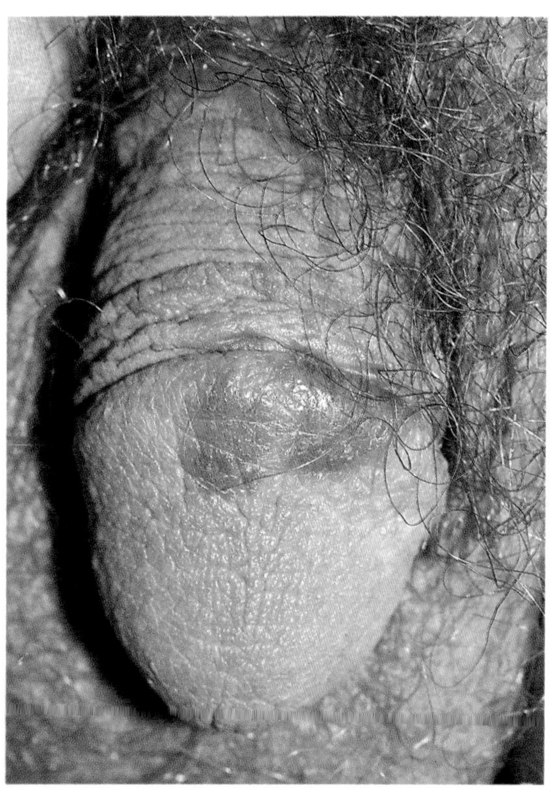

Fig. 6-2. Single skin lesion on a patient who subsequently developed other findings of psoriasis. The scaling nature of the plaque is subtle but detectable by the shininess of the surface produced by adherent scale.

mons pubis generally manifests as typical red, heavily scaling, and well-circumscribed plaques, although erythema is often obscured by hyperpigmentation in black skin. On the other hand, other affected genital skin often appears to be less thickened and to have less scale than is typical of affected exposed skin (Fig. 6-1). The occluded, damp nature of genital skin also renders scale less clinically obvious. The individual lesions generally remain well demarcated on non-mucous membrane skin. Psoriasis is common in the inguinal crease, upper inner thighs, perineum, and scrotum or hair-bearing portion of the vulva. Lesions are common on the shaft and especially on the glans penis, where they may be less well demarcated (Figs. 6-2 and 6-3). Mucous membrane and modified mucous membrane skin of the vulva is only rarely affected by psoriasis; when it does occur, it is usually associated with pustular psoriasis on surrounding non-mucous membrane skin.

Histology

Although old lesions may not show specific histologic findings, a biopsy of early or active areas is likely to exhibit diagnostic features. The epidermis shows acanthosis with regular elongation of the rete ridges and a loss of the granular layer with corresponding parakeratosis. A mild lymphocytic inflammatory infiltrate occurs in an edematous papillary dermis. Di-

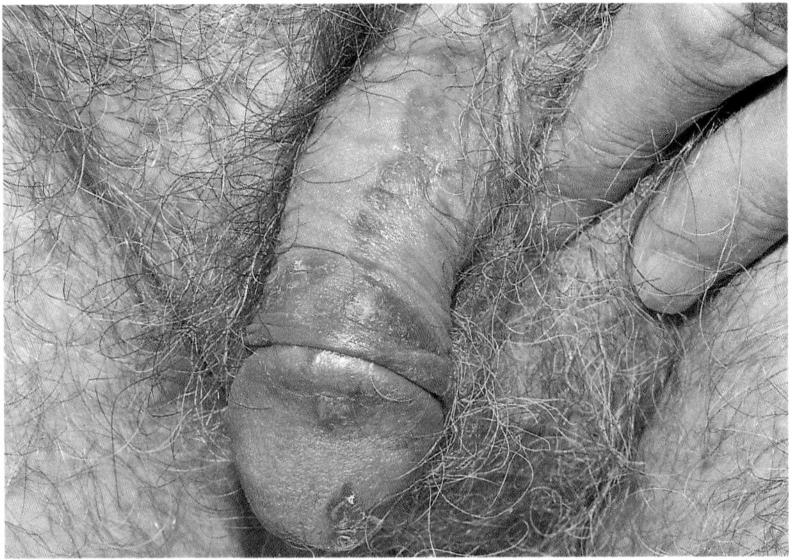

Fig. 6-3. Erythematous plaque with scale-crust and sharp borders typical of Reiter syndrome in a circumcised man and indistinguishable from psoriasis.

lated papillary dermal vessels show neutrophils migrating through the walls and into the epidermis, forming small microabscesses just below and within the stratum corneum. These neutrophilic abscesses are sometimes quite large, producing the clinical picture of pustular psoriasis.

Diagnosis

The diagnosis is usually easily established on the basis of the extremely typical clinical characteristics. When skin lesions are not specific, the differential diagnosis of genital psoriasis includes other erythematous, scaling, or pustular, crusting diseases such as seborrheic dermatitis, *Candida* or dermatophyte infection, lichenified eczema, Paget's disease, Bowen's disease, contact dermatitis, Zoon's balanitis, and (especially in men) nonerosive lichen planus. However, an examination of other skin surfaces of patients with genital psoriasis usually reveals typical lesions elsewhere. The distribution of the lesions and the presence and nature of psoriatic nail changes and arthritis can be useful in differentiating genital psoriasis from these other diseases of the genitalia. The elbows and knees are usually affected. Scalp involvement is nearly always present in patients with psoriasis and may resemble seborrheic dermatitis, although psoriatic plaques are thicker and more sharply demarcated, and the scale is denser. Psoriasis generally spares the face except when precipitated by seborrheic dermatitis as a result of Köbner's phenomenon. Psoriasis of the nails is common, presenting as random pits, onycholysis (lifting of the nail from underlying skin), or red-brown spots (oil-drop spots) under the nails.

If an examination of these other areas of the skin and nails does not yield a firm diagnosis of psoriasis, a potassium hydroxide preparation of scale or a biopsy should be performed to rule out yeast or fungal organisms as a cause of the eruption. A biopsy may also be necessary to rule out malignant changes such as Bowen's disease or Paget's disease, both of which may improve somewhat with corticosteroid ointment despite the fact that they are tumors rather than inflammatory diseases. Reiter syndrome is easily confused with pustular psoriasis. In fact, shared similarities such as identical histology, arthritis, nail abnormalities, family history for either psoriasis or Reiter syndome, and eye findings indicate that these diseases are related and exist on a spectrum. At times they cannot be absolutely distinguished. This is discussed in more detail below.

Course and Prognosis

Psoriasis is a chronic disease that exhibits waxing and waning of activity but is usually controlled with the measures discussed below. There are no long-term physical sequelae such as scarring in the genital area, but emotional repercussions are common, and patients often have difficultly coping with their disease.

Pathogenesis

The etiology of psoriasis is not known. Psoriasis is a disease of epidermal hyperproliferation and dermal inflammation. Epidermal cell turnover is much increased, with the transit time of a keratinocyte from the basal cell layer to the mature stratum corneum decreased from about 36 days to about 7 days.[1] Histologically, dermal inflammation is marked, with neutrophils producing microabscesses even in clinically nonpustular forms. Although the neutrophils themselves are probably normal, chemotactic factors such as microbial products, complement components, epidermal proteases, and arachidonic acid products may play a role.[2,3] Disordered immunity may be important as well. There are abnormalities in the number and distribution of cutaneous antigen-presenting cells (Langerhans cells),[4] and there is expression of adhesion molecules by affected keratinocytes.[5,6] Like many other inflammatory diseases, psoriatic plaques show a preponderance of T cells, and there are several HLA associations, the strongest being with the HLA-CW6 haplotype.[7] As with many other diseases that show HLA associations, at least a tendency for psoriasis is familial. The inheritance pattern is probably multifactorial, with about one third of patients having a family history of the disease.

Treatment

The treatment of psoriasis is dictated by the severity and extent of the disease. Unfortunately, some of the best therapies are not useful in the genital area because of its relative inaccessibility and its tendency to be easily irritated. Chronic topical corticosteroid therapy is usually a first-line treatment for psoriasis, including genital psoriasis, because of simplicity and safety, but the effectiveness is limited. However, in the genital area, where the skin is thin and occluded by skin folds and clothing, this therapy is often adequate. Although a low-potency corticosteroid is sufficient in some patients, psoriasis is only moderately responsive to steroids and a mid- or high-potency steroid is often necessary, occasionally even with condom occlusion when the penis is involved. Often a cream vehicle is best accepted and minimizes maceration, but patients with pustular disease or intense inflammation should receive an ointment base because the alcohols in creams produce burning.

Although the thicker psoriatic lesions of the genitalia are less likely to atrophy than normal genital skin, topical medications are notorious for spreading to adjacent areas. Care should be taken to educate the patient about local side effects of topical steroid therapy and to evaluate the entire area carefully and regularly for atrophy and other local side effects.

Tar and anthralin are often used topically for psoriasis, but these should be used with caution on genital skin because of the risk of irritation. Perianal and intergluteal psoriasis may respond to short contact with anthralin at a concentration of 0.1 to 0.2 percent for 10 to 20 minutes, followed by complete removal of the medication with mineral oil and application of an emollient. Permanent staining of fabrics and temporary discoloration of the skin occurs, and the patient should be forewarned. Tar can be used in a bath or in the form of 5 percent liquor carbonis detergens (LCD) mixed with a topical corticosteroid cream and applied twice daily. For those patients with significant scale in the hairy areas of the genitalia, keratolytic or tar-containing shampoos can be useful. Calcipotriol, the active form of vitamin D_3, is an effective topical therapy widely used in Europe but has just become available in the United States as calcipotriene (Dovonex).

Ultraviolet light [both ultraviolet B light alone and oral psoralen along with ultraviolet A light (PUVA)] is extremely effective in the treatment of psoriasis, but this therapy is logistically difficult to use for genital psoriasis. Many areas of frequently affected genital skin are not easily exposed to light while the patient is standing in a treatment box. Also, there is a marked increase in the incidence of penile and scrotal squamous cell carcinomas in men treated with PUVA when the genitalia are exposed to light.[8]

In patients who have severe or widespread disease that is unresponsive to or inappropriate for ultraviolet light therapy, other systemic therapy is indicated. These alternate systemic treatments have the disadvantages of expense and toxicity but also the advantage of effectiveness for the genital area without producing the local side effects common with topical medications. Weekly oral or intramuscular methotrexate, besides being very effective for skin lesions of psoriasis, usually improves nail disease and arthritis. Patients require careful monitoring of bone marrow and liver function while on this medication. Patients with pustular or erythrodermic disease usually respond well to oral etretinate. This vitamin A derivative, or retinoid, is expensive and produces cutaneous dryness, fragility, and an increased sensitivity to sunlight, as well as occasional arthralgias and bone pain. It is a potent teratogen with an extremely long half-life so that women may be unable to bear children safely for years, if ever. Monitoring bone films for hyperostoses and lipid levels for hypertriglyceridemia is mandatory.

Finally, in patients with severe psoriasis refractory to the above treatments, oral cyclosporine, although not yet Food and Drug Administration (FDA)-approved for this use, is very effective.[9] The extreme cost and renal toxicity of this medication as well as the threat of late malignancy makes this option a last resort. Although less effective than these systemic treatments, oral sulfasalazine is a moderately priced alternative with a reasonable safety profile that is beneficial to some patients.[10]

Local care of the genital area is important. The scaling and hyperkeratotic skin of psoriasis in intertriginous areas of the gentialia predispose to maceration, erosion, and superinfection, and incompletely removed feces and urine may worsen psoriasis secondary to irritation. The area should be kept as dry as possible by allowing skin folds to air-dry completely before dressing after bathing, by the sparing use of topical medications, by weight loss if obese, and by separating macerated skin folds by soft gauze or cotton fabric that is replaced as it becomes damp. A light dusting of powder can help minimize moisture.

Not only does the local maceration and corticosteroid use associated with psoriasis increase the risk of infection with *Candida* spp. or a dermatophyte, but the red, scaling appearance of psoriatic lesions can also mimic these infections, allowing them to coexist without detection in the patient of the unsuspicious physician. A search for these infections should be done in patients resistant to treatment or those experiencing a flare of their disease.

Patients who experience itching with their disease benefit from nighttime sedation both to enable an adequate night's sleep and to prevent nocturnal scratching that may worsen the disease. Short-term relief of pruritus is sometimes afforded by a colloidal oatmeal (Aveeno) bath; one packet of oatmeal is added to bath water.

Patients with psoriasis often have difficulty dealing emotionally with their disfigurement; their depression and dissatisfaction may seem out of proportion to the degree of their skin disease. This unhappiness can be magnified in the patient who has genital psoriasis, especially in patients who are or wish to be sexually active. Recognizing and dealing with this aspect of the disease may enable patients to tolerate their psoriasis better.

REITER SYNDROME

Reiter syndrome is a skin, joint, and eye disease with such clinical and histologic similarity to psoriasis that these diseases are felt to be closely related, existing on a disease spectrum. The extracutaneous manifestations of arthritis, urethritis, cervicitis, iritis, and conjunctivitis are much more common and often more severe in patients with Reiter syndrome than with psoriasis. The disease occurs almost exclusively in men.

Clinical Presentation

Skin lesions identical to those of pustular psoriasis occur on the penis, especially the glans, or on the vulva, with the most noticeable disease on the hair-bearing areas. In circumcised men and on the hair-bearing portion of the vulva, the plaques are red, well demarcated, and exhibit scale/crust (Figs. 6-3 and 6-4). Black skin often appears hyperpigmented rather than red. In uncircumcised men, skin lesions of the glans consist of small, white, annular or arcuate papules and plaques (Fig. 6-5). Similar lesions may occur on the mucous membrane and modified mucous membrane portion of the vulva, vagina, and cervix. The hands and feet, particularly the palmar and plantar aspects, are usually affected. Asymmetrical arthritis of large, weight-bearing joints such as the knee or ankle is usual. Heel pain due to inflammation at the insertion of the Achilles tendon is common. Conjunctivitis, iritis, and urethritis occur in most patients. Although Reiter syndrome is defined by the presence of arthritis of more than 1 month's duration in association with conjunctivitis and urethritis or cervicitis, most patients present with incomplete Reiter syndrome.

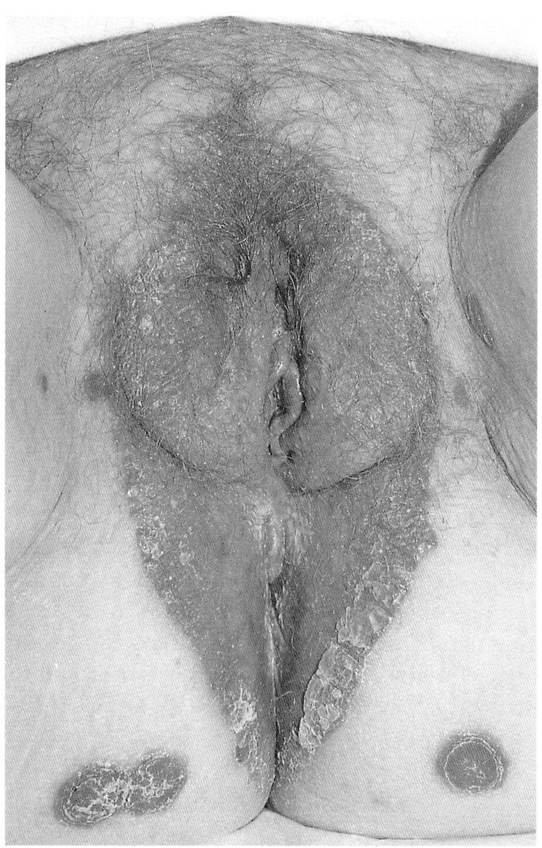

Fig. 6-4. Well-demarcated plaque with scale/crust over the vulva is typical for psoriasis or Reiter syndrome in this patient with Reiter syndrome. (From Edwards,[12a] with permission.)

Histology

The skin biopsy of Reiter syndrome is indistinguishable from that of pustular psoriasis.

Diagnosis

The diagnosis of Reiter syndrome is made by the constellation of clinical findings. The urethritis of early Reiter syndrome occurring before the development of significant skin findings may mimic gonorrhea, so exclusion of this disease in some patients is necessary. The disease most easily confused with Reiter syndrome is pustular psoriasis, and sometimes the distinction cannot be made absolutely. HLA-B27 positivity is more common in patients with Reiter syndrome and patients with psoriasis are more likely to have generalized skin disease with less likelihood of eye findings, urethritis, or cervicitis.

Course and Prognosis

Reiter syndrome is a chronic disease that requires ongoing therapy. Although many patients are relatively well controlled on medications, most experience persistent symptoms and skin findings to some degree. Disabling arthritis can occur in some but can be minimized with aggressive management.

Pathogenesis

Reiter syndrome is a reactive process most often found in genetically susceptible individuals and often associated with an infection. The most commonly implicated organisms include those that cause dysentery or urethritis including *Yersinia enterocolitica, Y. pseudotuberculosis, Shigella flexneri, Salmonella typhimurium,* and *S. enteritidis* and its subtypes *muenchen* and *heidelberg. Ureaplasma urealyticum, Campylobacter fetus, Neisseria gonorrhoea,* and *Chlamydia trachomatis* are also known to precipitate this disease. More recently, an association with human immunodeficiency virus (HIV) infection has been realized, but whether the virus directly provokes the

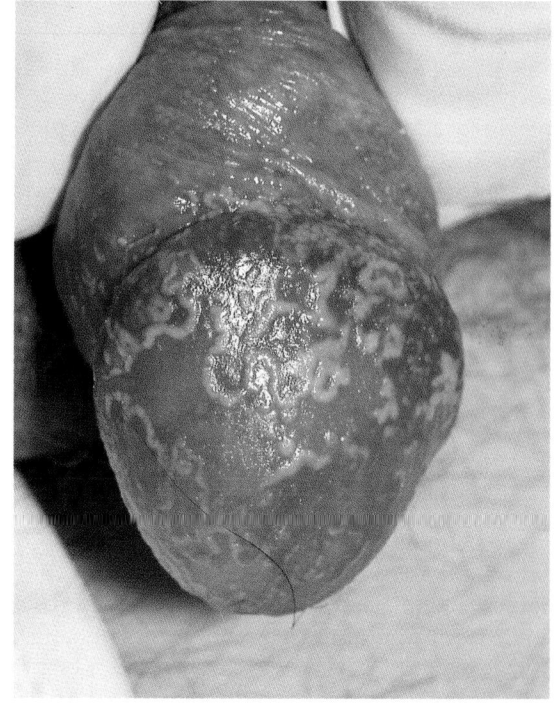

Fig. 6-5. Classic white, circinate papules over the glans of an uncircumcised male with Reiter syndrome.

disease or whether the immune changes associated with HIV disease create a susceptibility to Reiter syndrome is not known. Patients with and without HIV disease usually show HLA-B27 positivity.[11]

Treatment

Since the differentiation of Reiter syndrome and psoriasis can be difficult or impossible, it is fortunate that the treatment of these two diseases is the same. Topical corticosteroids are useful in the immediate amelioration of the skin disease. In all but mild disease, treatment with systemic weekly methotrexate or daily oral etretinate is necessary. Those with significant arthritis are best treated with methotrexate. Oral etretinate produces excellent results in many but is not very effective for the arthritis and, because it is a teratogen stored for years in the body fat, it should be avoided in women who may wish to bear children some day. Evidence of an obvious precipitating infection should be pursued. When diarrhea is present, fecal material should be cultured and patients treated for any infections identified. Although most organisms will have disappeared, *Chlamydia* is the most notable infectious agent likely to play an ongoing role, and it should be actively sought.[12] Because of the association of Reiter syndrome and HIV disease, an evaluation of HIV status should be considered in patients with new onset of this disease.

The few case reports of women with Reiter syndrome have described clinical confusion of this condition with a yeast infection or an increased frequency of recurrent vulvovaginal *Candida* infections. The clinician should be careful not to mistake the adherent, potassium hydroxide (KOH)-negative, white papules of the vulva, vagina, or cervix seen in Reiter syndrome for yeast. Also, the physician should not dismiss all white lesions in women with Reiter syndrome as indicative of the underlying disease instead of considering superimposed yeast.

LICHEN PLANUS

Lichen planus is a relatively common mucocutaneous disease that sometimes affects the genitalia. Approximately 25 percent of men with typical cutaneous lichen planus exhibit genital lesions, most often on the glans, but the frequency of genital lichen planus in women is not known.

Clinical Presentation

The classic lesions of cutaneous lichen planus are well-circumscribed, violaceous, flat-topped papules. Scale is present, but its adherent nature results in a shiny surface rather than obvious scale. Keratinized skin lesions may include other morphologic variants that exhibit hyperkeratosis, blistering, annularity, or more obvious scaling. Genital non-mucous membrane lesions usually conform to the classic violaceous (Fig. 6-6) or brown, flat-topped appearance, although lesions of the glans penis and shaft are sometimes annular (Figs. 6-6 and 6-7). Black patients often exhibit lesions that appear extremely dark rather than inflammatory, and lesions are often thick with heavy scale.

Mucous membrane lichen planus may be nonerosive or erosive. Nonerosive lesions anywhere on moist skin such as the labia minora or the uncircumcised glans penis are white papules or poorly marginated plaques; many are linear, fernlike, or reticular in

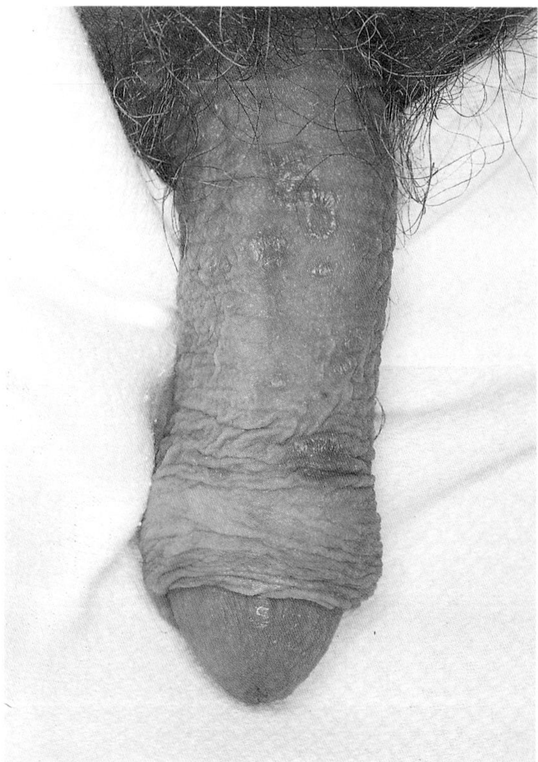

Fig. 6-6. Violaceous annular papules of lichen planus with overlying white Wickham's striae.

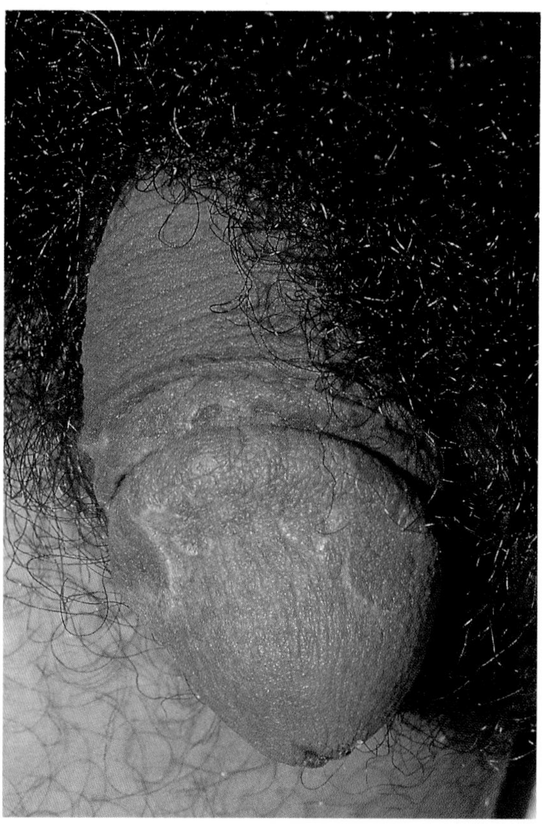

Fig. 6-7. White, annular plaques of annular lichen planus.

pattern (Figs. 6-8 and 6-9). Erosive lichen planus occurs primarily in the vestibule (Figs. 6-10 and 6-11) and vagina, and sometimes on the glans penis. Erosive disease of the vulva is generally accompanied by vaginal disease, which nearly always shows nonspecific erosions or ulcerations, sometimes with white hyperkeratosis. Erosive lichen planus may occur in the vagina without vulvar lesions and without other typical lesions of lichen planus, making diagnosis difficult. While lichen planus may not be the only disease that produces this nonspecific picture of desquamative vaginitis, it is certainly the most common cause known. Close examination of the vulva and mouth often reveals involvement with more typical lichen planus. In men, ulcerative lesions are usually limited to the glans. On careful examination, patients with ulcerative disease usually exhibit surrounding areas of abnormal skin, sometimes nonspecific-appearing hyperkeratosis, and often lesions suggestive of lichen planus. Advanced disease results in progressive scarring and a clinically nonspecific end-stage appearance of smooth, often atrophic skin with loss of normal genital landmarks (Figs. 6-12 through 6-14). Erosions of the vaginal walls sometimes result in bleeding, superinfections, and scarring with adhesions and obliteration of the vaginal space, preventing intercourse and the introduction of an examining speculum.

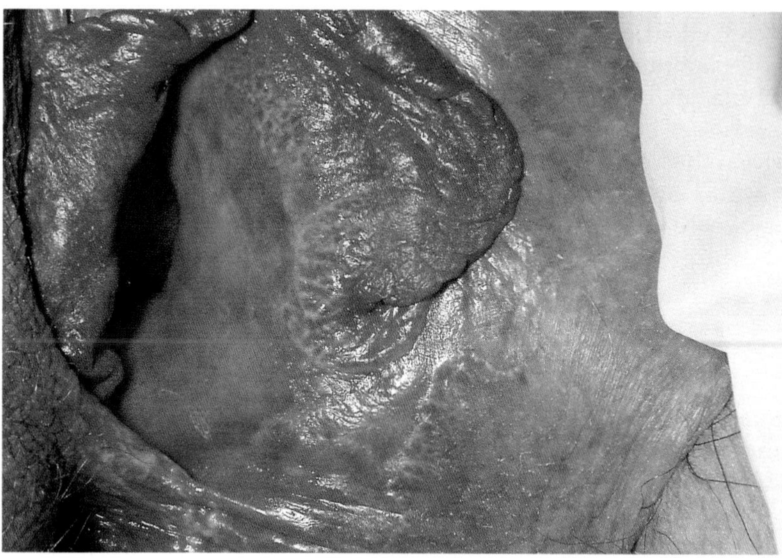

Fig. 6-8. Classic fernlike white papules over the inner aspect of the labium minus surround superficial erosions of the vestibule in this patient with lichen planus.

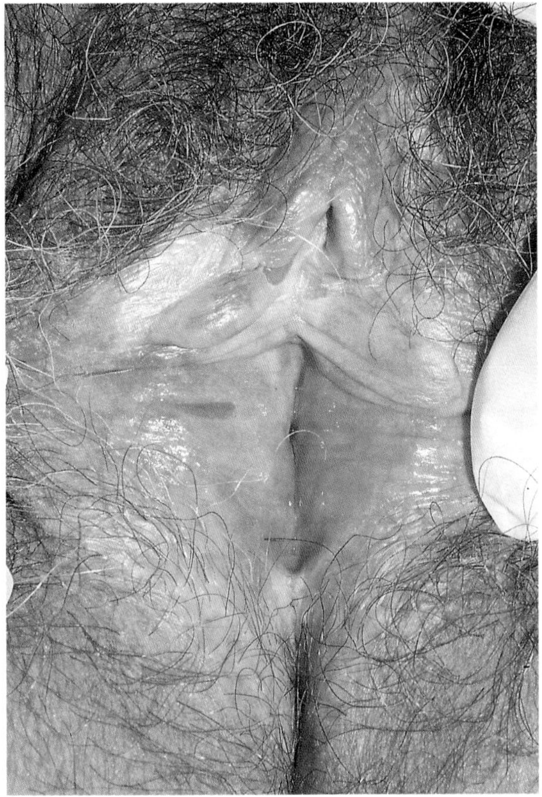

Fig. 6-9. Mildly erosive lichen planus easily recognized by the white surface epithelial change.

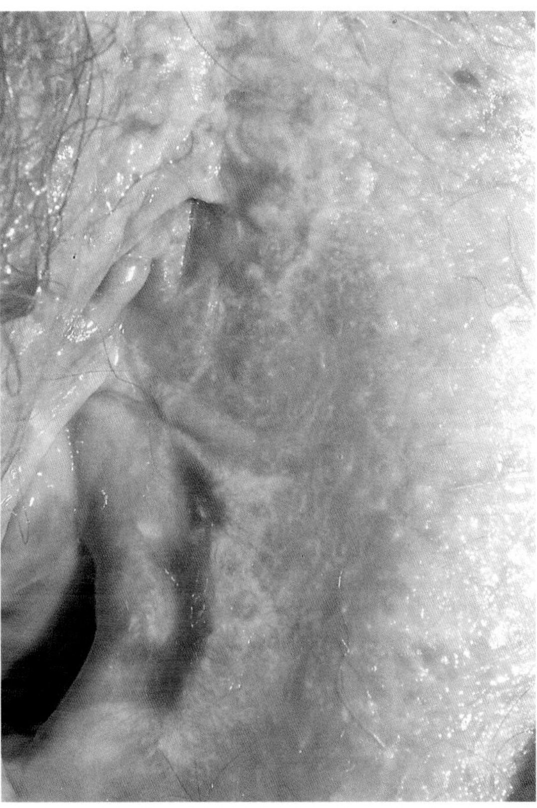

Fig. 6-11. Although this white hyperkeratotic epithelium surrounding linear erosions resembles neurodermatitis, the white papules are reticulate, suggesting the correct diagnosis of lichen planus. Compare with Figures 5-8 and 11-6.

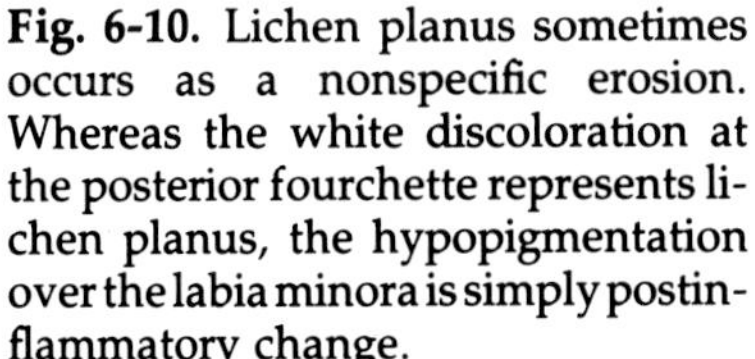

Fig. 6-10. Lichen planus sometimes occurs as a nonspecific erosion. Whereas the white discoloration at the posterior fourchette represents lichen planus, the hypopigmentation over the labia minora is simply postinflammatory change.

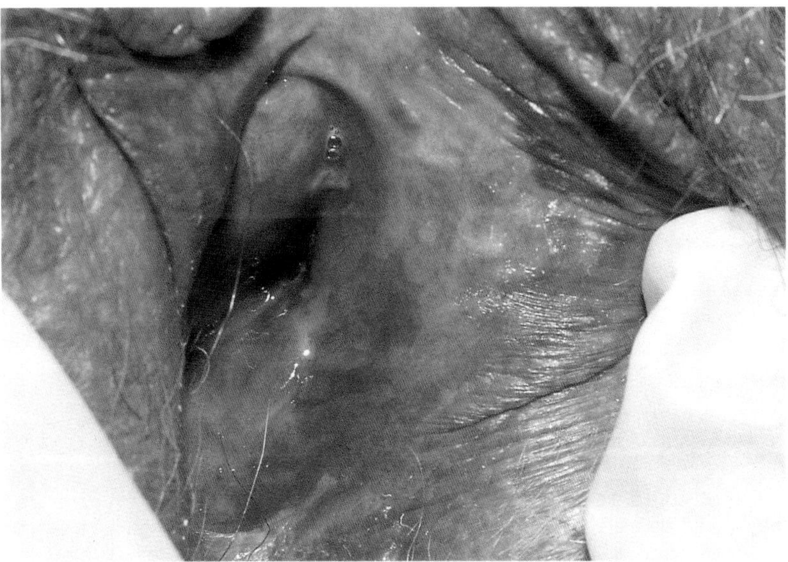

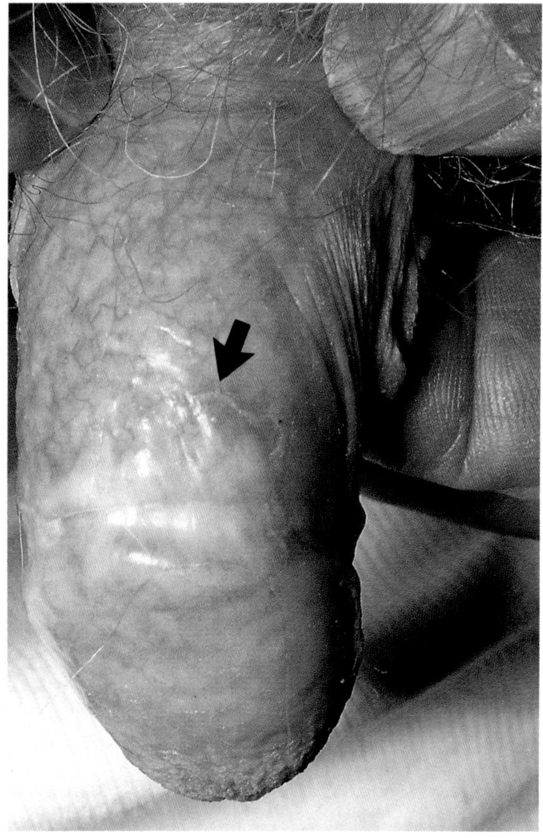

Fig. 6-12. Although erosive lichen planus with scarring is more common in women, this occurs also in men, with the only specific clue in this patient the fine white stria over the distal shaft *(arrow).*

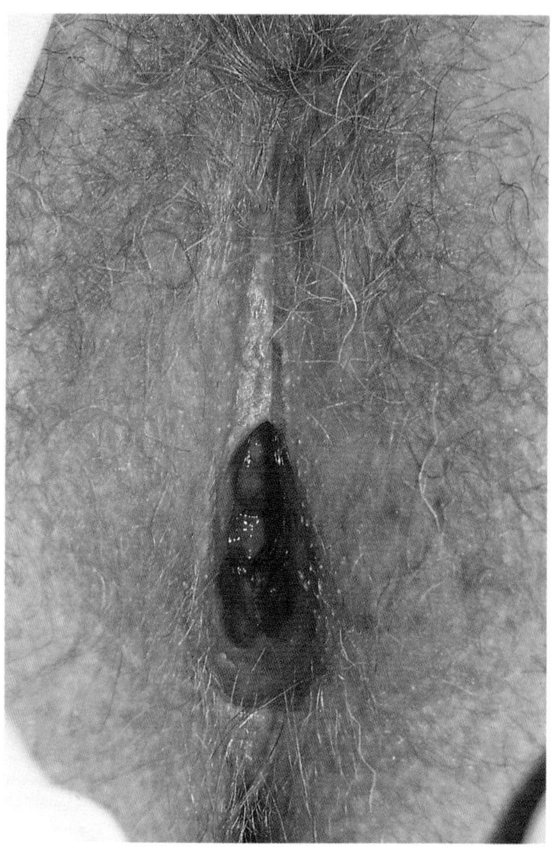

Fig. 6-13. Loss of labia minora, agglutination of clitoral hood, and introital erosions in a young woman with lichen planus incorrectly diagnosed as having dyspareunia on the basis of psychosexual maladjustment.

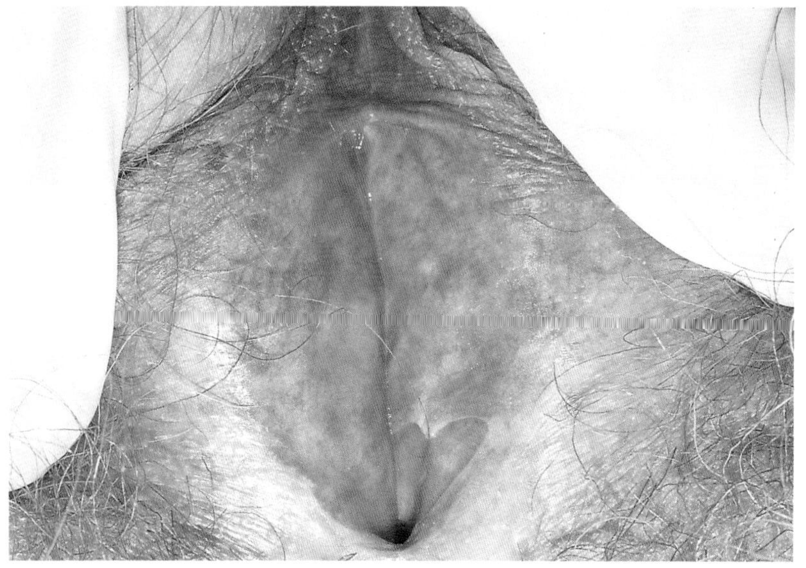

Fig. 6-14. Severe scarring with a loss of normal skin texture, disappearance of the labia minora, and obliteration of the vaginal space are the most striking feature of this patient with lichen planus, but the more specific findings are the erosion over the anterior left vulva and the surrounding white epithelium. Compare with Figures 11-12 and 16-9.

Most patients with erosive genital lichen planus do not have skin lesions elsewhere, but oral involvement is usual. Ulcerative genital lesions are generally accompanied by ulcerative oral disease, and nonerosive disease of the genitalia is usually accompanied by white, linear or reticulate morphology in the mouth (Fig. 6-15). The posterior buccal mucosa and gingivae are the areas of the mouth most likely to be affected. Although lesions of the bladder and rectal mucosa have been reported, these are rare and do not require evaluation beyond a directed review of systems.

Patients with ulcerative lichen planus complain primarily of pain and itching, whereas those with nonerosive disease usually describe only pruritus. Women with erosive disease often experience recurrent episodes of a purulent, painful, or irritating vaginal discharge. The secretions exhibit a pH greater than 5 and multiple white blood cells on microscopic examination. This discharge is often precipitated or worsened by a bacterial superinfection of eroded vaginal epithelium. The presence of this discharge should alert the clinician to the probable presence of active, significant vaginal disease.

Histology

Histologically, lichen planus shows irregular thickening of the epidermis and hyperkeratosis, except on mucous membrane, where thinning can occur. Focal accentuation of the granular cell layer of the epidermis is present, as well as a dense mononuclear infiltrate in the upper dermis. This inflammation extends to the basal cell layer of the epidermis and produces damage manifested by necrotic keratinocytes and evidence of disruption of the basement membrane. Mucous membrane lesions of the genitalia may show parakeratosis rather than hypergranulosis, and epidermal necrosis or subepithelial blistering are likely to produce erosions. When erosive disease is sampled, the biopsy should be performed from the edge of an erosion where epithelium is present, since the histologic diagnosis of lichen planus requires the epidermal changes described above.

Diagnosis

The diagnosis of lichen planus is made on clinical grounds and confirmed histologically. The dusky red, sharply circumscribed, and often very subtly scaling papules of non-mucous membrane skin may be difficult to differentiate from psoriasis, a dermatophyte infection, or neurodermatitis. However, these diseases usually present with larger plaques than found with lichen planus, and they can be further differentiated from lichen planus by distribution and a potassium hydroxide examination. When nonerosive lichen planus occurs on the glans, differentiation from psoriasis, plasma cell balanitis, Bowen's disease, and yeast infection can be difficult. If a potassium hydroxide preparation of the lesion and an examina-

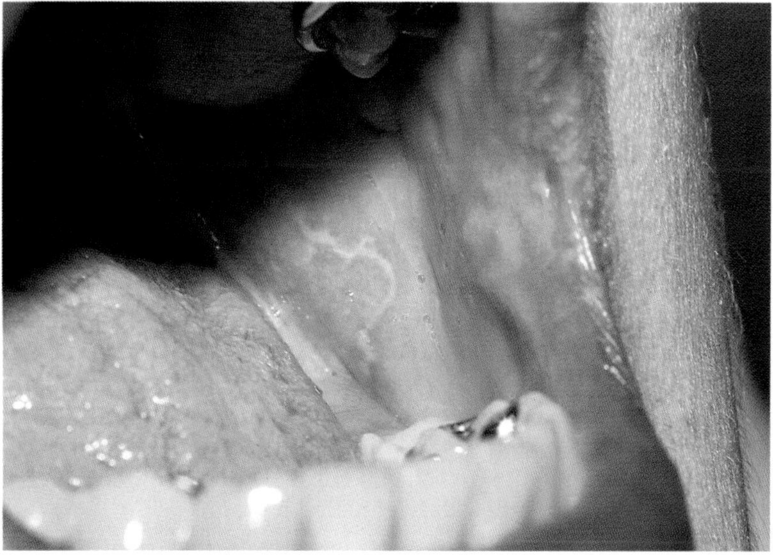

Fig. 6-15. Irregular white striae of lichen planus in the posterior buccal mucosa. Either this nonerosive form of the disease or oral erosions are nearly always present in association with genital lichen planus and provide valuable confirmation of the diagnosis.

tion of the mouth for lichen planus are not helpful, a biopsy often yields a definitive diagnosis. Although the white, linear papules of typical mucous membrane lichen planus are easily recognized and specific, the diagnosis of very subtle or erosive lichen planus can be difficult, especially for the clinician without a high index of suspicion. The white lesions may be inconspicuous or hidden within vulvar folds and not easily visualized unless the examiner is looking specifically and carefully for these changes. These white changes can be confused with *Candida* infection or nonspecific hyperkeratosis from inflammation or scratching.

Erosive lichen planus occasionally presents with no surrounding typical lesions. Although these erosions are generally easily differentiated from infectious causes by their chronic course, their lack of indurated borders and base, and their superficial nature, differentiation from other inflammatory or blistering diseases may be difficult. Those diseases likely to present diagnostic difficulties are summarized in Table 6-1. These especially include plasma cell vulvitis and balanitis, cicatricial pemphigoid, and pemphigus vulgaris. If mouth lesions are not present or are not clinically identifiable, then a biopsy is necessary.

The differentiation of late or advanced disease characterized by nonspecific scarring and loss of genital landmarks from several other inflammatory and blistering diseases can be difficult. This clinical picture is characterized by adhesions and disappearance of normal external architecture, including loss of the labia minora; agglutination of the clitoral prepuce with covering of the clitoris under scar; narrowing of the introitus; and, in men, loss of the sharp demarcation of the corona from the shaft. Lichen sclerosus and cicatrical pemphigoid especially can be indistinguishable from lichen planus at this stage disease. In addition, the skin is smooth and lacks normal sebaceous glands, skin markings, folds, and irregularities. The most common diagnostic dilemma in late disease is the differentiation of lichen planus from the much more common lichen sclerosus. However, lichen sclerosus never occurs in the vagina or mouth, whereas lichen planus regularly occurs in these areas, and in many patients clinically diagnostic lesions of lichen planus or the white, finely crinkled papules of lichen sclerosus can be identified on careful examination. Scarring and erosive lichen sclerosus and lichen planus may lose their differentiating morphologic and histologic features. Also, the coexistence of lichen planus and lichen sclerosus has been noted by many clinicians, and both diseases may be present. Careful follow-up of patients and several biopsies may be necessary to make the correct diagnosis.

Course and Prognosis

Symptoms of patients with nonerosive lichen planus are often well controlled with topical corticosteroids, and the disease may remit spontaneously. However, erosive disease is chronic, recalcitrant, and scarring, producing pain or pruritus that is only partially ameliorated by therapy. Although mild disease is sometimes controlled with topical corticosteroids, the course of usual erosive lichen planus is one of exacerbations with slow healing, recurrent secondary infections, and expensive or dangerous therapies.

Pathogenesis

The cause of lichen planus is not known. Evidence indicates a probable role for an autoimmune disorder of cellular immunity.[13] Also, the histologic features of lichen planus closely resemble those of graft-versus-host disease, another condition of immune origin.

Treatment

The treatment of erosive lichen planus is difficult, although many patients with nonerosive disease do well using only topical corticosteroids. A midpotency corticosteroid ointment applied twice a day is necessary, and a higher potency can be substituted for patients with a poor response. Men with recalcitrant erosive penile disease may benefit from a corticosteroid ointment under condom occlusion to enhance the potency of the medication. Those using long-term or high-potency corticosteroids should be followed carefully for atrophy in the affected area and surrounding skin since medication generally spreads to unaffected skin. In nonerosive disease, a cream base is often tolerated better than an ointment. Severely eroded skin cannot be treated well with topical medication because of local pain, and medication does not remain on exudative skin. Open areas of limited size can often be healed with intralesional triamcinolone acetonide injections at a concentration of 3 mg/ml. When the area of involvement is too great for intralesional therapy to be practical, oral prednisone at a dose of 40 mg each morning until healing has occurred allows better management with topical agents. As the skin heals, topical corticosteroids may be added as prednisone is tapered. Those patients whose disease cannot be maintained satisfactorily on the topical corticosteroids normally deemed appropriate in the genital area may be given a careful and closely monitored trial of an ultrahigh-potency corticosteroid such as clobetasol propionate 0.05 percent.

For patients not controlled by safe doses of corticosteroids, topical cyclosporine provides a safe and often effective albeit extraordinarily expensive alternative for mucous membrane disease. (Pelisse et al, personal communication, 1991). The oral or injectable form of the medication is applied in 100 mg amounts directly to the affected skin four times a day initially. If several mucous membranes are affected, for example, 100 mg is applied to the vulva, 100 mg inserted in the vagina, and 100 mg held in the mouth for as long as tolerated before spitting. In penile disease, cyclosporine can be placed under condom occlusion for enhanced absorption. As disease is controlled, the frequency of application can be tapered. Occasionally, in patients with debilitating and painful disease not adequately treated by therapies discussed above, oral cyclosporine may be used.[14] This medication should be used only by physicians experienced in its use and willing to exercise extreme caution and care in ongoing evaluations of organ systems, especially renal function. Also, this medication confers an increased risk of late lymphoma. Cyclosporine should be started at a dose of 3 mg/kg and increased only as needed to 5 mg/kg. Above this dose, the risk of toxicity becomes much greater.

For those patients who do not respond to topical or intralesional corticosteroids or cyclosporine, several other medications may occasionally be useful. Retinoids, especially topical tretinoin, have been used in the treatment of oral mucous membrane disease. Unfortunately, this medication is too irritating to be tolerated in the genital area by most patients, especially in those with preexisting painful disease. Oral retinoids at a standard dose of 40 mg twice a day (isotretinoin) or 25 mg twice a day (etretinate) may be tried.[15] The effectiveness of retinoids for oral lichen planus has been described in small series. The information available on the activity of retinoids in genital lichen planus is scant but indicates no marked favorable effect. Oral griseofulvin has been reported useful in the treatment of lichen planus,[16] but significant improvements have only occasionally been described in women with erosive genital disease.[17] One small and unconfirmed series found dapsone useful for lichen planus, but this medication was not effective for a small group of women with erosive vulvovaginal disease.[17] Finally, in severe disease, oral cyclophosphamide or azathioprine have been reported to be useful.

Local and supportive care are important in the management of genital lichen planus. Women with erosive vaginal disease are especially likely to develop superinfections, both bacterial and, with subsequent antibiotic therapy, *Candida*. The presence of a yellow or green vaginal discharge characterized microscopically by multiple white blood cells indicates the need for a vaginal culture and antibiotic treatment. Careful and frequent examination of the vagina for early adhesions is important, and patients who do not have regular intercourse should use vaginal dilators to maintain patency of the vagina. The use of hydrocortisone acetate suppositories, 25 mg, at bedtime can also be useful in minimizing vaginal scarring by providing a space-occupying delivery of medication.

Those women who experience scarring that results in introital stenosis and vaginal adhesions sometimes benefit from the use of vaginal dilators at home in graduated sizes or surgical release of scars. Surgery should only be performed after active disease is controlled; otherwise, scarring rapidly recurs. Following surgery, patients must use vaginal dilators daily to maintain adequate patency of the introitus and vagina during healing. These women should be followed carefully to separate early re-forming adhesions manually, treat secondary infections, and offer moral support.

Important in the management of patients with gential lichen planus, especially erosive disease, is patient education and support. Patients with scarring, painful, and often recalcitrant gential disease not only must deal with the obvious discomfort of the disease and the expense and side effects of therapy, but also with problems of self-image and sexuality. Many people with erosive lichen planus are unable to engage in sexual intercourse either because of pain or scarring, particularly of the vagina. Some patients

Table 6-1. Comparison of Characteristics of More Common Noninfectious Erosive and Bullous Diseases

Disease	*Clinical Manifestations*					*Biopsy*	*Treatment*	*Course*
	Genital	*Oral*	*Other*	*Age*	*Onset*			
Lichen planus	Red-lavender papules with white striae over glans and shaft of penis, or white reticulate striae over modified mucous membranes of vulva; or erosions of glans, vulva (especially vestibule), and vagina Late, sometimes severe scarring	White striae or erosions over posterior buccal mucosa; erosive genital lesions often associated with desquamative gingivitis	Other lesions occur but are rare	40+ years	Slow	Chronic bandlike upper dermal inflammatory infiltrate with liquefaction degeneration of basal cell layer	Topical corticosteroids, cyclosporine for severe, recalcitrant disease	Chronic, poor response to therapy
Lichen sclerosus	White, crinkled plaques with fragility manifested by purpura, erosions; located over modified mucous membranes of vulva, perineum, perianal area of women, glans of men No vaginal involvement Gradual sometimes severe scarring	None	Approximately 20% of women have distant keratinized skin involvement	Any	Slow	Flattening of epidermis, homogenization of upper dermis, liquefaction degeneration of basal cell layer, upper dermal chronic inflammatory infiltrate	Topical corticosteroids, topical testosterone	Chronic but excellent response to therapy with cessation of scarring
Cicatricial pemphigoid	Nonspecific erosions, especially over glans penis, modified mucous membranes of vulva, vestibule, and vagina Sometimes blisters or erosions of surrounding, keratinized skin. Severe scarring possible	Oral erosions usual	Conjunctival lesions usual, other mucous membrane involvement common; keratinized skin blisters and erosions in 10–30%	60+ years	Slow or relatively fast over several weeks	Subepidermal blister, lymphocytic infiltrate, often also eosinophils or neutrophils	Systemic corticosteroids; azathioprine or cyclophosphamide	Chronic; sometimes poor response to therapy

Bullous pemphigoid	Erosions and blisters usually limited to keratinized skin, without scarring	Up to ⅓ of patients with oral lesions	Bullae of distant keratinized skin usual	60+ years	Variable	Subepidermal blisters, lymphocytic inflammation, often also eosinophils or neutrophils	Systemic corticosteroids; azathioprine or cyclophosphamide	Chronic, usually responsive to therapy Often self-limited
Pemphigus vulgaris/vegetans	Nonspecific erosions, usually modified mucous membranes and vagina first, then surrounding keratinized skin Sometimes scarring	Usual	Mucous membranes common, keratinized skin erosions and bullae follow	30–50 years	Over weeks	Intraepithelial suprabasilar acantholytic blister	Systemic corticosteroids; azathioprine or cyclophosphamide	Chronic, sometimes remission with therapy
Acute contact dermatitis	Vesiculation, erosion; location depending on distribution of contactant No scarring	None	Depends on distribution of contact, inner thighs common	Any	Sudden	Spongiosis, epidermal necrosis, erosion	Withdrawal of contactant, soaks, sometimes oral corticosteroids	Self-limited
Erythema multiforme/Stevens-Johnson syndrome	Erosions of vagina and modified mucous membranes of vulva and glans penis, sometimes with surrounding keratinized skin involvement Sometimes scarring	Usual, often including lips	Usually palm and sole lesions, often generalized red plaques or blistering	Any, often young adults	Sudden	Epidermal spongiosis and necrosis, liquefaction degeneration of basal cell layer, lymphohistiocytic dermal infiltrate	Withdrawal of antigen, supportive care and soaks, sometimes oral corticosteroids early	Self-limited
Fixed drug eruption	Modified mucous membranes of vulva, glans; usually 1–3-cm erosions, limited number	Often	Lesions of distant keratinized skin often	Any	Sudden	Epidermal spongiosis and necrosis, liquefaction degeneration of basal cell layer, superficial and deep lymphohistiocytic dermal infiltrate	Withdrawal of offending medication, soaks	Recurrent with use of offending agent

have difficulty sitting and walking, making activities of daily living difficult. Severe genital disease is often associated with severe mouth disease that can make eating and talking painful. Many patients are understandably depressed, and supplying them with both emotional support and antidepressant therapy when indicated is a major component of the management of lichen planus. These patients also need education about their disease, treatment options, and expectations. Those patients expecting an inexpensive cure will be disappointed and frustrated. When they are counseled about the trial-and-error nature of therapy and the goal of control rather than cure, patients are much more tolerant of side effects, slow healing, and multiple and frequent interventions.

LUPUS ERYTHEMATOSUS

There are few reports of genital involvement in lupus erythematosus, although lesions of the mucous membranes of the mouth are well described. It is likely that relatively asymptomatic or unrecognized lesions of genital lupus erythematosus are more common than realized.

Clinical Presentation

Lupus erythematosus is an autoimmune disease that exists on a spectrum from mild disease with only minor skin lesions to multisystem, life-threatening illness. The skin lesions of lupus erythematosus are divided into morphologic types that generally correlate with the presence and degree of systemic involvement.

Chronic cutaneous lupus erythematosus (CCLE), or discoid lupus erythematosus, is most often associated with minimal or no systemic symptoms. Skin lesions are characterized by well-demarcated, deeply erythematous (or, in black patients, dark brown) plaques with scale and sometimes crusting. Central healing follows with scarring and depigmentation, while active peripheral disease shows surrounding hyperpigmentation that is much more marked and common in dark skin. CCLE first occurs on the face, especially the lateral aspects, and often remains limited to this area. In more severe disease, lesions develop over the central face, scalp, and upper chest and extremities and are more likely to be associated with systemic evidence of disease. Subacute cutaneous lupus erythematosus (SCLE) generally is associated with systemic disease but usually without severe renal or central nervous system involvement. These skin lesions show solid or annular red, sharply marginated, scaling papules and plaques that heal without scarring. Lesions typically develop over the upper trunk and dorsal aspect of the upper extremities. The skin lesions of systemic lupus erythematosus are red, nonscarring, less well-demarcated plaques, often with edema and sometimes with fine scale, primarily located over the face.

The prevalence of genital lesions of lupus erythematosus is not known because physicians do not routinely examine the genitalia for lesions. Oral mucous membrane involvement occurs in up to 45 percent of patients, most often in those with systemic disease; many fewer discoid lupus erythematosus patients are affected. It is likely that genital mucous membrane lesions follow this general pattern. The only study that has specifically examined the prevalence of genital lesions of lupus erythematosus examined 90 women with CCLE and SCLE; two had genital lesions and one patient had symptoms but no specific lesion.[18]

Most reports of genital lupus erythematosus have documented its existence but not characterized its morphologic appearance. Those genital lesions that have been described are usually erosions or ulcers with surrounding inflammation. These punched-out, well-demarcated lesions are often painful. More superficial, erosive plaques resembling erosive lichen planus have been described on the mucous membrane portion of the vulva, and white, lacy plaques resembling typical mucous membrane lichen planus have also been reported.[19] Lesions in the vulvar area may also be circinate.[19] Both ulcers and erosive disease of the vagina have also been reported, and scarring may occur but vaginal synechiae and loss of vulvar architecture apparently do not develop.

Histology

The histologic appearance of lupus erythematosus is specific, although, like the clinical appearance, there are strong similarities to lichen planus. Epithelial thinning with liquefaction degeneration of the basal cell layer is present, or, in old disease, thickening of the basement membrane indicative of past injury occurs. A patchy superficial and deep lymphocytic infiltrate in the dermis with periadnexal and perivascular distribution is characteristic of lupus. Hair-bearing skin shows hyperkeratosis and follicular plugging.

Diagnosis

The diagnosis of genital cutaneous lupus erythematosus is generally made by correlation with nongenital findings or a skin biopsy, or both. Examination of other skin surfaces often reveals other evidence of cutaneous lupus erythematosus and more specific signs to aid in the diagnosis. The genital ulcers of lupus erythematosus may mimic those found in Behçet's disease, aphthous ulcers, and ulcers produced by sexually transmitted diseases such as primary syphilis, chancroid, granuloma inguinale, and herpes simplex virus infection. Erosive lesions may be confused with erosive lichen planus, fixed drug eruption, erythema multiforme, or immunobullous diseases, and the white mucous membrane lesions should also be differentiated from lichen planus. If specific evidence of lupus erythematosus is lacking in other aspects of the physical examination, a biopsy is usually helpful.

Course and Prognosis

Patients with genital lupus erythematosus often have systemic disease requiring systemic treatment. The local disease is chronic, but fairly good control is generally obtained with therapy.

Pathogenesis

Lupus erythematosus is an autoimmune disease characterized by the presence of multiple autoantibodies that probably are important in the pathogenesis of the disease. Both hereditary and environmental factors are responsible for the production of these antibodies and the subsequent development of the disorder.

Treatment

Patients with significant systemic signs require oral corticosteroid therapy that also often controls skin disease, including genital disease. Others need safer, chronic measures to control their genital lesions. Those with very localized genital disease can be treated with intralesional triamcinolone acetonide at a concentration of 3 mg/ml. For ulcerative disease not improved with intralesional corticosteroids, a short burst of oral prednisone at 40 mg each morning for 1 to 3 weeks may encourage healing and allow institution of topical corticosteroids or safer but slower oral medications to control lesions over the long term. Lesions that are not ulcerative in nature may improve with the application of a topical, usually high-potency and occasionally superpotent, corticosteroid with careful monitoring for surrounding cutaneous atrophy. Vaginal lesions of any type may be treated with a corticosteroid inserted in the vagina at bedtime. Hydrocortisone acetate rectal suppositories, 25 mg, are usually well tolerated, but other corticosteroid creams or ointments can also be inserted vaginally. Recalcitrant penile lesions may improve if treated with corticosteroids; sometimes they require either condom occlusion or a superpotent class of medication.

If these measures are ineffective, oral antimalarial medications such as chronic oral hydroxychloroquine at 200 mg twice a day or chloroquine at 500 mg/day may be beneficial. As long as careful and regular examinations of the retinas and monitoring of liver functions are performed, these medications are safe and well tolerated. Genital lesions recalcitrant to these measures often can be controlled with oral retinoids such as isotretinoin 40 mg bid. Cost, teratogenicity, and cutaneous dryness and chapping are the primary disadvantages of this therapy that otherwise may be very effective. Other alternatives in patients with unusually difficult disease include combinations of more than one of the therapies discussed, including a combination of more than one antimalarial agent.

In the genital area, care should be taken to maximize the healing conditions of the local environment. Genital bacterial or fungal superinfections should be treated. The vagina should be examined routinely for the presence of significant scarring or a superimposed bacterial vaginitis. In some cases, an antibiotic ointment may decrease pain by virtue of its emollient properties and may minimize the risk of infection.

Patient education and emotional support are important in the management of patients with genital lesions of lupus erythematosus. Since these patients often have systemic disease, there are usually many issues that need to be addressed, and a multidisplinary approach may be required.

PITYRIASIS ROSEA

Pityriasis rosea is a common condition. It occurs primarily in late childhood through early adult life. The trunk is always involved, but extension occurs onto the proximal extremities with appreciable frequency. For this reason, the anogenital region may be involved.

Clinical Presentation

Pityriasis rosea is an easily recognized disease when it presents in its most classical form. Typically 50 to 100 small (1- to 2-cm) flat lesions are noted over the trunk and proximal extremities. The individual lesions are oval or elliptical in shape, and all of the lesions are situated with their long axes parallel both to each other and to the rib lines (Fig. 6-16). This pattern, when viewed on the patient's back, suggests the branches of a spruce ("Christmas") tree extending laterally from the spine. All of the lesions (except the herald patch) are approximately the same size; this feature causes the eruption to appear somewhat "monotonous." Scale is scanty if present at all. The lesions are usually asymptomatic, but occasionally itching is troublesome.

The so-called herald patch, which occurs in about one half of the patients, is also a characteristic feature of the disease. It is a solitary, large (4 to 8 cm) patch that precedes the development of the smaller lesions. This larger lesion is usually more round than oval and very frequently has an annular outline. The herald patch, in contrast to the smaller, oval lesions described above, often has a scaling border.

The herald patch, with its ringlike configuration, may occur on the lower trunk, the perigenital area, or the upper thighs. In these areas it may assume the appearance of tinea cruris or tinea corporis. Distinction is possible on the basis of either a KOH preparation (see Ch. 2) or biopsy.

Pityriasis rosea is improved with exposure to ultraviolet light. Conversely, in a well-tanned individual lesions may not occur on sunexposed areas of skin. For this reason it is not terribly uncommon for the majority of lesions to be found only on the skin covered by the lower half of a swimsuit. In such cases the disease, lacking the classic features described above, can be quite difficult to recognize.

Differential Diagnoses

Diseases to be considered in the list of differential diagnoses include secondary syphilis, guttate psoriasis, and fungal infection. Lack of involvement of the face, scalp (patchy hair loss), palms, and soles helps to exclude secondary syphilis; it can be totally ruled out if a syphilis serologic test is negative. The lesions of guttate psoriasis are round rather than oval and are generally covered with appreciable scale. Tinea corporis and cruris are excluded on the basis of KOH

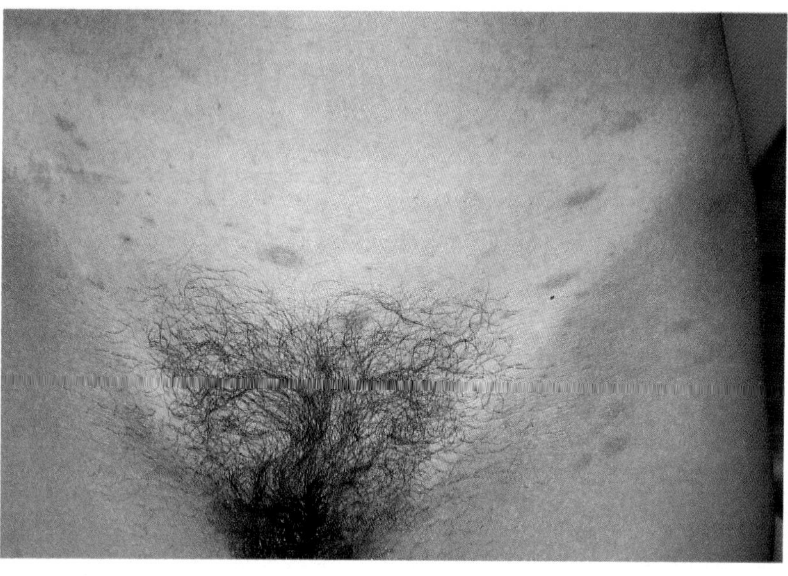

Fig. 6-16. Characteristic oval, pink, minimally scaling papules of pityriasis rosea.

examination as described above. The lesions of tinea (pityriasis) versicolor are not oval and vary appreciably in size from one lesion to another; a KOH preparation reveals typical mycelia and spores. The histologic appearance of these diseases is distinctive enough to allow biopsy identification when the clinical picture is confusing.

Course and Prognosis

Pityriasis rosea is a totally benign disease that runs its complete course in 6 to 12 weeks. The herald patch, if one occurs, precedes the development of the remainder of the eruption by 7 to 14 days. Most of the smaller lesions tend to develop in a crop over just a few days. However, new individual lesions may continue to appear during the first 3 to 4 weeks. Once the resolution phase begins, lesions disappear insidiously over about a week; no scarring or pigmentary change remains. Recurrence of the disease develops in about 5 percent of patients.

Pathogenesis

The cause of pityriasis rosea is unknown. About 20 percent of the time it follows a preceding pharyngitis or upper respiratory infection, suggesting that it may be a postinfectious exanthem. The infrequency of recurrence suggests a viral etiology. On the other hand, the lack of clustered cases in families and among school children argues against infection as a cause of the disease.

Treatment

Since the disease resolves spontaneously, treatment is not necessary. Some patients experience troublesome itching. In such cases, topical steroids and orally administered antihistamines (as described in Ch. 3) can be used. Ultraviolet light therapy is somewhat effective but is rarely indicated.

BOWEN'S DISEASE, BOWENOID PAPULOSIS, AND ERYTHROPLASIA OF QUEYRAT

The diseases discussed in this section represent clinically distinguishable forms of squamous cell carcinoma in situ (SCCIS). However, biologically and histologically they are for practical purposes indistinguishable. Because of these similarities, many argue that the old eponymous terminology should be replaced with the term *intraepithelial neoplasia,* preceded by the anatomic site. Thus, Bowen's disease of the genitalia would become vulvar intraepithelial neoplasia (VIN) and penile intraepithelial neoplasia (PIN). Gynecologists, pathologists, and some dermatologists believe that this terminology best describes the nature of the problem in terms understandable to all.

The use of this *intraepithelial neoplasia* terminology also allows for grading the degree of dysplasia present. Thus VIN I indicates mild dysplasia, VIN II indicates moderate dysplasia, and VIN III indicates severe, full-thickness dysplasia. Others, mostly dermatologists, have been slow to accept this view not only for reasons of tradition but also because the nomenclature becomes unwieldy when the concept is extended to in situ carcinoma of the perigenital skin. An excellent discussion of these terminology problems can be found in the 1989 International Society for the Study of Vulvar Disease (ISSVD) presidential address by Edward Wilkinson.[20]

Although the lesions of SCCIS are clinically distinctive, biopsy is always required for confirmation of diagnosis. A small lesion with uniform color and elevation usually requires only a single biopsy from a randomly chosen site. However, when the surface of a single lesion is heterogenous it is best to carry out several biopsies (especially from eroded or ulcerated areas) in order that areas of invasion can be identified. Multifocal disease poses a greater problem. Three or four biopsies from scattered lesions are desirable when multiple lesion are present since one or more of the sites may demonstrate focal areas of invasion.

In the past, 1 or 2 percent toluidine blue solution was used as a diagnostic aid in choosing the site for biopsy. Those areas retaining the dye after acetic acid wash were considered as most likely to reveal microscopic evidence of malignancy. More recently 3 to 5 percent acetic acid application has been suggested as a helpful way of identifying lesions that contain human papillomavirus (HPV) DNA. Since the presence of HPV DNA is associated with the potential development of SCCIS, biopsies would be taken from areas that became aceto-white. The use of acetic acid for the purposes of identifying wart virus infection is further considered in the section on genital

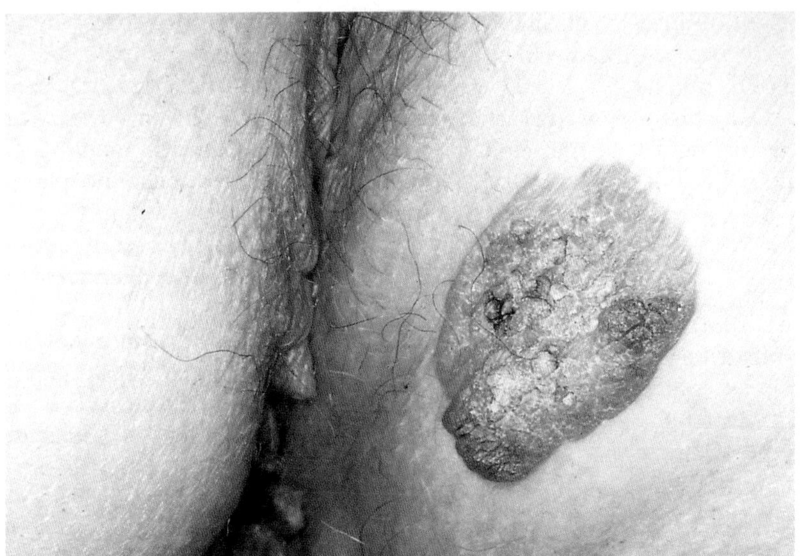

Fig. 6-17. Sharply demarcated, keratotic plaque of Bowen's disease.

warts (see Ch. 9), but in our opinion neither acetic acid or toluidine blue have sufficient sensitivity or specificity to warrant their use for purposes of identifying malignancy. Instead, we believe that any lesion that cannot be positively identified as benign deserves biopsy.

Clinical Presentation

Bowen's Disease

Bowen's disease is clinically distinctive. It occurs as a dusky red, sharply marginated plaque that is round to somewhat gyrate in configuration (Figs. 6-17 and 6-18). Scale may or may not be present on the surface. Lesions vary in size from 2 to 10 cm in diameter; lesions smaller in diameter are sometimes termed Bowenoid papulosis (see below). In most instances only a single lesion is present. The clinical entity recognized as Bowen's disease is located primarily on perigenital skin and on nonmucosal aspects of the genitalia. Bowen's disease is rarely encountered before the age of 50 years.[21]

Patients with Bowen's disease are slow to seek medical attention because of the insidious onset and the stability of lesional size. When asked about such lesions the patient commonly replies, "It's nothing; I've had it for years and it's never changed or grown." Itching is present in about 50 percent of women and in a somewhat smaller percentage of men. The pres-

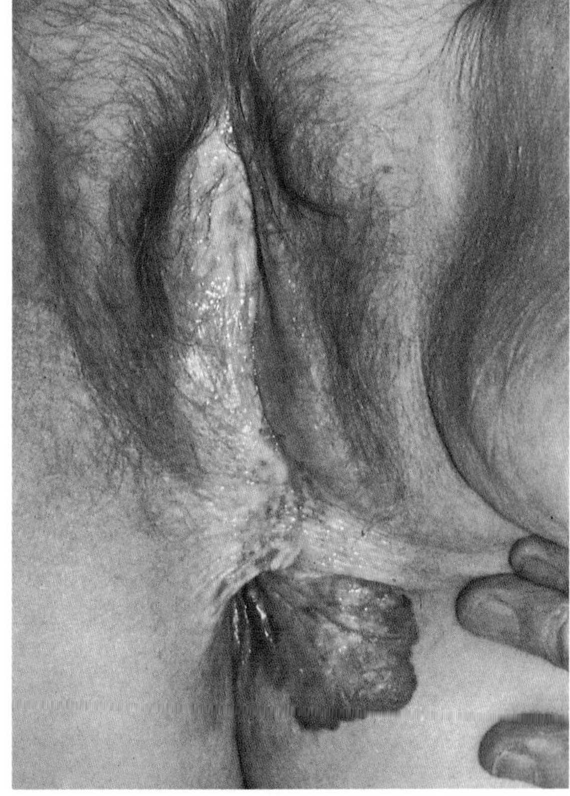

Fig. 6-18. Erythematous, moist plaque of perianal Bowen's disease with peripheral hyperpigmentation.

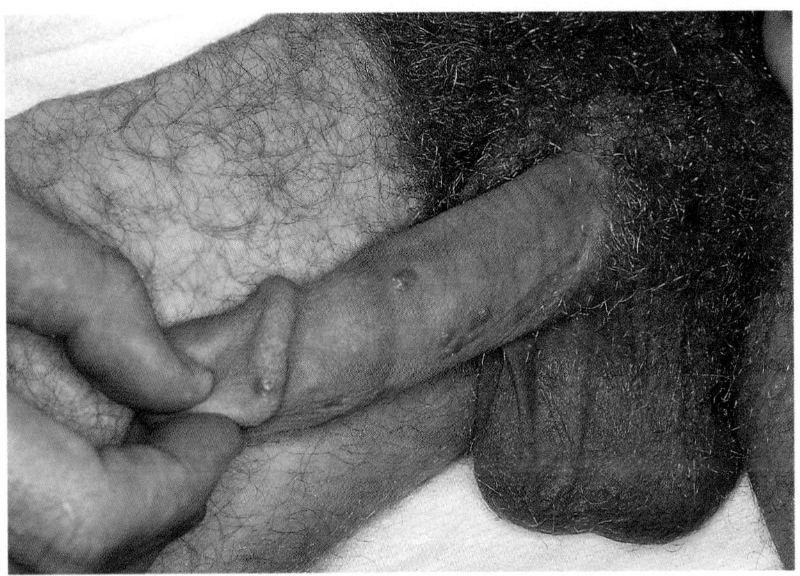

Fig. 6-19. Flat, pink papules of Bowenoid papulosis.

ence of pruritus is often the main reason for a patient's decision to seek medical care.

Bowenoid Papulosis

Bowenoid papulosis is a term coined by Wade, Kopf, and Ackerman in 1978[22] when they described a multifocal, papular form of carcinoma in situ occuring on the penis in young men. Similar lesions had been noted in women some years earlier, and in 1979, the term *Bowenoid papulosis* was extended to include vulvar lesions.[23] While *Bowenoid papulosis* appeals to dermatologists,[24] it does not to gynecologists, who generally prefer the ISSVD terminology, multifocal VIN.

The lesions of Bowenoid papulosis are sharply marginated, flat-topped papules or small plaques. In men, the lesions tend to be small, often no more than 4 or 5 mm in diameter (Fig. 6-19). In women the lesions are more variable in size, with diameters as large as 2 or 3 cm. The color is also quite variable. Pink and red hues (hence the discussion in this section) are most common, but nearly an equal number will be hyperpigmented, with shades ranging from tan to dark gray-brown (Figs. 6-20 and 6-21). Lesions on the moist areas of the vulva may even be white in color.

In men, 5 to 10 lesions are usually found, whereas in women the range is greater; sometimes as many as

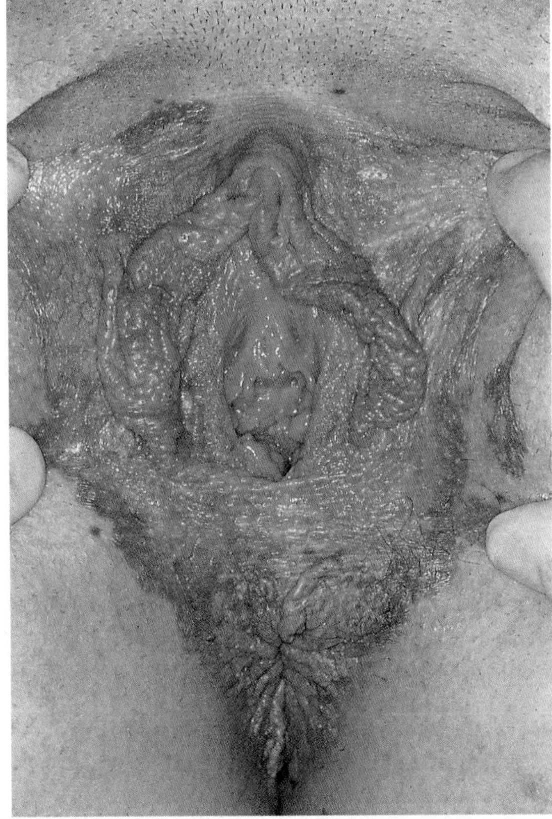

Fig. 6-20. Extensive, erythematous, and hyperpigmented plaque and papules of multifocal VIN of Bowen's disease.

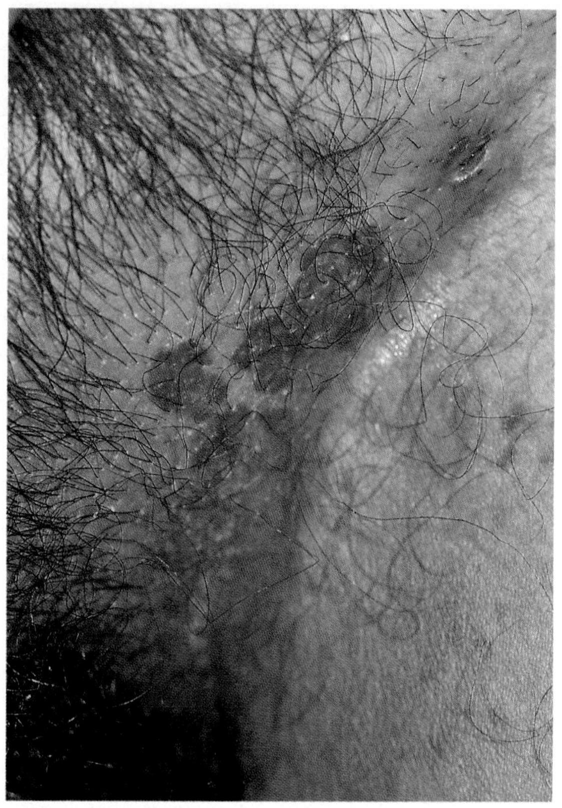

Fig. 6-21. Flat-topped, brown, sharply demarcated papules of multifocal Bowen's disease.

25 lesions may be present. The distribution is remarkably widespread. In women the vestibule, the outer aspects of the labia minora, and the labia majora are most often involved. In men, the glans penis, prepuce, and shaft of the penis are the favored locations. Perianal lesions are also commonly encountered in both sexes. Lesions may be discrete and at some distance from one another, but, especially in women, confluence of lesions can occur, in which case larger plaques with gyrate borders are noted.

The average age of onset for multifocal carcinoma in situ is much younger than that for unifocal disease.[21] Most commonly, patients are 20 to 40 years of age, but lesions have been found in children as young as 2 years of age. The onset is also more sudden than that for unifocal disease; often the full complement of papules and plaques will develop in a matter of weeks or months. This explosive onset is particularly common in pregnancy. In men the lesions are usually asymptomatic; in women, pruritus occurs about 30 to 50 percent of the time.[25]

Erythroplasia of Queyrat

The term *erythroplasia of Queyrat* (EQ) has historically been used for unifocal carcinoma in situ when it occurs on the inner aspects of the prepuce (Fig. 6-22) or on the glans penis (Fig. 6-23). As the name implies, it appears as a sharply marginated red patch or slightly elevated plaque. Occasionally in uncircumcised men the surface is white when the lesion is occluded by the foreskin. However, within minutes of foreskin retraction, moisture evaporates, leaving the characteristic red color. Scale is not clinically apparent.

The average size of EQ is 1 to 2 cm in diameter. Generally, a single lesion is present. Onset is insidious, and inasmuch as the process is usually asymptomatic, the lesion will usually have been present for a year or more at the time the patient first presents for examination.

Lesions entirely similar to EQ may be found on the inner aspects of the labia minora in women. In this setting, for no reason other than convention, the term *Bowen's disease* has been used instead of *erythroplasia.* Interestingly, similar lesions, termed *erythroplakia,* also occur on the mucous membranes of the mouth.

Course and Prognosis

As indicated above, SCCIS of the unifocal type has an insidious onset over a matter of many months. Moreover, enlargement occurs so slowly as to be almost imperceptible. On the other hand SCCIS of the multifocal type begins earlier in life and evolves more rapidly. Both types of lesions have the biologic potential for local invasion and eventual metastatic spread, but in almost all instances in men, and in most instances in women, this potential is never expressed.[24,25] In fact, in some patients with multifocal disease, spontaneous regression of one or more lesions definitely occurs.[23,26]

Several factors are important in determining the outcome of patients with SCCIS. Of these, the degree to which the patient is immunocompetent is probably the most important. For instance, notably rapid progression toward invasive disease has been observed in patients with acquired immunodeficiency syn-

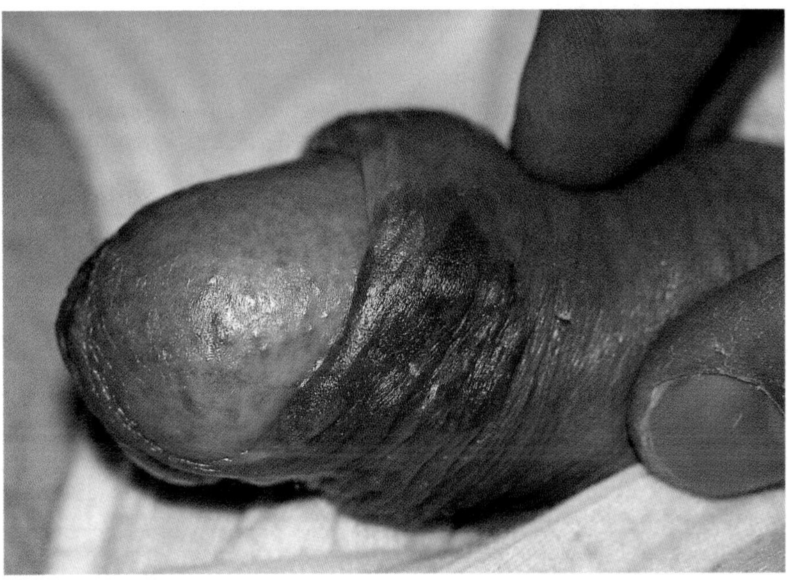

Fig. 6-22. Well-demarcated, shiny, red plaque of Bowen's disease on the foreskin (erythroplasia of Queyrat).

drome (AIDS). Age may be a factor for related reasons; immune responsiveness decreases with aging. Thus, younger patients seem at less risk for development of invasive disease than do the elderly.[27] A third factor is the site of the lesions. Those occurring on keratinizing epithelium seem less likely to become invasive than those occurring on mucosal surfaces. Most importantly, lesions occuring at transformation zones (the cervix and the anus) have a rather high risk of invasion and metastasis. Several cofactors (cocarcinogens or promoters) may worsen the prognosis. The best studied of these is cigarette smoking, which has been well documented as having a detrimental effect.[28,29] Other factors such as therapeutic use of corticosteroids and sex hormones are somewhat less clearly involved.

The course of anogenital squamous cell carcinoma, once it has become invasive or metastatic, lies beyond the scope of this book.

Pathogenesis

Much excitement exists regarding the role that virus infection, particularly that due to HPV infection, plays in the development of SCCIS.[30,31] This subject will be specifically covered in this section on genital warts, but suffice it to say that HPV infection seems critically important in the etiology of multifo-

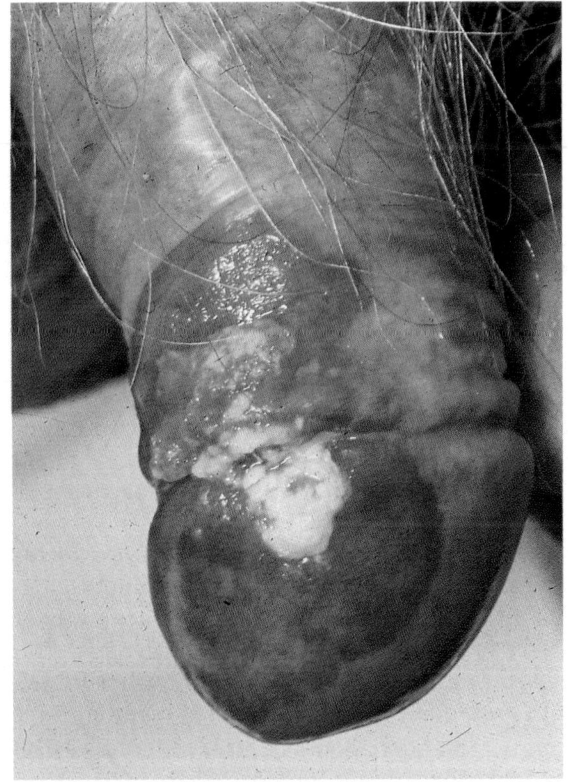

Fig. 6-23. Red, glistening, well-demarcated plaque of erythroplasia of Queyrat (Bowen's disease).

cal SCCIS, whereas its role in unifocal disease, if any, is much less clear. Interestingly, and by analogy with cervical carcinoma, the p53 tumor-suppressor gene (and its protein product) may play a role in both HPV-positive and HPV-negative types of disease. In HPV-positive disease the protein product of the HPV E6 gene binds and degrades normal p53 protein, thus preventing it from performing its tumor suppressor function. In HPV-negative cervical carcinoma, mutations are found in the p53 suppressor gene and, as a result, a faulty, inoperative protein is produced.[32]

Treatment

Treatment of SCCIS has become somewhat less agressive during the last 10 years. In the past, vulvectomies and penectomies were frequently carried out in belief that in situ disease would invariably, and possibly quickly, progress to invasive cancer. Cure rates were, in fact, quite good, but as the average age of patients with SCCIS decreased, there has been increasing pressure to use less radical procedures that preserve genital tissue. Today, most agree that if one or more biopsies reveal only in situ disease, local excision is sufficient. Margins used for local excision vary according to site, but generally at least 3 to 5 mm of clinically noninvolved tissue should be taken. Histologic examination of the margins is desirable because the local recurrence rate, not suprisingly, rises appreciably if marginal involvement is present. In most instances the use of margins of 5 mm or less will allow for primary closure, but obviously it is better to err on the side of adequate removal even if this requires grafting.

Recurrence rates are rather high even with wide local excision. These high rates occur for two reasons. First, HPV DNA is invisibly left in the margins of almost all excised lesions; this oncogenic agent can cause the development of additional dysplasia in these marginal sites months or years later. Second, new areas of SCCIS may arise near (but not contiguous with) the site of excised lesions; these new lesions will be thought of as recurrences even though technically they are not. Nevertheless, ultimate cure rates with excisional surgery approach 100 percent.

Special mention should be made of the advantages of Mohs micrographic surgery because of its remarkable tissue-sparing effect.[33,34] In simplistic terms this type of surgery can be considered as using frozen section observation of deep and lateral margins for every piece of tissue removed. Basically, extremely thin horizontal slices of tissue are removed, and the edges of the tissue are marked with dyes. Each of these sections is microscopically examined moments later. Additional sections are then excised at any mapped site that reveals tumor involvement. Micrographic surgery is more time consuming than simple excision, but this is balanced by the fact that tumor-free margins are ensured and by the fact that no unnecessary normal tissue has been removed.

More recently laser therapy has been recommended for SCCIS.[35] This approach does not, of course, result in the availability of tissue that can be examined for dermal invasion or marginal involvement. Nevertheless, if several pretreatment biopsies are taken and if sufficiently wide margins (0.5 to 1.0 cm) are treated, the cure rates are similar to those for local excision. Electrosurgical destruction can achieve these results with no more patient discomfort and a lesser expense.

Some dermatologists have advocated even less aggressive treatment for multifocal SCCIS in men with very small lesions. Eventual cure rates in these patients using cryotherapy, trichloracetic acid, and fluorouracil appear to be comparable to those obtained with excision and laser ablation. Local recurrence rates are probably higher; the superficial destructive effect of these agents presumably leaves foci of dysplasia in adnexal structures. In any event, the low risk of progression to invasive disease in men with small lesions probably makes these higher recurrence rates acceptable.

Treatment of invasive SCC extends beyond the scope of this chapter. Coverage of invasive and metastatic disease can be found in standard textbooks of gynecology and urology.

EXTRAMAMMARY PAGET'S DISEASE

Extramammary Paget's disease occurs less commonly than Paget's disease of the nipple, but since more than 250 cases have been reported, nearly all gynecologists, urologists, and dermatologists will end up encountering a case or two in the course of practice.

Clinical Presentation

Extramammary Paget's disease is found almost entirely in the elderly. The average age at the time of diagnosis is approximately 65, and only a rare case has been reported in anyone under 50. As for Paget's disease of the nipple, women are involved more frequently than men by a ratio of approximately 3:1.

Most instances of extramammary Paget's disease occur in the anogenital region, although there are scattered reports of cases involving the axillae and the remainder of the "milk line" along the anterior portion of the trunk. The most frequent extramammary site is the vulva (approximately 65 percent of reported cases) followed by an anal and perianal location in both sexes (about 20 percent of cases).[36,37] Involvement of the male genitalia occurs in the remaining 15 percent of cases.[38] Most often only a single plaque is present, but occasionally two or more plaques are found. When multiple plaques occur, they may assume a bilateral, symmetrical location.[39]

The lesions of extramammary Paget's disease are rather heterogeneous in appearance. As suggested by our placement of the disease in a chapter on papulosquamous diseases, lesions are erythematous slightly elevated plaques 1 to 10 cm in diameter with sharp margination along at least a portion of the circumference (Fig. 6-24). The surface may have an eczematous appearance with areas of erosion and mild crusting. However, early lesions, especially when located in dry areas, are slightly scaly or even smooth surfaced (Figs. 6-25 and 6-26). In moist areas the superficial scale can become hydrated such that there is a somewhat white surface.

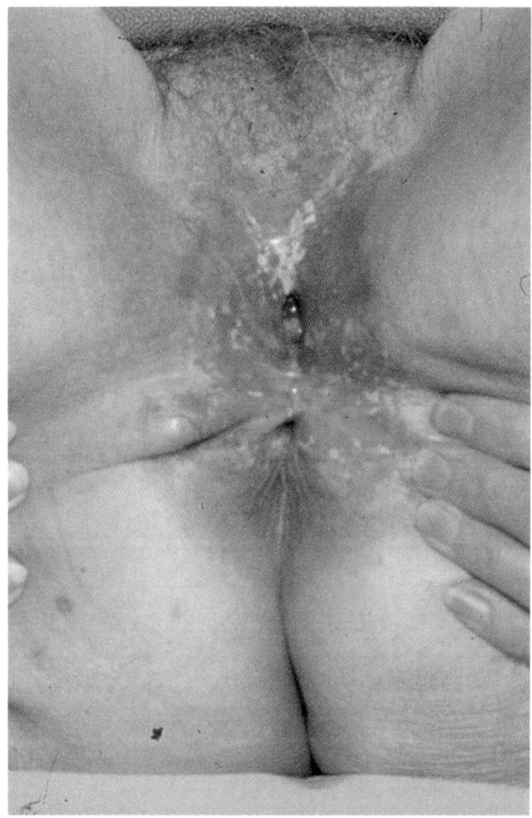

Fig. 6-24. Red, exudative plaque of extramammary Paget's disease on the moist surfaces of the vulva.

Fig. 6-25. Well-marginated, erythematous, irregular, multifocal plaques of extramammary Paget's disease over the mons pubis. These lesions represent recurrence. Note the surgical scar at the site of original removal.

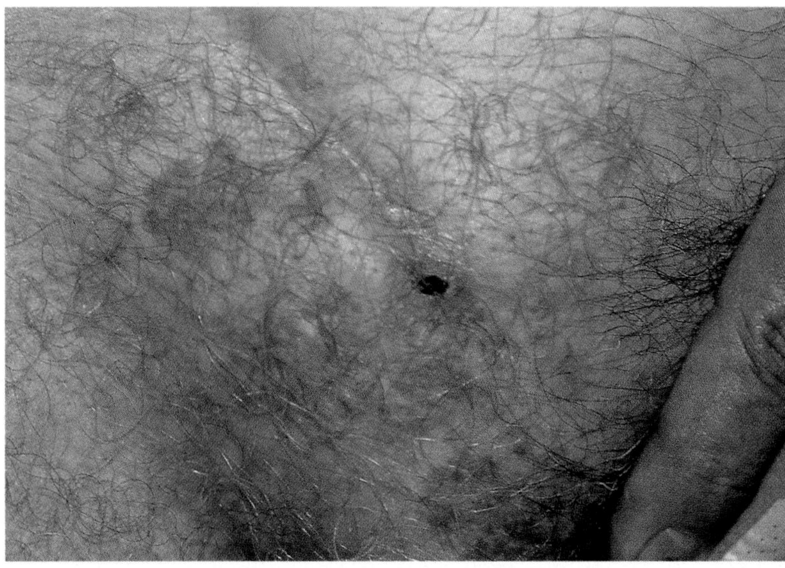

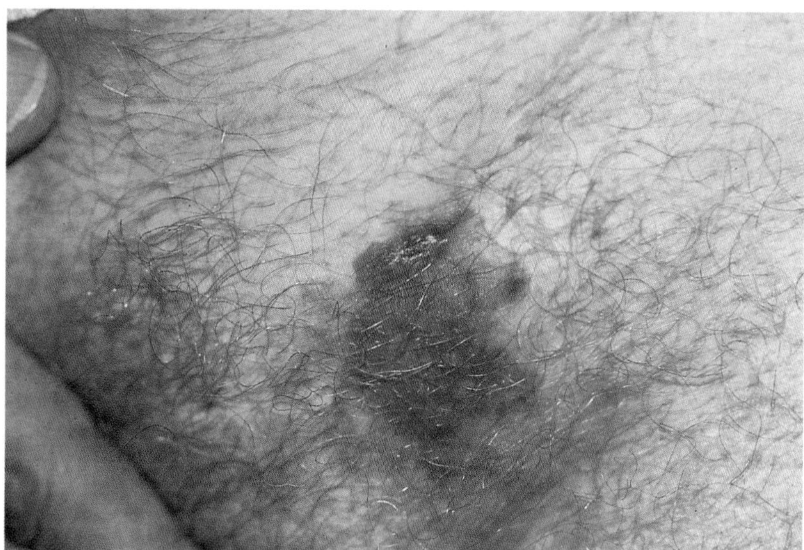

Fig. 6-26. Inflamed plaque of extramammary Paget's disease with uneven borders. This is the same patient as in Figure 6-25. The lesions were bilateral and fairly symmetrical.

Most of the plaques are approximately round in configuration, but occasionally, where nearby plaques have become confluent, gyrate outlines are noted. Sometimes the outline of the several plaques that have grown to confluence can still be detected within the central portion of the larger, gyrate plaque. This observation suggests that the process, at least at times, may represent a multifocal origin.

The plaques are usually asymptomatic, but mild to moderate pruritus can develop. In fact, the onset of pruritus may lead a patient to seek medical attention.

Histology

Biopsy provides for definitive diagnosis. The appearance of typical vacuolated Paget cells is usually quite distinctive, but occasionally special stains are necessary to exclude pagetoid squamous cell carcinoma and superficial spreading melanoma. The cells in Paget's disease stain positively for mucin and, on immunoperoxidase staining, they are positive for carcinoembryonic antigen (CEA).[40] The cells of melanoma fail to stain for these two products but are positive on immunoperoxidase staining for S-100 protein. The cells of pagetoid squamous cell carcinoma are negative with all of these stains.

Differential Diagnoses

Clinically, the differential diagnoses include eczematous disease, candidiasis, Bowen's disease, Darier's disease, and Hailey-Hailey disease. Eczematous disease can usually be ruled out because, in Paget's disease, the plaques are sharper in margination and are stable in size, shape, and color over months to years. Colonization with *Candida* spp. occurs with some frequency in Paget's disease; marginal improvement with anticandidal agents should not dissuade one from further considering Paget's disease. The sharp margination of the lesion and the failure to respond completely to steroid and anticandidal therapy should suggest the possibility of Darier's disease and Hailey-Hailey disease. Patients with these latter diseases will usually have lesions elsewhere on the body and will have a positive family history of similar disease.

Course and Prognosis

The lesions of extramammary Paget's disease develop slowly and insidiously. Centrifugal enlargement takes place over months to years. Gradually the plaques become thicker and deeper red. The surface of the lesion eventually demonstrates evidence of epithelial distintegration in the form of erosions and crusting. Because of this very slow pattern of change and relative lack of symptoms, patients are fooled into thinking that the process is benign in nature. For this reason, lesions will often have been present for years before a patient seeks medical attention.

In most cases, at the time of definitive diagnosis, Paget's cells have proliferated to the point at which 30 to 50 percent of the epithelial keratinocytes have been replaced with malignant cells. Invariably, the epithelial component of the adnexal structures has become involved. Originally the adnexal involvement was thought to represent "invasion," but now such involvement is understood to be in situ disease. This change in understanding, together with a trend toward earlier diagnosis, has changed the statistical data regarding the frequency with which "underlying sweat gland carcinoma" is found to be present. In the 1960s underlying carcinoma occurred in 25 to 30 percent of cases; today it is found in fewer than 10 to 15 percent of the patients.[36]

Extramammary Paget's disease is not only associated with underlying sweat gland carcinoma, as indicated above, but is also associated with other forms of carcinoma occurring at distant sites. Approximately 10 percent of the patients with vulvar Paget's disease also have breast or genitourinary carcinoma; a similar proportion of males have genitourinary carcinoma.[36,41] In both sexes, patients with anal or perianal involvement are sometimes found to have contiguous or distant colon carcinoma.

The overall fatality rate, due either to metastasis from underlying invasive sweat gland carcinoma or to associated carcinoma (as noted above), is said to be about 25 percent. However, because of very slow tumor growth, those with invasive disease have fairly high 5-year survival rates. The outlook for those without invasive sweat gland carcinoma or other associated malignancy is excellent; because of the advanced age of onset, most of these patients will die of intercurrent disease long before their Paget's disease becomes a threat to life.

Pathogenesis

Desmosomes are present on Paget cells, and keratin tonofilaments are present within the cells. These observations indicate that Paget's cells are of epithelial derivation. Special stains for CEA further indicate that these epithelial cells are of the apocrine type, and the nature of the specific cytokeratins that are present suggests that the cells stem from the apocrine gland rather than from the apocrine duct.

All of these facts correlate well with the knowledge that breast tissue is of apocrine origin (hence Paget's disease of the nipple) and that extramammary Paget's disease is usually located at sites (along the "milk line") where apocrine-derived cells may be found.[42] Interestingly, extramammary Paget's disease has been reported, albeit rarely, in the ceruminous glands of the ears and in Moll's glands of the eyelids; the cells of these glands are of apocrine origin.[42] Nagle et al[43] have recently provided evidence suggesting that both mammary and extramammary Paget's disease are derived from a characteristic clear cell that was originally described by Toker in the nipple. Presumably these cells are normal inhabitants of the milk line epithelium.

While there is general acceptance that Paget cells are apocrine in nature, it is much more controversial as to whether the process begins in adnexal precursor cells in the overlying, interadnexal epithelium or whether, by analogy with mammary Paget's disease, it extends upwards from underlying sweat gland adenocarcinoma of either the in situ or the invasive type. This argument cannot be settled with the knowledge available today, but perhaps two separate types of Paget's disease exist, with one type deriving from the former mechanism, and another from the latter.[44]

Clinically, extramammary Paget's disease appears, at least at times, to be multifocal. In fact, if total vulvectomy is carried out, multiple foci of apparently noncontiguous involvement can be demonstrated in areas where there were no corresponding visible clinical lesions.[45] In addition, preliminary laboratory data, carried out on breast tissue of mammary Paget's disease, do suggest that the process may be of a polyclonal rather than a monoclonal origin.

Treatment

When a diagnosis of extramammary Paget's disease has been confirmed by biopsy, the physician should carry out an evaluation of the breasts, genitourinary tract, and rectum. Any carcinoma found in these sites should, where possible, be treated.

Treatment of the extramammary Paget's disease itself consists of excision of all clinically involved tissue. This not only results in tumor removal but also allows for microscopic determination as to whether underlying sweat gland carcinoma exists. In the past, rather radical surgery was undertaken in an attempt to obtain microscopically clear margins; in spite of these efforts, local recurrences were very frequent. Now, with a better understanding of the multifocal nature of Paget's disease, narrow local resection is preferred. This can be done with conventional excision techniques or with Mohs micrographic surgery, in which case tumor-free margins are more likely to be obtained.[46]

No matter which surgical approach is used, the local recurrence rate is high. It appears, however, that these recurrences can be treated very conservatively with laser ablation or electrosurgery without increasing the eventual mortality due to the disease.[36] This can be explained by the fact that recurrences represent in situ disease, without underlying invasive sweat gland carcinoma, 99 percent of the time.

Treatment of extramammary Paget's disease associated with underlying invasive sweat gland carcinoma lies outside the scope of this textbook.

DERMATOPHYTE FUNGAL INFECTIONS

Dermatophyte infections of the genital skin, commonly referred to as tinea cruris, are a common condition produced by fungi that invade the stratum corneum, the most superficial portion of the epidermis.

Clinical Presentation

Tinea cruris occurs much more often in postpubertal men than in any other group; it is characterized by erythematous, scaling, sharply demarcated, and often pruritic plaques over the proximal, inner thighs to the crural crease. (Fig. 6-27). Black patients may present with striking hyperpigmentation rather than obvious erythema. Often, but not always, a peripheral border with overlying scale lends an annular "ringworm" appearance to the eruption (Fig. 6-28). Red papules and sometimes pustules may occur in the plaque, particularly within the leading edge (Fig. 6-29). These papules represent extension of the infection to the follicular epithelium and occur more often in patients with more or coarser hair in the area of involvement, and in those who have been treated with topical corticosteroids. Clinical evidence of the dermatophyte infection usually does not extend to the scrotum or penis in men unless they are immunosuppressed. On the other hand, this disease in women is likely to affect the hair-bearing portion of the vulva. Tinea cruris can extend to include the buttocks in both men and women. An examination of other areas of the body often reveals the lifted, thickened toenails of onychomycosis, or the red, scaling plaques of tinea pedis.

Histology

A biopsy is generally not performed for the diagnosis of a dermatophyte infection since this is usually accomplished by a direct examination of scale for the organism in a KOH preparation. For difficult cases, a skin biopsy using special stains may demonstrate the fungus in the stratum corneum, and sometimes in the hair follicles and hairs themselves. A perifolliculitis is common.

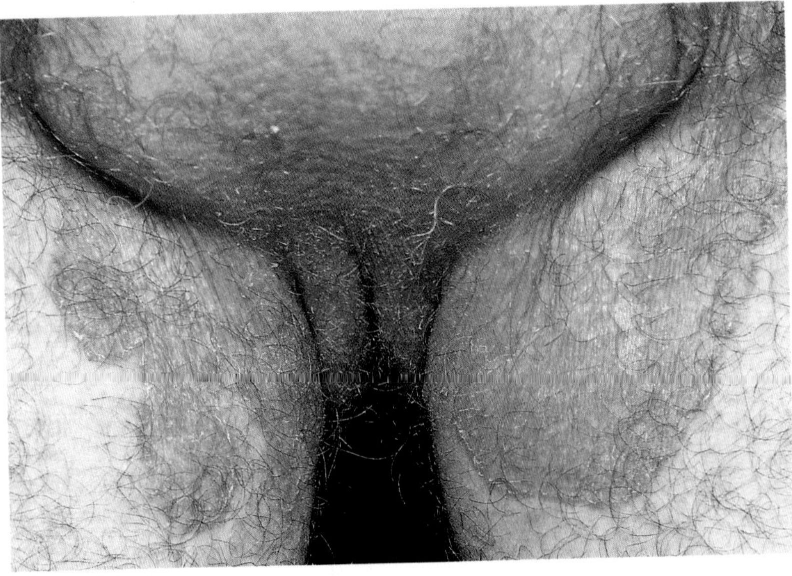

Fig. 6-27. Sharply demarcated, red, scaling plaque over the upper medial thigh, extending to the scrotum of a patient with tinea cruris.

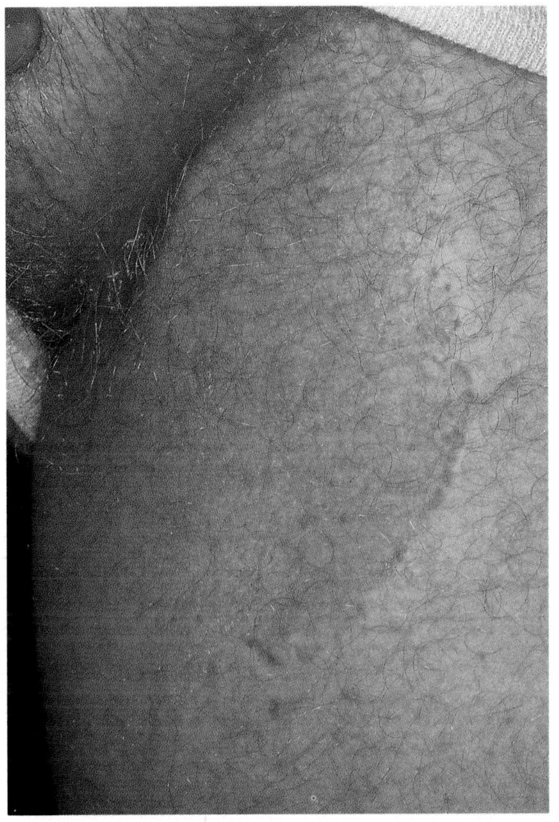

Fig. 6-28. Pink, scaling plaque over medial thigh exhibits a more prominent annular rim typical of tinea cruris.

Diagnosis

Tinea cruris can usually be diagnosed by its typical clinical appearance, especially in the setting of another dermatophyte infection. Differentiation from a *Candida* infection is important since nystatin, commonly used for *Candida*, is ineffective in the treatment of superficial dermatophyte infections. *Candida* in men occurs almost exclusively under the foreskin of uncircumsized patients or as an intertriginous eruption in incontinent patients. These patients show peripheral superficial pustules and collarettes that extend beyond the primary plaque. Psoriasis can mimic tinea cruris, including the sharp borders and peripheral scale, and the two may occur together, especially when psoriasis is treated with a topical corticosteroid. However, genital psoriasis is usually accompanied by other characteristic skin involvement. Like psoriasis, neurodermatitis may resemble a dermatophyte infection and may also coexist with it, either secondarily or as a primary disease with superinfection. Usually, the plaques of neurodermatitis are less well demarcated but thicker and without peripheral scale, and the scrotum is prominently affected. The diagnosis of tinea cruris can be confirmed by a potassium hydroxide examination or by a culture performed on the peripheral scale.

Fig. 6-29. Atypical erythematous plaques of tinea cruris with pustules of fungal folliculitis but minimal scale and loss of typical peripheral accentuation of a patient incorrectly treated with corticosteroid (tinea incognito). (Courtesy of Ronald C. Hansen, M.D.)

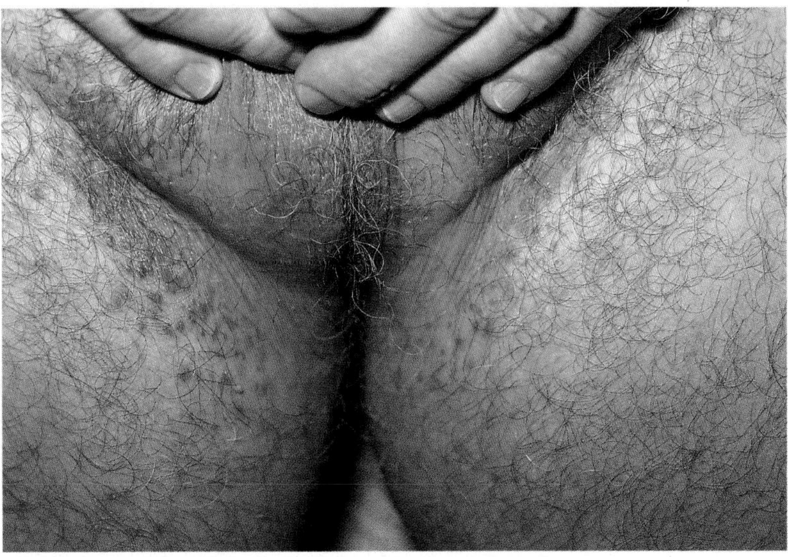

Course and Prognosis

Genital dermatophyte infections are temporarily eradicated with therapy. However, affected patients are at high risk for recurrence and should be forewarned. Some require ongoing use of topical antifungal preparations to prevent a return of the infection.

Pathogenesis

The most common organisms responsible for genital dermatophyte infections are *Trichophyton rubrum, Trichophyton mentagrophytes,* and *Epidermophyton floccosum.*

Treatment

Any one of several topical antifungal agents may be used (see also Topical Antifungal and Anticandidal Agents in Ch. 3). Because this is a recurring problem in many men, the effective over-the-counter medications clotrimazole (Lotrimin) and miconazole (Micatin) creams are practical. Other prescription choices include naftifine hydrochloride (Naftin), sulconazole nitrate (Excelderm), oxiconazole nitrate (Oxistat), econazole nitrate (Spectazole), haloprogin (Halotex), and ciclopirox olamine (Loprox). Naftifine hydrochloride, sulconazole nitrate, oxiconazole nitrate, and econazole nitrate have the advantage of once-a-day dosing. Nystatin is not effective in the treatment of dermatophyte infections.

When disease is extensive, occurs in a very hairy areas, or red, indurated papules indicate follicular involvement, topical medications may be only partially effective, and oral medication is indicated. Safety and cost make griseofulvin the first-line therapy against dermatophytes, although it is useless against *Candida.* Although the side effects of bone marrow failure and liver toxicity are the most well known and worrisome, these are extremely rare, whereas headache, nausea, and urticaria are relatively common and can be bothersome. Oral ketoconazole (Nizoral) at 200 mg a day is active against both dermatophytes and *Candida* and has fewer common side effects. Unfortunately, potentially life-threatening, idiosyncratic hepatotoxicity occurs (rarely), and liver functions should be monitored. Fluconazole (Diflucan) 100 mg a day is an effective but expensive alternative that is not yet approved for this indication by the Food and Drug Administration. It appears to have less hepatotoxicity, but monitoring of liver function tests is suggested with both medications, and both are very expensive. Recently, itraconazole (Sporanox) has become available and is extremely active and apparently safer, although very expensive.

PITYRIASIS (TINEA) VERSICOLOR

The yeast infection pityriasis (tinea) versicolor is not a dermatophyte infection but causes disease in its yeast form, so that the term *tinea* is a misnomer. Because it is a yeast infection, the classic dermatophyte therapy griseofulvin is not active.

Clinical Presentation

Pityriasis versicolor occurs most often on the trunk of young men. This disease acquires part of its name from its variable color on the skin. The round papules and small plaques may be pink, tan, or hypopigmented, and sometimes more than one color can occur in the same patient (Figs. 6-30 and 6-31). The lesions are more obvious in the summer, because a substance produced by the organism prevents tanning, and sun-exposed affected skin appears white against the tanned background of normal skin. Black skin sometimes exhibits extremely dark brown, heavily scaling, or small follicular papules of pityriasis versicolor. The lesions begin as barely elevated papules (with subtle, fine scale over the upper central back and chest) that coalesce and develop satellite lesions. Although generally limited to the trunk, neck, and upper arms, sometimes the genital area is involved, especially the mons pubis.

Differential Diagnoses

Pityriasis versicolor can be confused with secondary syphilis, pityriasis rosea, seborrheic dermatitis, and tinea cruris. An examination of the rest of the body shows typical lesions over the upper trunk, and a KOH examination shows the multiple short, curved hyphae and yeast forms of the organism *Malassezia furfur* (also called *Pityrosporum ovale,* and *P. orbiculare*) within the stratum corneum. A biopsy is not necessary.

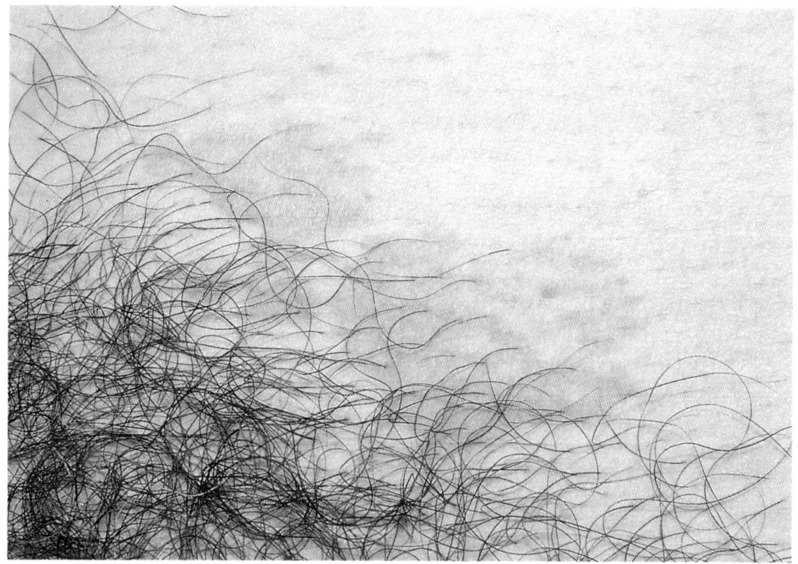

Fig. 6-30. Multiple subtle, light tan, finely scaling papules and small plaques of pityriasis (tinea) versicolor occuring on the mons pubis.

Treatment

Treatment can be oral or topical. In limited disease, topical antifungal agents such as miconazole, clotrimazole, naftifine hydrochloride, sulconazole nitrate, oxiconazole nitrate, econazole nitrate, haloprogin, and ciclopirox olamine are useful (see also the two sections on antifungal medication in Ch. 3). When larger areas are involved, selenium sulfide lotion 2.5 percent applied to the affected areas for 10 minutes daily for 1 week is effective but can be irritating. Alternatively, extensive disease can be treated with ketoconazole 200 mg each day for 5 days, with rare but reported hepatotoxicity after as few as 3 days of therapy. This yeast is ubiquitous and, after successful therapy, recurrence is extremely common in those who are susceptible to it. Therefore, prophylactic retreatment every 1 or 2 months is useful in preventing

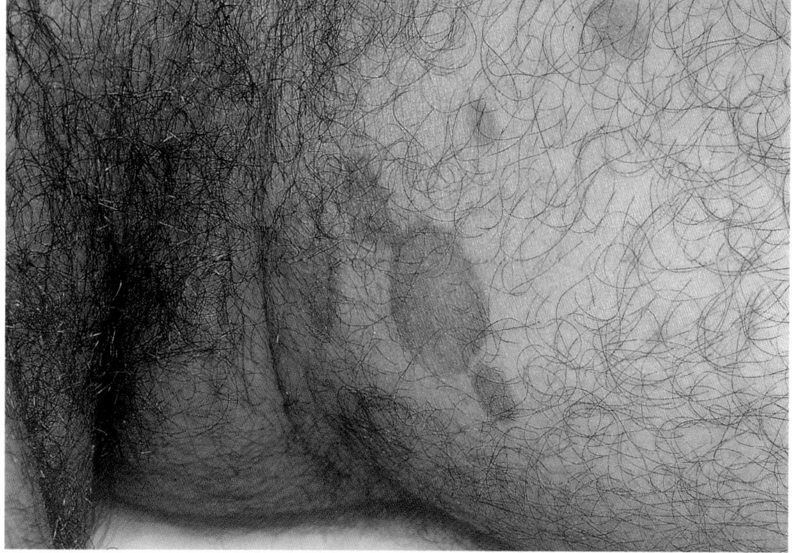

Fig. 6-31. Sharply marginated tan papules and plaques of pityriasis versicolor over inner thighs. As the name suggests, lesions can be brown, white, or red.

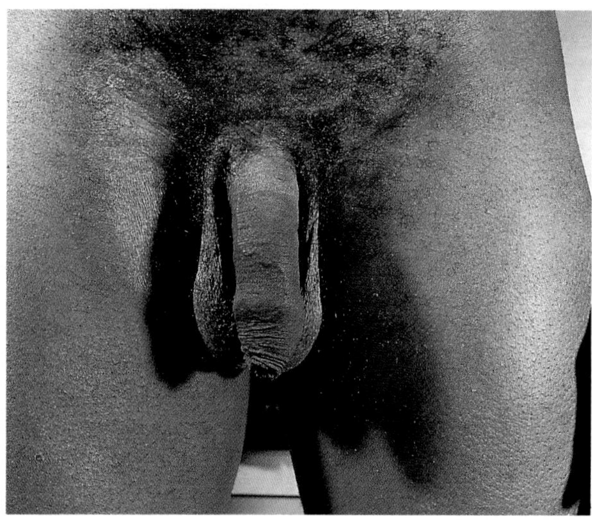

Fig. 6-32. Well-demarcated, hypopigmented, pink lightly scaling plaques of erythrasma over the upper medial thighs and proximal shaft of the penis.

these recurrences. This can be done with Selsun lotion or with a mixture of equal parts propylene glycol and water applied overnight.

ERYTHRASMA

Erythrasma is a red, scaling bacterial infection of the genital area that mimics tinea cruris. This eruption occurs most often in the summer and in warm, humid climates, especially in obese or debilitated patients. Some patients may complain of pruritus, although erythrasma is usually asymptomatic.

Clinical Presentation

The rash consists of pink-brown, lightly scaling patches or plaques over the proximal inner thighs, although the color may be hyperpigmented in black patients (Fig. 6-32). Older lesions may show fine wrinkling. Like tinea cruris, the plaques are sharply demarcated, but, unlike that disease, the lesions are solid without the raised border and prominent peripheral scale (Fig. 6-33). The scrotum and penis are generally unaffected. Toe web space involvement is common, and the axillae, intergluteal folds, and inframammary folds may occasionally show lesions. Rarely, plaques may become generalized.

Differential Diagnoses

This disease is easily confused with tinea cruris and, less often, with psoriasis and *Candida* infection. Neurodermatitis, with its poor margination, is less likely to mimic erythrasma. A potassium hydroxide examination is negative, but exposure of involved skin to a Wood's light produces a coral fluorescence. A biopsy is generally not performed but shows the organism as gram-positive rods in the stratum corneum. An examination of other skin surfaces also helps to evaluate the presence of psoriasis and neurodermatitis.

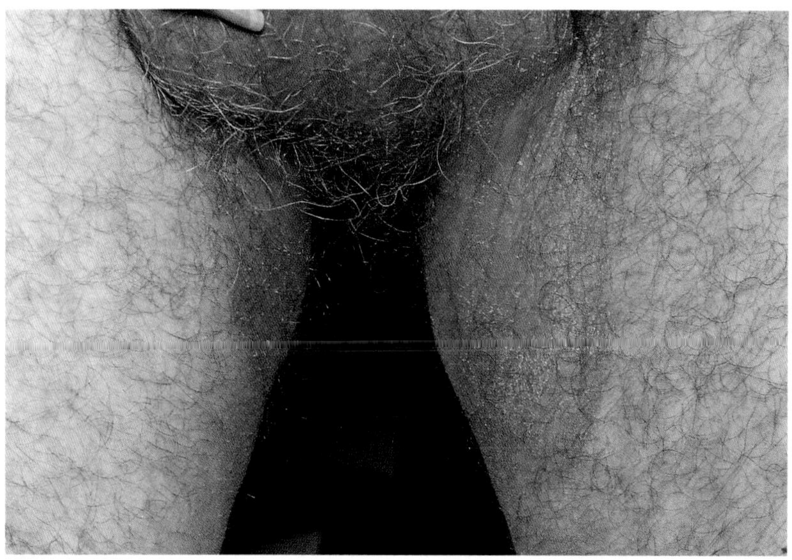

Fig. 6-33. Uniform, pink-brown plaque of erythrasma over medial thighs is easily confused with tinea cruris, which usually shows more peripheral accentuation and scale and, in light skin, less tan color.

Pathogenesis

Erythrasma is caused by *Corynebacterium minutissimum.* Heat and dampness promote growth of the organism and encourage disease.

Treatment

Erythrasma is treated with erythromycin, 500 mg twice daily for 7 to 14 days, or, in those intolerant to this medication orally, topical antibiotics and keratolytic agents can be used. Recurrence is common, and chronically recurrent disease can often be controlled by topical erythromycin, clindamycin, miconazole, or econazole.

SECONDARY-TYPE SYPHILIS

See Chapter 10 for a discussion of secondary-type syphilis.

REFERENCES

Psoriasis

1. Goodwin P, Hamilton S, Fry L: The cell cycle in psoriasis. Br J Dermatol 90:517, 1974
2. Christophers E et al: Identification of two endogenous neutrophil-activating peptides in psoriatic skin and inflammatory cells: C5ades arg and NAP. Dermatologica suppl. 1. 9:179, 1989
3. Voorhees JJ: Leukotrienes and other lipoxygenase products in the pathogenesis and therapy of psoriasis and other dermatoses. Arch Dermatol 119:541, 1983
4. Bieber T, Braun-Falco O: Distribution of CD1a-positive cells in psoriatic skin during the evolution of the lesions. Acta Derm Venereol (Stockh) 78:175, 1989
5. Griffiths CEM, Voorhees JJ, Nickoloff BJ: Characterization of intercellular adhesion molecule-1 and HLA-DR expression in normal and inflamed skin: modulation by recombinant gamma interferon and tumor necrosis factor. J Am Acad Dermatol 20:617, 1989
6. Kellner I et al: Overexpression of ECM-receptors (VLA-3, 5 and 6) on psoriatic keratinocytes. Br J Dermatol 125:211, 1992
7. McMichael AJ, Morhenn V, Payne R et al: HLa-C and D antigens associated with psoriasis. Br J Dermatol 98:287, 1978
8. Stern RS, members of the Photochemotherapy Follow-up Study: N Engl J Med 322:1093, 1990
9. Van Joost et al: Low-dose cyclosporin A in severe psoriasis. Br J Dermatol 118:183, 1988
10. Gupta AK, Ellis CN, Siegel MT et al: Sulfasalazine improves psoriasis. Arch Dermatol 126:487, 1990

Reiter Syndrome

11. Winchester et al: Implications from the occurrence of Reiter's syndrome and related disorders in association with advanced HIV infection. Scand J Rheumatol 74:89, 1988
12. Rahman MU, Hudson AP, Schumacher HR: Chlamydia and Reiter's syndrome (reactive arthritis). Rheum Dis Clin North Am 18:67, 1992

12a. Edwards L: Reiter's syndrome of the vulva: the psoriasis spectrum. Arch Dermatol 128:812, 1992

Lichen Planus

13. Morhenn VB: The etiology of lichen planus: a hypothesis. Am J Dermatopathol 8:154, 1986
14. Pigatto PD et al: Cyclosporin A for treatment of severe lichen planus. Br J Dermatol 122:121, 1990
15. Hersle K et al: Severe oral lichen planus: treatment with an aromatic retinoid (etretinate). Br J Dermatol 106:77, 1982
16. Massa MC, Rogers RS III: Griseofulvin therapy in lichen planus. Acta Derm Venerol (Stockh) 61:547, 1981
17. Edwards L, Friedrich EG Jr: Desquamative vaginitis: lichen planus in disguise. Obstet Gynecol 71:832, 1988

Lupus Erythematosus

18. Burge SM, Frith PA, Juniper RP et al: Mucosal involvement in systemic and chronic cutaneous lupus erythematosus. Br J Dermatol 121:727, 1989
19. Turner MLC: Vulvar manifestations of systemic diseases. Dermatol Clin 10:445, 1992

Bowen's Disease, Bowenoid Papulosis, and Erythroplasia of Queyrat

20. Wilkinson EJ: The 1989 Presidential address. International Society for the Study of Vulvar Disease. J Reprod Med 35:981, 1990
21. Bornstein J, Kaufman RH, Adam E et al: Multicentric intraepithelial neoplasia involving the vulva. Cancer 62:1601, 1988
22. Wade TR, Kopf AW, Ackerman AB: Bowenoid papulosis of the penis. Cancer 42:1890, 1978
23. Wade TR, Kopf AW, Ackerman AB: Bowenoid papulosis of the genitalia. Arch Dermatol 115:306, 1979
24. Schwartz, RA, Fanniger CK: Bowenoid papulosis. J Am Acad Dermatol 24:261, 1991
25. Barbero M, Micheletti L, Preti M et al: Vulvar intraepithelial neoplasia. A clinicopathologic study of 60 cases. J Reprod Med 35:1023, 1990
26. Planner RS, Hobbs JB: Intraepithelial and invasive neoplasia of the vulva in association with human papillomavirus infection. J Reprod Med 33:503, 1988
27. Barbero M, Micheletti L, Preti M et al: Biologic behavior of vulvar intraepithelial neoplasia. J Reprod Med 38:108, 1993
28. Hellberg D et al: Penile cancer: is there an epidemiological role for smoking and sexual behavior? Br Med J 295:1306, 1987
29. Daling JR et al: Cigarette smoking and the risk of anogenital cancer. Am J Epidemiol 135:180, 1992
30. Quan MB, Moy RL: The role of human papillomavirus in carcinoma. J Am Acad Dermatol 25:698, 1991
31. Park JS, Jones RW, McLean MR et al: Possible etiologic heterogeneity of vulvar intraepithelial neoplasia. Cancer 67:1599, 1991
32. Kaelbling M, Burk RD, Atkin NB et al: Loss of heterozygosity on chromosome 17p and mutant p53 in HPV-negative cervical carcinomas. Lancet 340:140, 1992
33. Brown MD, Zachary CB, Grekin RC, Swanson NA: Genital tumors: their management by micrographic surgery. J Am Acad Dermatol 18:115, 1988
34. Moritz DL, Lynch WS: Extensive Bowen's disease of the penile shaft treated with fresh tissue Mohs micrographic surgery in two separate operations. J Dermatol Surg Oncol 17:374, 1991
35. Shafi MI, Luesley DM, Byrne P et al: Vulval intraepithelial neoplasia—management and outcome. Br J Obstet Gynaecol 96:1339, 1989

Extramammary Paget's Disease

36. Paniel BJ, Lessana-Leibowitch M, Molinie V: Paget's disease of the vulva—46 cases. J Reprod Med 38:46, 1993
37. Schellenberger RR, Burford C, Kune GA: Perianal Paget's disease. Aust NZ J Surg 58:727, 1988
38. Perez MA, LaRossa DD, Tomaszewski JE: Paget's disease primarily involving the scrotum. Cancer 63:970, 1989
39. Imakado S, Abe M, Okuno T et al: Two cases of genital Paget's disease with bilateral axillary involvement: mutability of axillary lesions. Arch Dermatol 127:1243, 1991
40. Helm KF, Goellner JR, Peters, MS: Immunohistochemical stains in extramammary Paget's disease. Am J Dermatopathol 14:402, 1992
41. Powell FC, Bjornsson J, Doyle JA et al: Genital Paget's disease and urinary tract malignancy. J Am Acad Dermatol 13:84, 1985
42. Saida T, Iwata M: "Ectopic" extramammary Paget's disease affecting the lower anterior aspect of the chest. J Am Acad Dermatol 17:910, 1987
43. Nagle RB, Lucas DO, McDaniel KM et al: Paget's cells. New evidence linking mammary and extramammary Paget cells to a common cell phenotype. Am J Clin Pathol 83:431, 1985
44. Miller LR, McCunniff AJ, Randall ME: An immunohistochemical study of perianal Paget's disease. Possible origins and clinical implications. Cancer 69:2166, 1992
45. Gunn RA, Gallager HS: Vulvar Paget's disease. A topographic study. Cancer 46:590, 1980
46. Coldiron BM, Goldsmith BA, Robinson JK: Surgical treatment of extramammary Paget's disease. A report of six cases and a reexamination of Mohs micrographic surgery compared with conventional surgical excision. Cancer 67:933, 1991

SUGGESTED READINGS

Psoriasis

Farber EM, Nall L: Genital psoriasis. Cutis 50:263, 1992

Farber EM, Nall L: Perianal and intergluteal psoriasis. Cutis 50:336, 1992

These articles provide short reviews of the special issues of anogenital psoriasis, with suggestions for management.

Reiter Syndrome

Rothe MJ, Kerdel FA: Reiter Syndrome. Int J Dermatol 30:173, 1991

This article reviews the etiologies, clinical features, and therapy for Reiter's syndrome.

Lichen Planus

Boyd AS, Neldner KH: Lichen planus. J Am Acad Dermatol 25:593, 1991

This extensive and well-referenced review of lichen planus discusses the clinical appearances and variants of lichen planus, associated diseases, and therapy.

Edwards L: Vulvar lichen planus. Arch Dermatol 125:1677, 1989

This paper summarizes the clinical manifestations and response to therapy of seven patients with vulvar lichen planus and includes representative color photographs.

Pelisse M: The vulvo-vaginal-gingival syndrome: a new form of erosive lichen planus. Int J Dermatol 28:381, 1989

The author reviews the findings and course of erosive mucosal lichen planus of the vulva, vagina, and oral mucosa in 19 women.

Ridley CM: Chronic erosive vulval disease. Clin Exp Dermatol 15:245, 1990

This article reviews in table form the physical findings in 20 patients with lichen planus and discusses other causes of erosive vulvitis, as well as the management of these patients.

Lupus Erythematosus

Sontheimer RD, Euwer RL, Geppert TD, Cohen SB: Connective tissue disease. p. 1217. In Moschella SL, Hurley HJ (eds): Dermatology. WB Saunders, Philadelphia, 1992

Pityriasis Rosea

Parsons JM: Pityriasis rosea update: 1986: J Am Acad Dermatol 15:159, 1986

This is a good review article and is up to date, since little new has been published in the last several years about this disease.

Extramammary Paget's Disease

Jones RE Jr, Austin C, Ackerman AB: Extramammary Paget's disease. A critical reexamination. Am J Dermatopathol 1:101, 1979

This is an extensive review with a great deal of discussion regarding the origin of the Paget's cell.

Helwig EB, Graham JH: Anogenital (extramammary) Paget's disease. A clinicopathological study. Cancer 16:387, 1963

This is the first (and classic) review of the subject; all the literature to this point is summarized.

Chanda JJ: Extramammary Paget's disease: prognosis and relationship to internal malignancy. J Am Acad Dermatol 13:1009, 1985

This review primarily discusses the relationship of Paget's disease to carcinomas found in association with the disease.

Dermatophyte Fungal Infections

Smith EB: Topical antifungal drugs in the treatment of tinea pedis, tinea cruris, and tinea corporis. J Am Acad Dermatol [illegible]

This article reviews and compares the different classes of topical antifungal medications, including recently available drugs.

Pityriasis (Tinea) Versicolor

Rippon JW: Medical Mycology. 3rd Ed. WB Saunders, Philadelphia, 1988

7 Vulvovaginitis and Balanitis

VULVOVAGINITIS

Inflammation of the vulva (vulvitis) and vagina (vaginitis) often occur together either because the same process affects both areas, or because an irritating vaginal discharge produces an irritant contact dermatitis as it touches the vulva. The management of vulvitis requires investigation for (and treatment of) any possible vaginal abnormalities as well. Dermatologists often forget to look for and treat *Candida* vaginitis in the setting of *Candida* vulvitis, while gynecologists are more likely to overlook treatment of the external genitalia while treating the vagina. The most common symptoms of vaginitis are discharge, odor, itching or burning, and dyspareunia.

An evaluation for vaginitis requires a knowledge of normal findings on clinical examination and routine office procedures. The vagina is normally pink, with rugae of the walls. A thin, white discharge with minimal odor and a pH of about 3.5 to 4.5 is normally present. The pH may vary considerably in asymptomatic women, and it rises with contamination by blood, semen, or water from the speculum. A saline wet preparation shows multiple, large, flattened squamous epithelial cells with sharply defined borders and small nuclei. White blood cells are common but should not outnumber epithelial cells, and *Lactobacilli* are numerous. Low estrogen levels as seen in children, breastfeeding women, and postmenopausal patients produce thinner vaginal walls, higher pH measurements, and epithelial cells that are smaller and rounder, with larger nuclei. *Lactobacilli* are fewer.

The symptoms of vaginitis are most often attributable to bacterial vaginosis, candidasis, trichomoniasis, cytolytic vaginosis, and atrophic vaginitis. Less common are condylomatous vaginitis, vaginal herpes simplex infection, ulcerations of any cause, and desquamative vaginitis, or sloughing of vaginal walls usually as a result of erosive lichen planus. *Lactobacillus* vaginitis has recently been proposed as a cause of vaginitis symptoms (Horowitz B, personal communication, 1993). *Lactobacilli* adhere end to end to form filaments formerly called leptothrix. Treatment consists of oral Augmentin or doxycycline. A copious or malodorous vaginal discharge is not always attributable to vaginitis. Cervicitis may cause a purulent vaginal discharge, and some patients simply have an excess of normally desquamated vaginal epithelial cells that clump together in a white paste. Besides documented infectious agents, the multiple aerobic and anerobic bacteria in varying proportions that form the normal ecology of the vagina affect odor, as do hormones and secretions of vulvar apocrine glands.

Some differentiating features of the most common

causes of a vaginal discharge are compared in Table 7-1. *Candida* vaginitis and balanitis are discussed in Chapter 5.

BACTERIAL VAGINOSIS

Clinical Presentation

The most common cause of an increased vaginal discharge with odor is bacterial vaginosis (*Gardnerella* vaginitis, *Haemophilus vaginalis* vaginitis, nonspecific vaginitis), so named because inflammation and therefore symptoms such as itching, burning, and dyspareunia were originally believed to be absent. This polymicrobial syndrome occurs with such subtle changes in vaginal secretions that about half of patients notice no symptoms. However, many patients complain of discharge and a characteristic fishy odor, especially after intercourse, and some complain of irritation or pruritus. Because bacterial vaginosis may increase the risk of pelvic inflammatory disease and premature rupture of membranes or labor in pregnant patients, it should probably be treated even when asymptomatic.

Diagnosis

The diagnosis of bacterial vaginosis is made on the basis of the microscopic appearance of vaginal secretions as well as the high pH and distinctive odor released in the presence of KOH. The discharge is most often gray-white, thin, and homogeneous and exhibits a pH greater than 4.5. The secretions are characterized microscopically by clue cells, which are epithelial cells covered with bacteria so that the cytoplasm appears granular and borders are obscured. White blood cells and lactobacilli are lacking, and when a KOH mount is prepared or KOH is dropped on the speculum, a fishy odor is emitted.

Pathogenesis

The cause of bacterial vaginosis is uncertain, although increased numbers of some normal vaginal flora have been identified. *Gardnerella vaginalis, Mobiluncus* spp., *Bacteroides* spp., *Mycoplasma hominis,* and anaerobic gram-positive cocci probably interact to produce this condition. Polyamines produced by anaerobic bacteria produce the fishy odor when they are exposed to an alkaline pH such as potassium hydroxide (KOH) or semen. Some investigators feel that bacterial vaginosis is a sexually transmitted disease, but the fact that the responsible organisms are normal inhabitants of the vagina and that treatment of sexual partners does not seem to influence the recurrence rates suggest otherwise.

Table 7-1. Causes of Vaginal Discharge

Diagnosis	*Appearance of Discharge*	*pH*	*Microscopic Examination*
Normal	Thin, white, homogeneous	<4.5	Mature epithelial cells, *Lactobacilli,* few WBCs
Bacterial vaginosis	White-gray, homogeneous	>4.5	Clue cells, decreased *Lactobacilli*
Trichomoniasis	White-gray, homogeneous	>4.5	Flagellate protozoa, WBCs
Candidiasis	Thick, white, curdlike	<4.5	Budding yeast, usually hyphae
Atrophic vaginitis	Purulent	>5	WBCs, decreased *Lactobacilli,* immature epithelial cells
Cytolytic (Döderlein) vaginosis	Increased, white	<4.5	Increased epithelial cells, irregular loss of cytoplasm, increased *Lactobacilli*
Desquamative vaginitis, ulcers	Thin, serosanguineous, or purulent	>4.5	Multiple WBCs, RBCs
Cervicitis	Mucopurulent	>4.5	Multiple WBCs
Increased normal secretions and condylomatous	Thick, white	<4.5	Multiple epithelial cells, *Lactobacilli*

Abbreviations: RBCs, red blood cells; WBCs, white blood cells.

Treatment

The treatment of choice is metronidazole, either oral or topical. Oral metronidazole is effective either at a dose of 500 mg twice a day for 1 week or as a one-time dose of 2 g with higher recurrence rates. Recently, topical metronidazole vaginal gel 0.75 percent inserted in the vagina twice a day for 5 days has been shown to be effective with fewer side effects. Oral clindamycin 300 mg twice a day for 1 week is also useful, as is topical clindamycin vaginal cream 2 percent once daily for a week.

The recurrence rate of bacterial vaginosis within the first year is very high, for unknown reasons. In addition to frequent or chronic treatment, some physicians feel that vaginal douching with hydrogen peroxide-producing *Lactobacillus* spp. may reestablish this normal flora and help maintain a low vaginal pH. However, recent evidence suggests that commercially available *Lactobacillus* preparations are too dissimilar to the vaginal organisms to affect repopulation.

TRICHOMONIASIS

Clinical Presentation

Trichomoniasis is a sexually transmitted protozoal disease that often produces a copious vaginal discharge associated with vulvar pruritus, although many patients are totally asymptomatic.

Symptomatic patients exhibit a profuse malodorous vaginal discharge that can be gray, white, yellow, or green, sometimes with a foamy texture. Erythema and edema of the vulvar vestibule and the vagina are usual. A nonspecific, common sign of vaginal and cervical inflammation that may occur in trichomoniasis is the presence of multiple, punctate, red papules. Vulvar burning, dyspareunia, and pruritus may occur, and dysuria develops in a minority. Chronic disease may be associated only with an objectionable vaginal odor.

Diagnosis

Diagnosis rests with identification of the organism on a wet mount of vaginal secretions, which also shows a high pH. The microscopic examination shows multiple white blood cells and epithelial cells, as well as teardrop-shaped, motile protozoa with anterior flagellae. The trichomonads are usually easily seen because of their jerky, rapid movements in an otherwise relatively still microscopic field. If the slide dries or becomes cold, the organism becomes more spherical and immobile, making identification much more difficult. Those patients with symptoms and signs suggestive of trichomoniasis but with a negative wet mount can be cultured for the protozoa using Diamond's culture media, which detects about 95 percent of cases. A diagnosis made on a Papanicolaou (Pap) smear should be suspect because of the false negatives and false positives that can occur.

Pathogenesis

The cause of trichomoniasis is the flagellate protozoan *Trichomonas vaginalis.* Although the parasite is hardy and can live on fomites, the size of the inoculum necessary to cause disease dictates that this is a sexually transmitted disease. The organism resides in the vagina, urethra, and paraurethral glands and regularly exists chronically and asymptomatically in some poorly estrogenized women. Men may also be colonized with trichomonads. The incubation period is from 4 to 28 days.

Treatment

The treatment for trichomoniasis is oral metronidazole in a one-time dose of 2 g orally. Although several different dosing regimens are used, this schedule has an equivalent cure rate and the benefit of increased compliance with less cost.[1] Topical treatment should be avoided because of the inaccessibility of organisms in the paraurethral ducts and urethra to topical agents. Sexual partners should be treated also. Occasional patients exhibit persistence of the organism, and a higher and longer dosing regimen may be required.

ATROPHIC VAGINITIS

Clinical Presentation

Atrophic vaginitis occurs in the setting of, but does not result solely from, thinned, poorly estrogenized vaginal epithelium. Inflammation generally caused by secondary infection or an inflammatory response to erosions in friable tissue then produces symptoms of irritation and pruritus.

Diagnosis

Relative estrogen deficiency occurs before menarche, during pregnancy and breastfeeding, and after surgical or natural menopause. Milder changes occur with oral contraceptive use. Women often complain of dryness and (with increasing inflammation) soreness and dyspareunia when sexually active. A discharge ranging from serous or serosanguinous to purulent may occur. A physical examination shows a loss of vaginal rugae, with pink, smooth mucosa and variable inflammation. The pH of vaginal secretions is high, and a wet mount shows white blood cells and immature oval and round epithelial cells showing relatively large nuclei (see also Maturation Index in Ch. 2). *Lactobacilli* are usually lacking.

Pathogenesis

Atrophic changes occur because of the decreased glycogen content of the vaginal mucosa and poor maturation of the epithelium with secondary thinning and fragility from estrogen deficiency. Secondary bacterial infection or erosions produce inflammation and discharge.

Treatment

Treatment should address both the estrogen deficiency and any secondary processes. In postmenopausal women, oral estrogen replacement confers the advantage of systemic benefits such as minimizing osteoporosis. Topical estrogen therapy provides relief much faster and may produce better local effects, and it is certainly preferred to systemic therapy in prepubertal patients. For postmenopausal women, concomitant administration of both oral and topical estrogen provides rapid improvement in symptoms until the systemic effects of the oral preparation take effect. Topical conjugated estrogen cream (Premarin) 0.625 mg/g applied intravaginally and over the vestibule nightly for 3 weeks, and then twice a week, usually effects improvement in weeks, and then therapy may be further tapered to the most infrequent dosing that maintains healthy epithelium. For patients who experience irritation with application of the cream, estradiol cream (Estrace) 0.01 percent may be better tolerated, especially if the patient pretreats with triamcinolone ointment 0.1 percent twice daily for several days initially to decrease inflammation. Some patients, however, may find any topical medication other than bland petrolatum irritating, and in those women oral therapy may be all that is tolerated.

Women with symptoms resulting from breastfeeding also improve with topical estrogen therapy, but this is contraindicated in pregnant patients.

Women who are symptomatic as a result of oral contraceptives generally must discontinue the medication and use estrogen topically. When symptoms have abated, most can tolerate reinstitution of oral contraceptives. Those preparations less likely to produce vulvovaginal atrophy include the high-estrogen contraceptives Demulen, Loestrin, Cyclen, and Tricyclen. Alternatively, the patient can take ethinyl estradiol 50 μg daily with her oral contraceptive. Oral contraceptives best avoided in these patients include levonorgestrel, Ovral, Lo/Ovral, and any with less than 30 μg of ethinyl estradiol. In children, the physician should remember that foreign bodies and pinworms may be complicating factors (see also Ch. 22). A vaginal culture should be performed for those with a purulent discharge. Treatment of any secondary infections and the use of a vaginal lubricant such as Replens is useful in those with a complaint of dryness.

CYTOLYTIC VAGINOSIS

Clinical Presentation

Cytolytic vaginosis (Döderlein cytolysis) is felt by some to represent an unusually thick but normal physiologic discharge, and by others to describe a symptomatic pathologic discharge suggestive of chronic vulvovaginal candidiasis but caused by excess shedding and disruption of vaginal epithelial cells. Although Cibley and Cibley[2] believe that this entity is very common, we have not seen this disease as described with symptoms and naked epithelial nuclei.

Patients report cyclic symptoms of a cheesy, white vaginal discharge associated with itching, burning, and dyspareunia unresponsive to multiple medical interventions.

Diagnosis

A diagnosis is made by examination of the vaginal secretions. Secretions show a normally acid pH, and a KOH preparation is negative for *Candida*. A wet mount is negative for trichomonads, clue cells, and significant numbers of white blood cells, but it shows increased numbers of lactobacilli and epithelial cells, many with cytoplasm stripped from the nucleus.

Pathogenesis

The cause of this condition is unknown but it is postulated to result from abnormalities in the quantity or type of resident *Lactobacilli.*

Treatment

The treatment of cytolytic vaginosis consists of alkalinization of the vagina with sodium bicarbonate douches.

LACTOBACILLUS VAGINOSIS

Recently Horowitz et al have reported a possible new cause of vaginitis produced by *Lactobacillus,* which they have called "lactobacillus vaginosis" (Horowitz et al, personal communication, 1993). *Lactobacillus* spp., under certain conditions (particularly in response to anticandidal therapy) line up end to end to form long filaments formerly believed to represent leptothrix. They believe that this phenomenon produces symptoms of irritation, and that both the symptoms and the filaments on a saline preparation disappear following therapy with oral amoxacillin-clavulanate potassium or doxycycline. These findings have not been confirmed by others.

DESQUAMATIVE VAGINITIS

Desquamative, or erosive, vaginitis (purulent vaginitis) refers to fragility and resulting inflammation of the vagina that is usually due to lichen planus. Just as the term *desquamative gingivitis* refers to nonspecific erosions of the gingivae of several different causes, any erosive or blistering epithelial disease that occurs in the vagina may produce desquamative vaginitis. These diseases can affect the vulva, other mucous membranes, and often non-mucous membrane skin as well as the vagina, producing more specific and easily diagnosed lesions in these areas. Plasma cell vulvitis and balanitis (Zoon's) may likewise represent a nonspecific, common appearance of any of these diseases in a less erosive form.

Clinical Presentation

Patients present with vulvar burning, itching, discharge, and dyspareunia. They may or may not be aware of other areas of involvement and, even if other lesions are present, patients may not associate them with their genital symptoms. A physical examination shows patchy erythema and erosions of the vagina and sometimes cervix. Vaginal secretions usually exhibit a high pH and microscopically show multiple white blood cells, varying numbers of red blood cells, and a paucity of *Lactobacilli.* In late disease, vaginal synechiae may prevent the introduction of a speculum and careful inspection. Specific other abnormalities of the vulva, mouth, eyes, and keratinized skin depend upon the underlying etiology and stage of disease. Some causative diseases are summarized in Table 6-1 in Chapter 6.

Treatment

Treatment depends upon the cause of the erosive process and is discussed under the specific disease. However, local care of the vagina in addition to treatment of the underlying disease is important and can be generalized. Secondary infection is common. When the discharge is purulent, a vaginal culture should be performed and antibiotics prescribed as directed by the results. Often, even in the absence of identifiable pathogens, empiric antibiotic treatment with a wide-spectrum antibiotic that has good coverage against *Escherichia coli, Streptococcus,* and *Staphylococcus* spp. decreases the amount and purulent nature of the discharge, and symptoms decrease. Erythromycin should be avoided because the possible ineffectiveness of this medication in the low-pH environment of the vagina.[3] Because women with erosions of the vagina are at risk of scarring, with loss of patency of the vagina, care should be taken to expand the vagina daily with a dilator, hydrocortisone acetate suppository 25 mg, or intercourse to help prevent this side effect. With antibiotic and local corticosteroid therapy, *Candida* infection is likely. Any flare of symptoms in patients with desquamative vaginitis deserves reevaluation for a correctable, superimposed process.

CERVICITIS

Clinical Presentation

Sometimes a purulent vaginal discharge is actually produced by infection of the cervix. Patients complain of a mucopurulent discharge and spotting, usually without odor or vulvar symptoms unless the infecting organism also affects the vagina or vulva, as is common with herpes simplex virus infection.

Diagnosis, Pathogenesis, and Treatment

A physical examination shows the cervix to be friable. Vaginal pH is high, and a wet smear reveals multiple white blood cells and often red blood cells.

The most common infecting organisms are *Neisseria gonorrhea, Chlamydia trachomatis, Trichomonas vaginalis,* and herpes simplex virus. The diagnosis is by identification of the organism by the appropriate testing technique for the particular agent, and treatment depends upon the etiology.

CONDYLOMATOUS VAGINITIS

An exuberant vaginal wart infection with the human papillomavirus sometimes produces a vaginal discharge that can produce vulvar irritation.

Clinical Presentation

The patient is most often a young woman who complains of an increased vaginal discharge, often with vulvar pruritus but sometimes with burning and dyspareunia. A physical examination shows whitened, hyperkeratotic vaginal epithelium often with obvious patches of warts or generalized disease. The vaginal discharge is thick and white, often adhering to the vaginal walls. The pH is low, and the only microscopic abnormality is a greatly increased number of normal-appearing epithelial cells. Often, typical vulvar condylomata acuminata can be identified.

Diagnosis

The diagnosis is on the basis of the clinical picture with histologic confirmation, since some patients show an idiopathic leukokeratosis of the vagina.

Treatment

Treatment is addressed fully under Anogenital Warts in Chapter 9. In the vagina, the primary modes of treatment are topical fluorouracil and laser. Fluorouracil cream 2 percent inserted in the vagina nightly or weekly (less resulting inflammation) has the advantage of home treatment, low cost, and effectiveness. Patients should be followed carefully with dosing titrated as necessary to minimize tissue destruction. Unfortunately, fluorouracil is a teratogen that is not approved by the Food and Drug Administration for this indication, so use requires very careful patient education, birth control, and a reliable patient. Laser therapy can be effective and fast, but it is expensive, and slow and painful healing occurs in many patients. Those patients who present with burning pain as a result of their condylomatous vaginitis risk worsening of their pain by this treatment.

PLASMA CELL VULVITIS

Plasma cell vulvitis appears to be the female counterpart of balanitis circumscripta plasmacellularis or Zoon's balanitis (see below). The first cases in women were recognized at about the time of Zoon's original description, but the initial description in English was not published until 1957.[4] Since then fewer than 20 additional women, ranging from 20 to 70 years old, have been reported as having this condition. These cases were reviewed by Davis et al in 1983[5] and Scurry et al in 1993.[6]

Clinical Presentation

Vulvar lesions are similar to those that occur in men and appear as dusky red macules or patches with a glistening surface (Fig. 7-1). Several lesions may be present on the inner surface of the labia minora, whereas in men, only a single lesion is generally found. The vulvar lesions are usually asymptomatic, though dyspareunia has been noted.

Histology

On biopsy there is thinning (and sometimes absence) of the epidermis. A dense inflammatory infiltrate consisting primarily of lymphocytes and plasma cells abuts the involved epidermis. Capillaries are increased in number; erythrocyte extravasation and hemosiderin deposition are usually present. These changes rule out vulvar intraepithelial neoplasia (VIN) and Paget's disease, but they are similar to the lichenoid changes found in the mucosal expression of lichen planus, lichen sclerosus, lupus erythematosus, and cicatricial pemphigoid.

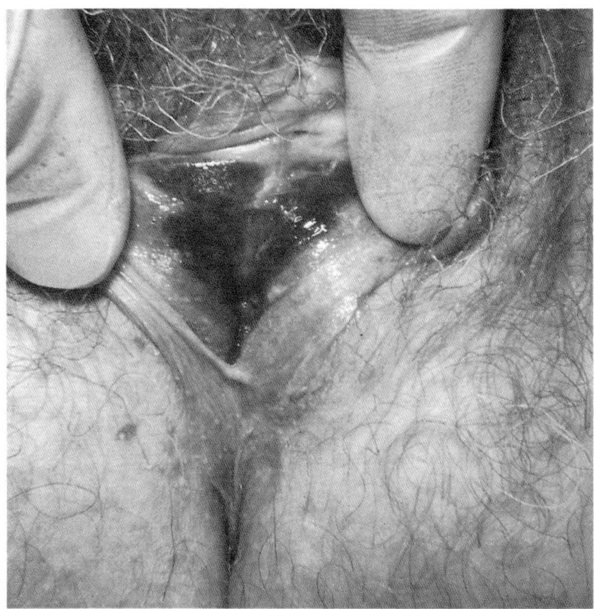

Fig. 7-1. Inflamed, moist plaque of plasma cell vulvitis over the modified mucous membrane skin of the vulva.

Differential Diagnoses

Diseases to be considered in the differential diagnosis include lichen planus, lupus erythematosus, cicatricial pemphigoid, VIN, and vulvar Paget's disease. In fact, as noted in the section on plasma cell balanitis, plasma cell vulvitis probably represents a nonspecific clinical and histologic presentation that occurs in common for all of these conditions except VIN and Paget's disease.

Course and Prognosis

The process is chronic. Lesions may slowly enlarge or may remain stable in size for many years with little change in the color or thickness. Malignant transformation has not been reported.

Pathogenesis

The cause is unknown. One reported patient may have had lupus erythematosus, and another had desquamative vaginitis that was probably a form of lichen planus.[6]

Treatment

Treatment is difficult or even impossible. High-potency topical steroids may produce some improvement, but clearing is not complete and exacerbation occurs as soon as the steroids are discontinued. Topical application of tretinoin (Retin-A) cream 0.025 percent applied daily for 6 weeks was helpful in several cases of plasma cell balanitis that we have treated and thus might be worth trying for this form of vulvitis. Others have used laser ablation, but recurrence following laser therapy has been observed.

PLASMA CELL BALANITIS

Plasma cell balanitis (balanitis circumscripta plasmacellularis, Zoon's balanitis) has been reported rarely; only about 50 cases have been noted in the English literature. Nevertheless, discussion with colleagues, together with our own experience, suggests that it is much more common than the paucity of reports suggest. Similar changes occur both on the vulva (see above) and on the oral mucous membranes; for this reason the more encompassing term *plasma cell mucositis* has been suggested as appropriate for the disease in any of its mucosal locations.[7]

Clinical Presentation

The disease in men seems to occur only in those who are uncircumcised. Lesions are located on the glans penis and the inner surface of the prepuce, where they present as bright red, fairly sharply marginated patches (Figs. 7-2 and 7-3). Most lesions are 1.5 cm or more in diameter. The surface is moist, and in long-standing, severe cases the surface may be visibly eroded. In nearly all cases only a single patch is present. The lesion is usually asymptomatic.

Histology

The diagnosis is established by biopsy. The microscopic picture consists of a thinned or even absent epithelium; epithelial cells when present may appear elongated, degenerated, or necrotic. Immediately under the epidermis there is a bandlike infiltrate consisting of lymphocytes and plasma cells. Extravasation of erythrocytes and deposition of hemosiderin may also be present in the upper dermis. While the

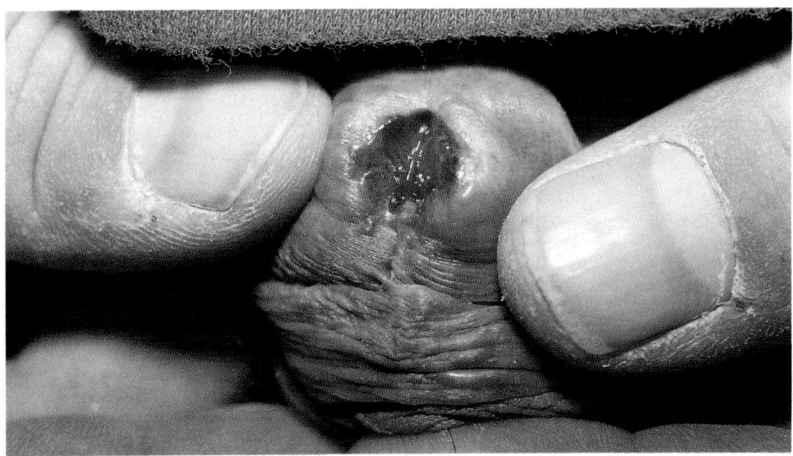

Fig. 7-2. Red, glistening periurethral plaque of plasma cell (Zoon's) balanitis.

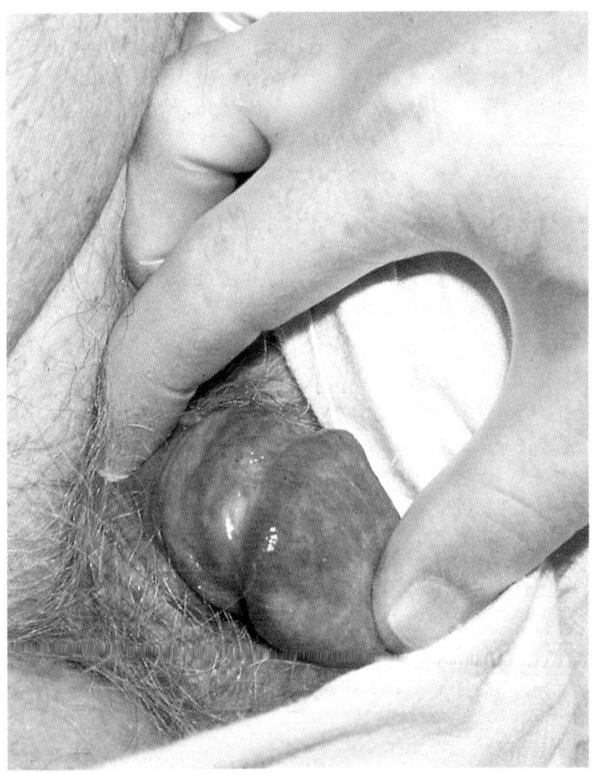

Fig. 7-3. Erythematous, moist plaque of plasma cell (Zoon's) balanitis.

histologic appearance is quite distinctive, large numbers of plasma cells are present in almost all instances of chronic inflammation involving mucous membranes; thus the presence of plasma cells alone is a nonspecific finding.

Differential Diagnoses

Diseases to be considered include candidal balanitis and erythroplasia of Queyrat. Candidal balanitis is an acute process and will have been present only a short time. Also the borders of candidal lesions are less sharply marginated, and the surface is often studded with minute pustules. Biopsy is usually required to differentiate between erythroplasia of Queyrat (squamous cell carcinoma in situ) and plasma cell balanitis.

Course and Prognosis

The course of the disease is unremitting and quite chronic; patients sometimes report that the lesion has been present for several years. It is not known whether the disease eventually resolves, evolves into recognizable lichen planus or other disease, or persists indefinitely.

Pathogenesis

The cause of plasma cell balanitis is unknown, and it may well be more than a single process. Thus, plasma cell balanitis could possibly represent a nonspecific clinical morphology for erosive lichen planus, lupus erythematosus, cicatricial pemphigoid, and other similar immunologically mediated diseases. As such, it would be analogous to the condition known as oral desquamative gingivitis or desquamative vaginitis (discussed above).

Treatment

Circumcision is the treatment of choice for plasma cell balanitis.[8] Removal of the foreskin regularly results in improvement and sometimes complete cure. Circumcision is also the treatment of choice for lichen sclerosus of the penis; this therapeutic observation suggests that the two diseases may be somewhat similar in nature. Surprisingly, there is very little response to topically applied corticosteroids, but long-term application of tretinoin (Retin-A) cream, 0.025 percent although uncomfortable for the patient, can be quite helpful. Recently, application of a new anti-inflammatory product, fusidic acid, was reported to be useful in treating eight patients.[9]

REFERENCES

Trichomoniasis

1. Eschenbach D. A.: Treatment of vaginitis. p. 195. In Horowitz BJ, Mardh PA (eds): Vaginitis and Vaginosis. Wiley-Liss, New York, 1991

Cytolytic Vaginosis

2. Cibley LJ, Cibley LJ: Cytolytic vaginosis: a common cause of vaginitis. p. 181. In Horowitz BJ, Mardh PA (eds): Vaginitis and Vaginosis. Wiley-Liss, New York, 1991

Desquamative Vaginitis

3. Durfee MA, Forsyth PS, Hale JA et al: Ineffectiveness of erythromycin for treatment of Haemophilus vaginalis associated vaginitis: possible relationship to acidity of vaginal secretion. Antimicrob Agents Chemother 16:635, 1979

Plasma Cell Vulvitis

4. Garnier G: Benign plasma-cell erythroplasia. Br J Dermatol 69:77, 1957
5. Davis J, Shapiro L, Baral J: Vulvitis circumscripta plasmacellularis. J Am Acad Dermatol 8:413, 1983
6. Scurry J, Dennerstein G, Brenan J et al: Vulvitis circumscripta plasmacellularis. A clinicopathologic entity? J Reprod Med 38:14, 1993

Plasma Cell Balanitis

7. White JW Jr, Olsen KD, Banks PM: Plasma cell orificial mucositis. Arch Dermatol 122:1321, 1986
8. Ferrandiz C, Ribera M: Zoon's balanitis treated by circumcision. J Dermatol Surg Oncol 10:622, 1984
9. Petersen CS, Thomsen K: Fusidic acid cream in the treatment of plasma cell balanitis. J Am Acad Dermatol 27:633, 1992

SUGGESTED READINGS

Vulvovaginitis

Sobel JD: Vulvovaginitis. Dermatol Clin 10:339, 1992

This practical article reviews the primary causes of vulvovaginitis as well as differentiating features, treatment, and prognosis.

Summers PR (ed): Vaginitis in 1993. Clin Obstet Gynecol 36:105, 1993

The chapters in this volume review the latest information on various infectious and inflammatory causes of vaginitis.

Sweet RL, Gibbs RS: Infectious vulvovaginitis. p. 216. In: Infectious Diseases of the Female Genital Tract. 2nd Ed. Williams & Wilkins. Baltimore, 1990

This chapter surveys the etiology, diagnosis, and treatment for the most common causes of infectious vaginitis.

Plasma Cell Balanitis

Souteyrand P, Wong E, MacDonald DM: Zoon's balanitis (balanitis circumscripta plasmacellularis). Br J Dermatol 105:195, 1981

This paper describes one of the largest series of patients and reviews the literature up to 1981.

8 Red Papules and Nodules

CONTACT URTICARIA

Some substances can produce a rapid, transient, cutaneous response to direct contact in the form of urticaria. Because allergic and irritant contact dermatitis of the genital area may manifest primarily through edema and erythema rather than visible scale, contact urticaria should be considered in some patients who report skin changes due to a contactant. The reaction may be either immunologic or a direct toxic effect.

Clinical Presentation

Patients are most often atopic and present with itching or burning, or describe recurrent dermatitis or generalized urticaria. Some patients will have systemic symptoms including asthma, angioedema, rhinitis, itching of the eyes, diarrhea, cramping, nausea, and occasionally even hypotension. Symptoms may not occur with every exposure, making a coherent history difficult.

Diagnosis

A physical examination may show no abnormalities, since the changes are usually transient and have disappeared by the time of the office visit. At times, poorly demarcated, erythematous, scaling, or lichenified plaques may be present as a dermatitis driven by the underlying urticarial reaction. The diseases most often confused with contact urticaria are common urticaria and dermatitis.

A skin biopsy shows only dermal edema and a mild perivascular mononuclear inflammatory infiltrate, sometimes with scattered eosinophils.

Pathogenesis

The pathogenesis of immunologically mediated (allergic) contact urticaria is that of an IgE immediate type I hypersensitivity or perhaps an IgM- or IgG-mediated activation of the complement cascade. Some responsible agents are also frequent causes of allergic contact dermatitis.

The most important substance that causes an immunologically mediated contact urticaria in the genital area is latex in examining gloves, condoms, and diaphragms. Latex may produce not only contact urticaria but also anaphylaxis. Some patients may have a delayed-type hypersensitivity in addition to contact urticaria. Medications such as neomycin, gentamicin, penicillin, and bacitracin may elicit contact urticaria in sensitive individuals. Preservatives and fragrances added to medications, soaps, shampoos, and perfumes such as benzoic acid, parabens, and many alcohols also can be offenders. Foods, flavorings, and preservatives in foods may be offenders and could conceivably produce genital disease in those practicing oral sex. Local vulvar contact urticaria to semen has been reported on a number of occasions.

The mechanism of nonimmunologic contact urticaria is unclear, and fortunately significant systemic reactions generally do not occur. A direct toxic effect on vessel walls or a nonspecific release of vasoactive substances is likely. High concentrations of some substances produce a nonimmunologically mediated contact urticaria in most normal individuals. These offenders include cinnamic acid and aldehyde, benzoic acid, sorbic acid, balsam of Peru, acetic acid, butyric acid, sodium benzoate, and many alcohols. However, some people are more sensitive, so lower concentrations can cause symptoms, and some agents can produce urticaria either immunologically or directly. Preservatives and flavorings that can produce direct, toxic urticaria include sorbic acid, formaldehyde, cinnamic acid and aldehyde, and balsam of Peru. Other offending agents are also responsible for irritant or allergic dermatitis (Table 8-1).

The evaluation of a patient for contact urticaria should be undertaken with care because of the unlikely but real possibility of a systemic reaction. This is best performed by a dermatologist or allergist experienced in the evaluation of immediate hypersensitivity and equipped to deal with systemic effects.

Table 8-1. Causes of Contact Urticaria

- Medications
  - Bacitracin
  - Benzocaine
  - Gentamicin
  - Neomycin
  - Penicillin
- Additives, preservatives, fragrances
  - Acetic acid
  - Many alcohols
  - Balsam of Peru
  - Benzoic acid
  - Butyric acid
  - Cinnamic aldehyde, acid
  - Formaldehyde
  - Lanolin
  - Lindane
  - Menthol
  - Parabens
  - Polyethylene glycol
  - Polysorbate 60
  - Sodium benzoate
- Other
  - Animal dander
  - Hair
  - Latex
  - Nickel
  - Placenta
  - Saliva
  - Semen

(From von Krogh G, Mailbach JI: The contact urticaria syndrome—1982. Semin Dermatol 1:59, 1982)

Treatment

The primary strategy in treatment of contact urticaria is avoidance of the responsible substance. Those with an allergy to latex should realize that nonlatex subsitutes are available and should be used. Oral antihistamines are sometimes useful in blunting the cutaneous response to the contactant. A patient who has systemic involvement should be aware of the potential dangers of the disease and should carry a bee sting kit containing injectable epinephrine.

CHERRY ANGIOMAS

Cherry angiomas (senile angiomas) occur on the hair-bearing skin of almost all white patients over 40 years of age. Some of these lesions may occur in the genital area or inner thighs, although this area is not affected preferentially. Most patients have only a few lesions, but some patients gradually develop hundreds of lesions, primarily over the trunk and proximal extremities.

Cherry angiomas are usually bright red in color, although some are deep red or purple (Fig. 8-1). They exhibit very sharply demarcated borders, unlike inflammatory papules that show peripheral fading of color. Very early lesions may be pinpoint in size and flat, mimicking petechiae, especially in those patients with multiple lesions. Some of these very tiny angiomas blanch with pressure, although larger papular angiomas do not blanch. Histologically, these first show a lobular proliferation of capillaries in the dermis, but the vessels of older lesions are dilated, with edematous stroma and homogenized collagen underlying a thinned epithelium.

Angiomas are asymptomatic, permanent, and require no treatment. Destruction would be necessary for elective removal. The passage of time usually brings increasing numbers of angiomas.

ANGIOKERATOMAS

Angiokeratomas (angiokeratomas of Fordyce) are small, benign, blood vessel tumors with overlying keratotic epithelium. They are very common on the

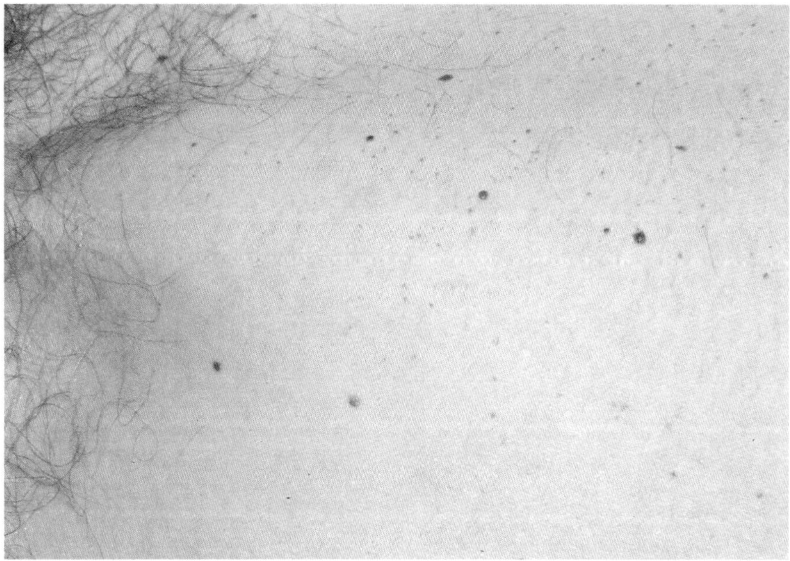

Fig. 8-1. Bright-red, well-demarcated, dome-shaped cherry angiomas.

genitalia and usually occur as a normal variant rather than disease.

Genital angiokeratomas are red to dark purple, firm, small papules clustered primarily over the scrotum or hair-bearing portion of the vulva although they may occasionally extend to the upper thighs or penile shaft (Figs. 8-2 and 8-3). They are usually multiple and range from 1 to 3 mm in diameter. Occasionally, angiokeratomas of the genital skin are single, larger, and irregular in shape, reminiscent of nodular malignant melanomas. As lesions age, they tend to become darker and occasionally clinically keratotic, although not generally appearing actually warty. They are usually asymptomatic. On biopsy, an angiokeratoma shows dilated capillaries in the upper dermis enclosed by the rete ridges of epidermis. The epidermis is hyperkeratotic, especially in older lesions.

Angiokeratomas are sometimes related to an increase in local venous pressure but more often have no medical implications. Even less often, extensive lesions appear as markers for several rare genetic inborn errors of metabolism, including Fabry's disease.

In general, treatment is not needed. Destruction or a biopsy may be indicated when an occasional angiokeratoma is pruritic, exophytic with bleeding, or mimics a cutaneous melanoma.

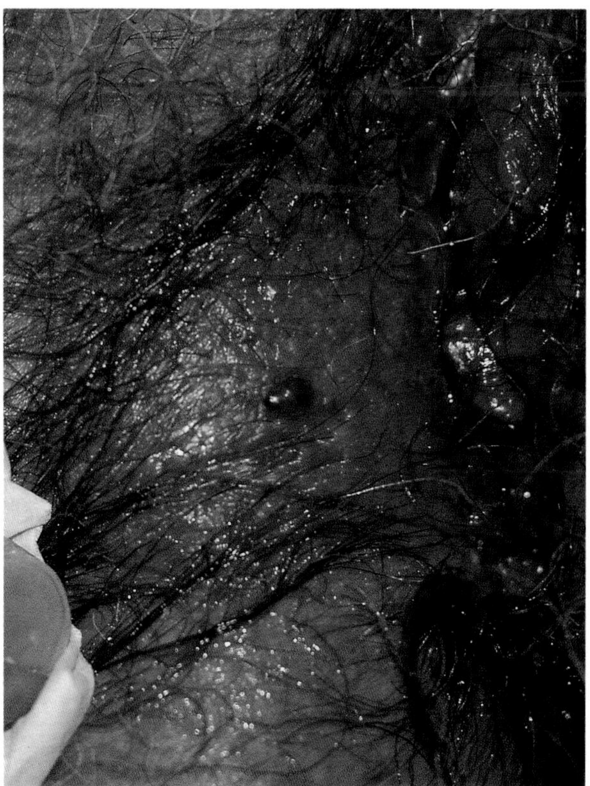

Fig. 8-2. Deep purple papule of a vulvar angiokeratoma.

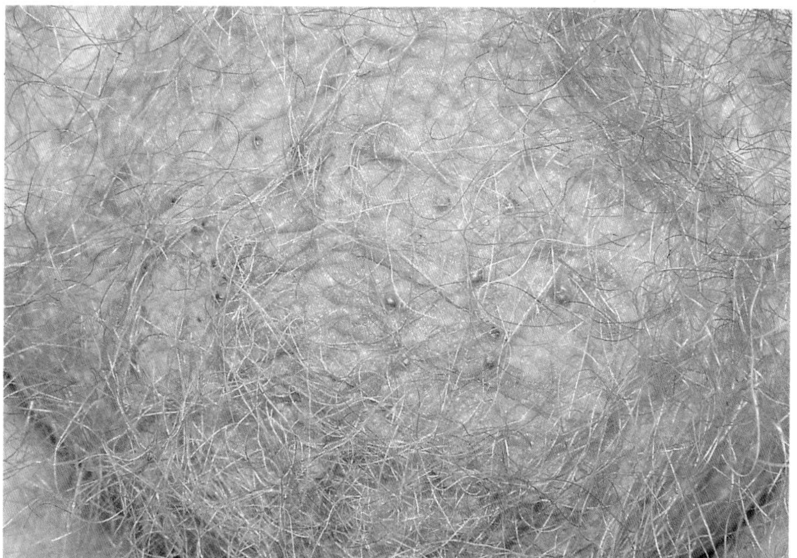

Fig. 8-3. Multiple, small, red and purple papules of angiokeratomata of Fordyce on a scrotum.

URETHRAL CARUNCLES

The urethral caruncle, an exophytic lesion at the urethral opening, is relatively common in older women.

This lesion may be asymptomatic and unnoticed by the patient or it may be a cause of pain and bleeding. The urethral caruncle appears as a bright red, glistening, polypoid papule or nodule of urethral mucosa extruding through the urethral meatal orifice (Fig. 8-4). It differs from urethral prolapse by its more polypoid surface and the histologic appearance. Dilated vessels with acute and chronic inflammation are usual. Infolding of epithelium and glandular structures may suggest an erroneous diagnosis of malignancy.

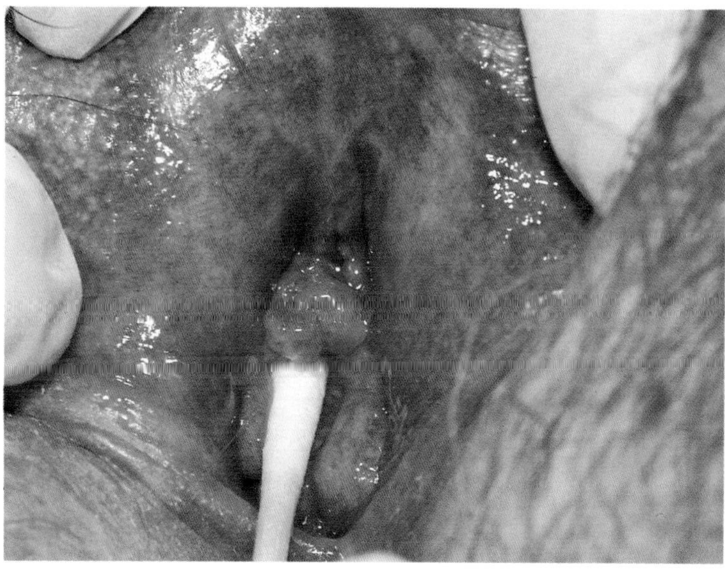

Fig. 8-4. Flesh-colored, polypoid tumor characteristic of a urethral caruncle.

Urethral caruncles should be differentiated from other tumors and biopsied when there is doubt. Topical estrogen cream to the area or oral estrogen may control symptoms and bleeding.[1] Otherwise, cryosurgery, laser vaporization, or surgical removal of the tumor including the meatus and surrounding urethral mucosa are required. Treatment is unnecessary when the patient is asymptomatic, and recurrences following treatment are common.

URETHRAL PROLAPSE

The urethral mucosa occasionally protrudes from the urethra of women with a resulting lesion very similar in appearance to a urethral caruncle. Occurring in postmenopausal women and girls before menarche, an erythematous, edematous ring of prolapsed tissue appears at the urethral orifice. Although it is usually painless, urinary retention may occur. The cause is not known, but urethral prolapse appears to be related to estrogen deficiency and increased intra-abdominal pressure. Histology shows edematous and inflamed mucosa with engorged and thrombosed vessels. The main lesions to be considered in the differential diagnosis are the urethral caruncle and other tumors. Treatment is usually by excision of the tissue, but ligation and cryotherapy are used by some clinicians.

ENDOMETRIOSIS

Endometriosis may occur on the vulva or cervix and in the vagina. Vulvar involvement, which is uncommon, most often develops after a surgical procedure or trauma that coincides with endometrial curettage, allowing implantation of endometrium within scar tissue. Vaginal and cervical disease also occurs as a result of implantation in areas of trauma, but occasionally endometriosis extends via blood or lymphatic vessels or by direct extension.

Patients may present with tenderness or dyspareunia, or with lesions that enlarge during menses. Superficial disease exhibits red, purple, or hyperpigmented macules, papules, or nodules that often deepen in color during menses. Those that reside deeper in the skin are bluish in color, and very deep lesions may be skin-colored.

The diagnosis is by biopsy, which shows typical endometrial tissue, often with fibrosis and hemosiderin within macrophages. Treatment, when required, consists of surgical excision, although recurrence is common.

SARCOIDOSIS

Sarcoidosis is an inflammatory granulomatous process of unknown etiology that most often affects the skin and lungs.

Clinical Presentation

Occurring most often in black patients in the southeastern United States, this disease mimics granulomatous infection clinically. Lesions are generally asymptomatic, but some patients may experience pruritus. Although cutaneous sarcoidosis displays a wide morphologic variety, the classic and most common lesions are erythematous, skin-colored, or lightly hyperpigmented papules, nodules, or plaques, sometimes with scarring[2] (Figs. 8-5 and 8-6). Most often the individual lesions are smooth, dome-shaped, and nonscaling, with surface shininess and a translucent character that may create the illusion of a blister. Less often, lesions are scaling or atrophic, and ulcerative anogenital lesions have also been reported.[3] Some variety of cutaneous sarcoidosis can be included in the differential diagnosis of almost any skin disease. Lesions are most often located on the face, especially over the cheeks and nares, but sarcoidosis can also affect any area of the skin, including the genital area. Thickening or nodules of the epididymis may occasionally occur.

Systemic disease is common. The lungs are most often affected, with hilar adenopathy and infiltrates that are detectable by chest radiographs when present. Iridocyclitis, retinitis, keratoconjunctivitis, liver and spleen involvement, arthritis, heart disease, and parotid involvement may occur.

Diagnosis

The diagnosis is made clinically from the nature of the skin lesions, but it should be confirmed histologically to rule out various granulomatous infections. A skin biopsy of sarcoidosis shows well-demarcated, noncaseating granulomas composed of epithelioid histiocytes, with only mild surrounding lymphocytic inflammation. At times, routine histology cannot absolutely differentiate between infection and sarcoidosis, in which case special stains, cultures, and a search for typical systemic disease are necessary.

Treatment

The treatment of cutaneous sarcoidosis is difficult. Initially, an evaluation for significant systemic disease is essential. Skin lesions are most predictably responsive to oral prednisone at a dose of 40 to 60 mg each day, but recurrence is probable with cessation of therapy. Mid- and high-potency topical corticosteroids are useful for symptomatic improvement of pruritic skin lesions and sometimes decrease the size of the lesions, but surrounding steroid-induced hypopigmentation of the lesions sometimes occurs and

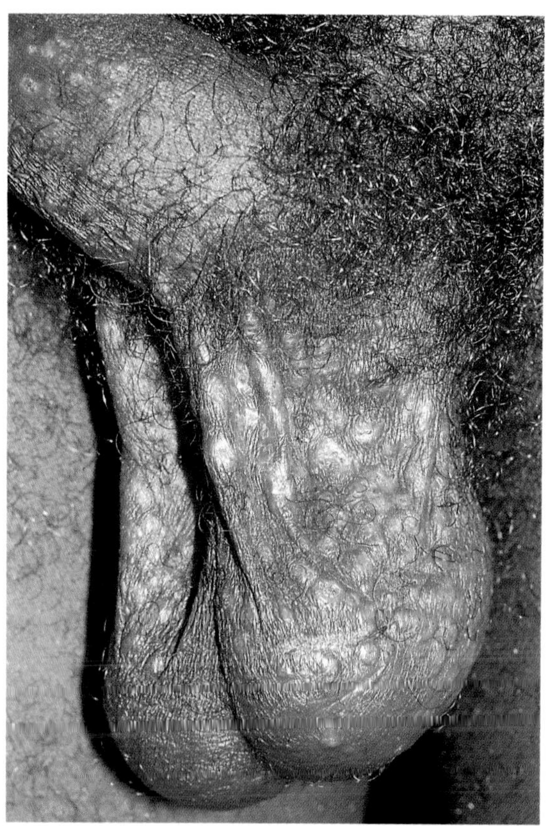

Fig. 8-5. Hypopigmented, pink, scaling papules, some with erosions, in a patient with sarcoidosis.

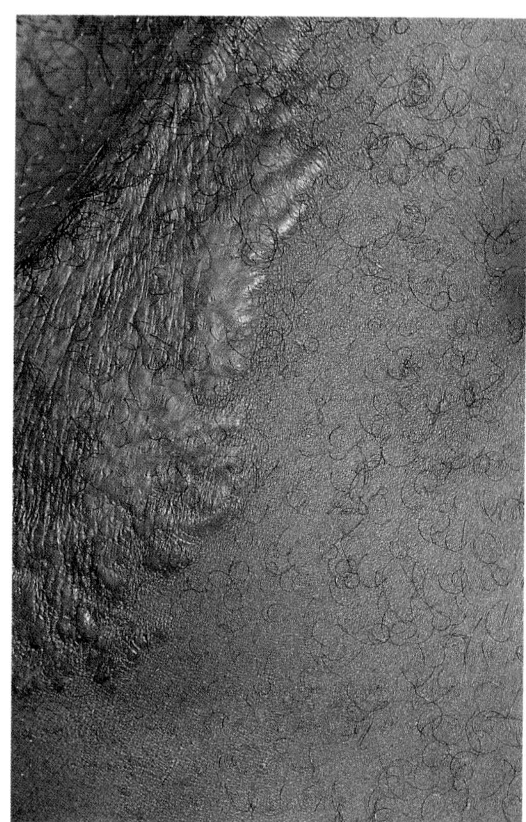

Fig. 8-6. Hyperpigmented, smooth, indurated, nodular plaque of sarcoidosis of the upper inner thigh.

may be unattractive. Intralesional corticosteroids in the form of triamcinolone acetonide 3 mg/ml are often useful in individual lesions.

For patients with widespread or cosmetically disfiguring disease who require additional therapy, oral hydroxychloroquine is safe and sometimes effective at a dose of 200 mg bid, especially as a long-term control following initial treatment with oral steroids. In recalcitrant patients, weekly oral methotrexate in low doses can sometimes be beneficial. Oral isotretinoin and chlorambucil also have been reported useful.

FURUNCULOSIS

Furunculosis is a deep, suppurative, bacterial infection of the hair follicles.

Clinical Presentation

Patients with furunculosis complain of painful boils and may experience fever and malaise. Physical examination reveals erythematous nodules that eventually drain (Fig. 8-7). Often, this is a chronic process, with healing lesions replaced by new lesions elsewhere. On occasion, several nearby affected follicles may coalesce and develop multiple sinus tracts to the surface, producing a carbuncle. These occur most often in very hairy areas and in skin exposed to friction, occlusion, and moisture, including the buttocks and genital area.

Diagnosis

The diagnosis of furunculosis is made by the clinical examination and bacterial culture. It is important to differentiate this disease from hidradenitis suppurativa, an initially sterile, deep inflammatory reaction to occlusion of the apocrine-associated follicle, resulting in nearly indistinguishable genital, buttock, or axillary lesions. In hidradenitis suppurativa, lesions are limited to these areas, and chronic, draining sinus tracts in the midst of scars are common. Histologically, a furuncle shows acute perifollicular inflammation and abscess formation.

Treatment

The causative organism of furunculosis is *Staphylococcus aureus.* Treatment requires systemic antistaphylococcal antibiotics such as dicloxacillin, cephalexin, or erythromycin, and recurrences are common. Because many patients with furunculosis are carriers of *S. aureus,* some patients require prolonged antibacterial therapy, often with mupirocin ointment applied in the nares four times a day for 1 week to help eliminate this carrier state.

HIDRADENITIS SUPPURATIVA

Hidradenitis suppurativa is a cystic, purulent, draining, and scarring follicular disease that occurs primarily in the axillae and anogenital areas. Historically it was considered to be a bacterial infection, but it is now recognized as noninfectious and acneiform in nature. Mild disease is fairly common, but severe involvement is encountered rarely. The disease does not begin prior to puberty and is seen most frequently between the ages of 20 and 40 years. Women are affected much more commonly than men; black individuals have an appreciably higher incidence than those of other races. Patients with hidradenitis suppurativa may also have one or another of the related inflammatory follicular diseases: acne conglobata or dissecting cellulitis of the scalp.

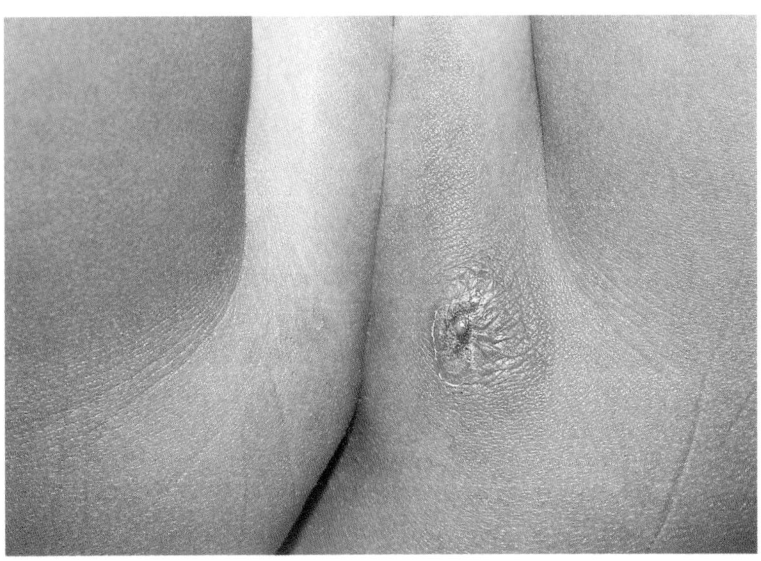

Fig. 8-7. Erythematous, indurated, ruptured nodule of Staphylococcal furunculosis.

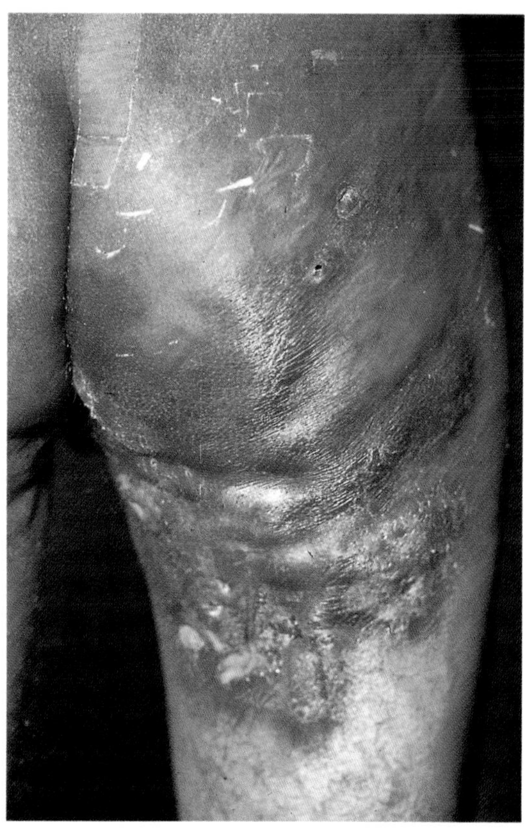

Fig. 8-8. Hidradenitis suppurativa demonstrating fluctuant nodules, draining sinus tracts, and hyperpigmentation from inflammation and postinflammatory changes.

Clinical Presentation

Hidradenitis suppurativa is extremely multiform in appearance. Early lesions consist of red papules that enlarge over days to become nodular or cystic. These lesions are essentially identical in appearance to staphylococcal furuncles ("boils") and are equally painful. Most of the inflammatory nodules eventually form a central pustule; these lesions subsequently rupture and form chronic draining sinuses (Figs. 8-8 and 8-9). Individual lesions eventually heal with scarring; sometimes the scarring is hypertrophic or even keloidal in type. The scarring can lead to impressive edema (Fig. 8-10) or architectural distortion of the genitalia, or both. Careful examination will usually reveal nearby follicles that are anatomically abnormal. These abnormal follicles are recognized by the presence of twin comedones that form in a Y-like split of the distal follicle as it emerges to the skin surface (Fig. 8-11). Twin comedones are pathognomonic for the disease.

The number of lesions is highly variable. In mild cases there may be only a few active lesions, whereas in severe cases they may be too numerous to count. Lesions occur most commonly in the axillae and in the perianal, genital, and perigenital skin. Specifically, the labia majora in women and the penis in men represent the most commonly involved sites. Lesions

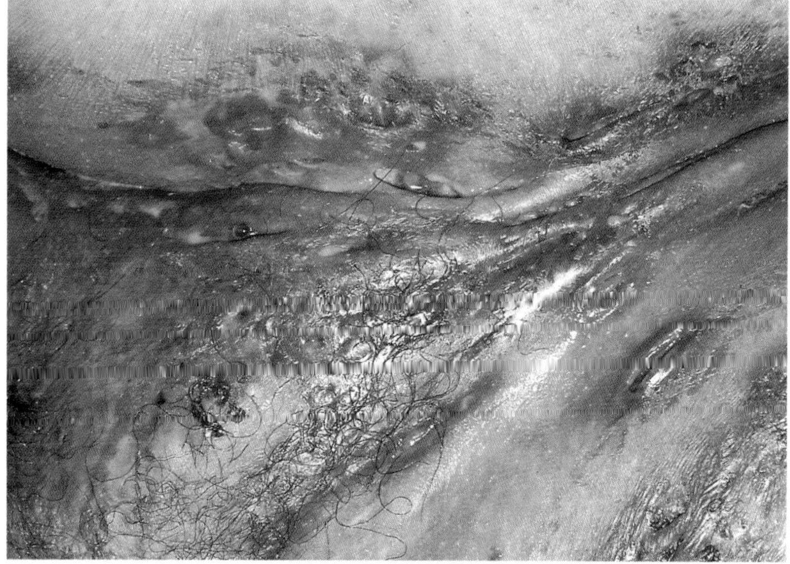

Fig. 8-9. Multiple ruptured inflammatory cysts and draining sinus tracts of hidradenitis suppurativa over the lower abdomen and inguinal area.

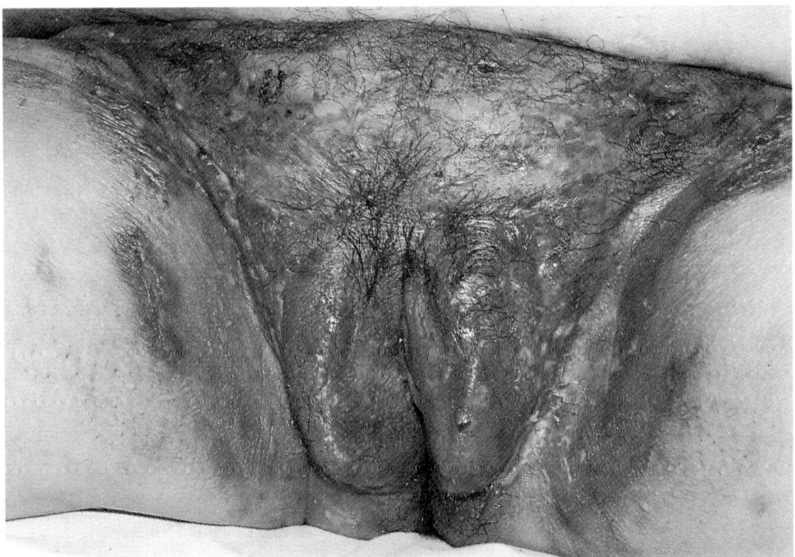

Fig. 8-10. The multiple chronic, draining cysts and inflammation of hidradenitis have resulted in permanent lymphedema of the vulva.

may also occur on the upper and inner thighs and on the buttocks.

Regional lymphadenopathy is often present. Patients with particularly severe disease may also develop fever, malaise, arthralgia, arthritis, and anemia. A few cases have been reported in patient's with Crohn's disease, but the link, if any, between these two diseases is not understood.[4]

Course and Prognosis

Hidradenitis suppurativa pursues a chronic course over many years, but there may be periods of months at a time when disease activity is minimal. Activity begins in isolated, single follicles, but commonly inflammation at one site "recruits" inflammation at nearby follicles, leading to the development of large,

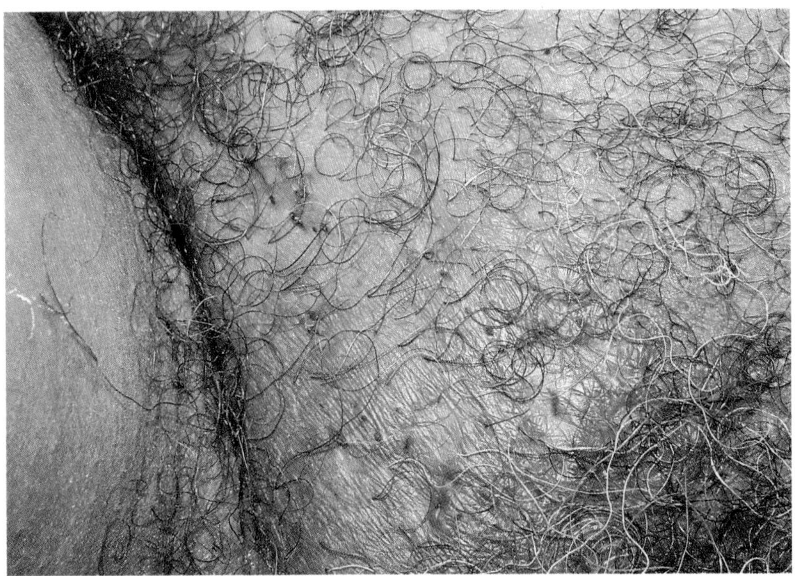

Fig. 8-11. This patient with hidradenitis suppurativa demonstrates the striking comedones, some with a double outlet, that represent the initial lesion of this disease. Keratin, sebum, and bacteria trapped below the comedones then expand the follicular epithelium into a cyst wall.

boggy, inflammatory plaques. Solitary small lesions undergo spontaneous resolution over 4 to 6 weeks; large nodules and inflammatory plaques may remain active for months.

Redevelopment of an inflammatory nodule at a previously involved site occurs frequently, but eventually scarring results in destruction of the affected follicle. As the involved follicles gradually are replaced with scarlike fibrosis, there is a gradual "burning out" of the disease process. The scarring can be severe and extensive; in such instances grotesque distortion of the genitalia may develop. Hidradenitis suppurativa of the perigenital skin sometimes results in rather massive edema of the genitalia even in the absence of direct involvement of the genital tissue.

About 15 cases of squamous cell carcinoma have been reported in old, scarred lesions,[5] presumably like the development of carcinoma in chronic stasis ulcers (Marjolin's ulcer). It may relate to the oncogenic effect of constant stimulation of epithelial cells by growth factors.

Pathogenesis

The distribution of lesions is rather sharply limited to areas of the body where apocrine glands are known to be situated. The initiating event, noted histologically, is the appearance of an acute inflammatory reaction in and around the apocrine gland and duct. The most likely explanation for the development of this inflammation is blockage at the ostium of the follicle just distal to the point at which the apocrine duct joins the hair follicle.[6] The blockage may occur for two reasons: anatomically defective follicles (see discussion of Y-like follicles above) or keratin buildup within the follicular outlet, or both. The keratin plug then acts as a dam that causes "downstream" follicular distention and subsequent leakage of material from the follicle and apocrine gland into the surrounding connective tissue. The material extruded from the blocked apocrine follicles includes apocrine sweat, keratinous material, and follicular bacteria. These materials, when present in the perifollicular tissue, act as foreign bodies inciting first an acute neutrophilic response and later a granulomatous response. The inflammation incorporates the entire involved follicle and may spread to adjacent follicles as well. The inflammation, if massive enough, can then even dissect into the subcutaneous tissue, where it calls forth a systemic, toxic response.

Originally the disease was thought to be a bacterial infection of apocrine-bearing hair follicles; more recent evidence suggests that the bacteria causes inflammation because of a foreign body reaction rather than true infection. Of course, once a lesion ruptures to the surface, there is likely to be colonization with nonfollicular varieties of bacteria. Evidence that hidradenitis suppurativa is not truly an infectious process includes the fact that (1) antibiotic treatment rarely results in rapid or complete resolution, (2) cultures reveal a mixture of organisms rather than a single dominant one, and (3) repetitive cultures rarely reveal consistency in the types of organisms recovered. It is possible that true secondary infection (as opposed to simple colonization) occurs, but, again, the failure to respond to antibacterial therapy suggests that these organisms are not acting as primary pathogens.

Many factors lead to the events described above. A genetic factor certainly plays a role since the disease sometimes occurs in an autosomal dominant fashion.[7] On the other hand, a positive family history is only found in about half of the cases. Whether inherited or not, the primary abnormality appears to be the presence of anatomically abnormal follicles as manifested by the presence of the "twin" comedones mentioned above. Racial factors also seem to be important. Hidradenitis suppurativa occurs much more frequently in blacks than in those of other races; this is most likely because blacks have more numerous apocrine gland-associated hair follicles.

Environmental factors probably play a role as well. The disease is more common and more severe in those who are obese. The obesity probably results in sweat trapping and maceration. The maceration, in turn, causes mechanical obstruction of the follicular orifices even as a similar mechanism seems to cause eccrine miliaria (prickly heat).

Hormonal factors are quite important. Hidradenitis suppurativa does not begin prior to puberty, is most active in young adult life, and, in women, is associated with premenstrual flare and menstrual irregularity. These factors fit both with observed (albeit minimal) androgen abnormalities[8] and the fact that apocrine glands are known to be androgen dependent. One might then expect that men would be more frequently affected (as they are in acne vulgaris), but in fact women outnumber men by a 3:1 ratio. Perhaps this can be explained by the observation that women have more numerous and more widely distributed apocrine gland-associated hair follicles.

Treatment

Topical treatment similar to that used for acne is often recommended for hidradenitis suppurativa. Unfortunately, support for the efficacy claimed is essentially anecdotal, and these agents have not proved very helpful in our hands. Medical therapy is, instead, based primarily on systemically administered agents. The medications described in the paragraphs that follow are discussed more thoroughly in the section on general systemic therapy in Chapter 3.

Orally administered antibiotics have historically represented the treatment of choice in hidradenitis suppurativa. Originally they were used in the belief that the disease was a bacterial infection. Today antibiotics are used as they are for acne: they act pharmacologically as nonsteroidal anti-inflammatory agents, and they reduce the number of normally present follicular bacteria such that there is less foreign protein available to incite an inflammatory reaction. Tetracycline and erythromycin are most often used. They are taken in a dosage of 500 mg bid and must be used for months before any significant degree of effectiveness can be demonstrated.

Alternatively, cultures are taken from involved lesions and antibiotic treatment is planned around the determined sensitivities.[9] Since the bacteria recovered from anogenital lesions probably derive from the rectum, it is not surprising that they are diverse in type and resistant to the most common inexpensive antibiotics. It is our belief that the cost of such treatment rarely results in improvement greater than that achieved with tetracycline and erythromycin.

Steroids are, of course, highly effective anti-inflammatory agents. Most often intralesional injections of triamcinalone acetonide (Kenalog 10) are used. Individual lesions are injected with about 0.5 ml of the stock 10 mg/ml solution. Unfortunately, the frequency and discomfort of these injections limit their usefulness. Orally administered prednisone can quiet a severe flare, but risks of long-term treatment limit this approach to infrequent "bursts" of 20 to 40 mg/day for 7 to 14 days.

Hormonal treatment is helpful for hidradenitis suppurativa just as it is for acne vulgaris. Oral contraceptives containing 50 μg of estrogen combined with those progestins that have minimal androgenic effects are quite effective and can be used for long periods of time. Demulen 1/50 represents a good choice in this regard. Spironolactone (50 mg two or three times daily) and cyproterone (which is not available in the United States) are effective antiandrogens and can be used in men as well as women. Data supporting their usefulness in hidradenitis suppurativa are not extensive,[10] but, based on more widespread experience with their use in acne, these antiandrogens seem to represent a reasonable therapeutic option.

Orally administered retinoids, especially isotretinoin, work extremely well in acne, and expectations that they would be equally useful in hidradenitis suppurativa have been high. Unfortunately, only about 50 percent of patients respond, and even then relapse occurs quickly when the retinoids are discontinued.[11,12] In addition, the troublesome side effects, the high cost, and the risk for teratogenesis when taken during pregnancy limit their therapeutic role.

Surgery is rapidly becoming the treatment of choice. Originally surgery was limited to incision and drainage or marsupialization; both "cold steel" and electrosurgical destructive approaches were used. These techniques remain effective if the number of lesions is small, but for most patients excision of involved tissue is more effective and requires less overall medical attention. The key to using surgical excision is an understanding that the process is not a bacterial infection. One can then carry out surgery in the presence of draining pus, and one can leave involved areas at the margin without interfering with good wound healing. Good results occur with either primary closure or with split-thickness skin grafting. The likelihood that new lesions will develop adjacent to the surgical site is rather high,[13,14] but most patients prefer surgery to ongoing medical treatment, and 70 to 90 percent of patients are highly satisfied with the results obtained.[15]

INFLAMED CYSTS

Cysts are nonsolid tumors that originate from various components of the skin, its appendages, or glandular structures. Although the color of various cysts depends upon their contents, any cyst may become inflamed, with a resulting red color predominating. The causes and clinical presentation of specific cysts are addressed in Chapter 10. The causes of inflammation of cysts include rupture, irritation from friction, or infection.

Clinical Presentation

Inflammation of the most common cysts (epidermal) is usually on the basis of rupture not on the presence of infection, as is assumed by many clinicians. An inflamed epidermal cyst is red, with a relatively small surrounding erythematous halo. When truly infected, there is usually a substantial degree of surrounding erythema. Pain, warmth, enlargement, and fluctuance are commonly seen with both infection and sterile inflammation. However, actual infection, sometimes recurrent, more often occurs in the cysts of Bartholin's gland (Fig. 8-12). In addition, Bartholin's glands may become infected, with resulting abscess formation in the absence of a preexisting cyst.

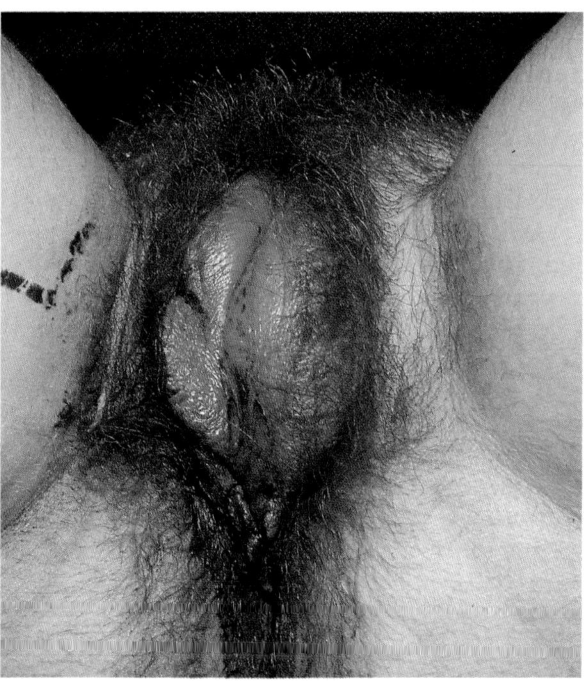

Fig. 8-12. Marked edema and erythema with distortion of the vulva from an inflamed Bartholin's gland duct cyst. (Courtesy from Raymond H. Kaufman, MD)

Pathogenesis

Gonorrhea is an important cause of Bartholin's gland abscesses and cyst infection. Other common etiologic agents include *Staphylococcus aureus, Escherichia coli, Streptococcus faecalis,* and *Pseudomonas aeruginosa.* Other types of cysts are less likely to become inflamed with either of these mechanisms, but some vestibular cysts and cysts of the canal of Nuck may be pedunculated, with resulting inflammation and necrosis after torsion of the stalk.

Treatment

Treatment of an inflamed cyst depends upon the cause of the inflammation. With any question of infection, culture and oral antibiotic treatment are indicated. If the cyst is fluctuant, incision and drainage should be performed. In the case of a Bartholin's gland cyst, repeated infection or inflammation may require marsupialization, in which the roof of the cyst is removed and the remainder of the cyst exteriorized to prevent recurrence. Alternatively, an inflatable bulb-tipped catheter (a Word catheter) can be introduced through a stab incision into the cyst; the bulb is then inflated to hold the catheter in place. When the stab opening has reepithialized to provide a permanent outlet for secretions, the catheter is removed.

An inflamed, uninfected epidermal cyst that is firm but nonfluctuant usually responds well and quickly to a small amount of intralesional triamcinolone acetonide at a concentration of 3 mg/ml injected with a 30-gauge needle into the cyst wall. In general, an inflamed cyst should not be surgically removed until the primary erythema and pain have improved because a larger incision is often required to remove the edematous and less well demarcated lesion, resulting in a larger scar. Patients often elect not to excise the lesion after it has returned to its asymptomatic state.

REFERENCES

Urethral Caruncle

1. Kaufman RH, Friedrich EG Jr, Gardner HL: Solid tumors. p. 194. In Kaufman RH, Friedrich EG Jr, Gardner HL (eds): Benign Diseases of the Vulva and Vagina. 3rd Ed. Year Book Medical Publishers, Chicago, 1989

Sarcoidosis

2. Tatnall FM, Barnes HM, Sarkany I: Sarcoidosis of the vulva. Clin Exp Dermatol 10:384, 1985
3. Neill SM, Smith NP, Eady RA: Ulcerative sarcoidosis: a rare manifestation of a common disease. Clin Exp Dermatol 9:277, 1984

Hidradenitis Suppurativa

4. Burrows NP, Jones RR: Crohn's disease in association with hidradenitis suppurativa. Br J Dermatol 126:523, 1992
5. Anstey AV, Wilkinson JD, Lord P: Squamous cell carcinoma complicating hidradenitis suppurativa. Br J Dermatol 123:527, 1990
6. Yu CCW, Cook MG: Hidradenitis suppurativa: a disease of follicular epithelium, rather than apocrine glands. Br J Dermatol 122:763, 1990
7. Fitzsimmons JS, Guilbert PR, Fitzsimmons EM: Evidence of genetic factors in hidradenitis suppurativa. Br J Dermatol 113:1, 1985
8. Mortimer PS, Dawber RPR, Gales MA, Moore RA: Mediation of hidradenitis suppurativa by androgens. Br Med J 292:245, 1986
9. Highet AS, Warren RE, Weekes AJ: Bacteriology and antibiotic treatment of perineal suppurative hidradenitis. Arch Dermatol 124:1047, 1988
10. Mortimer PS, Dawber RPRD, Gales MA, Moore RA: A double-blind controlled cross over trial of cyproterone acetate in females with hidradenitis suppurativa. Br J Dermatol 115:263, 1986
11. Hogan DJ, Light MJ: Successful treatment of hidradenitis suppurativa with acitretin. J Am Acad Dermatol 19:355, 1988
12. Norris JFB, Cunliffe WJ: Failure of treatment of familial widespread hidradenitis suppurativa with isotretinoin. Clin Exp Dermatol 11:579, 1986
13. Wiltz O, Schoetz DJ, Murray JJ et al: Perianal hidradenitis suppurativa: the Lahey Clinic experience. Dis Colon Rectum 33:731, 1990
14. Harrison BJ, Mudge M, Hughes LE: Recurrence after surgical treatment of hidradenitis suppurativa. Br Med J 294:487, 1987
15. Jemec GBE: Effect of localized surgical excisions in hidradenitis suppurativa. J Am Acad Dermatol 18:1103, 1988

SUGGESTED READINGS

Contact Urticaria

von Krogh G, Maibach JI: The contact urticaria syndrome—1982. Semin Dermatol 1:59, 1982

This review includes the pathogenesis, presentation, and etiologies of contact urticaria as well as a discussion of the evaluation of the patient.

Sarcoidosis

Sharma OP: Sarcoidosis of the skin. p. 2221. In Fitzpatrick TB, Eisen AZ, Wolff K et al (eds): Dermatology in General Medicine. McGraw-Hill, New York, 1993

This chapter is a concise summary of the clinical manifestations of sarcoidosis.

Hidradenitis Suppurativa

Ebling FJG: Apocrine glands in health and disorder. Int J Dermatol 28:508, 1989

Endometriosis, Urethral Prolapse, and Urethral Caruncle

Kaufman RH, Friedrich EG, Garnder HL: Benign diseases of the vulva and vagina. p. 224. 3rd Ed. Year Book Medical Publishers, Chicago, 1989

III Skin-Colored and White Lesions

9 Skin-Colored Papules

ANOGENITAL WARTS

The last two decades have witnessed the rise of viral infections as the most important, troublesome, studied, and discussed forms of sexually transmitted disease. One of these, human papillomavirus (HPV) infection, is particularly important because of its high prevalence and etiologic role in anogenital carcinoma.

Determination of HPV prevalence is problematic because of the absence of an acceptable serologic test and the fact that the virus can exist in a latent state identifiable only with molecular laboratory tests.[1] Clinically visible anogenital warts are present in about 1 percent of the adult population[2]; cytologic changes indicative of HPV infection of the cervix are found in 2 to 5 percent of women; hybridization studies detect genital HPV DNA in 10 to 20 percent of the adult population, and, when the polymerase chain reaction (PCR) is used to amplify HPV DNA, 30 to 60 percent of adults are found to be infected.[3,4]

The incidence of genital warts is said to be increasing rapidly, and, as is true for other genital viral infections, this is probably true. Some portion of the purported increase, however, is probably related to increased awareness and better diagnostic tools.

Men and women are presumably affected at similar rates, although most of the prevalence studies have been carried out in women. Infection can occur at any age from birth (as a result of maternal contagion) to death. Visible lesions in the form of anogenital warts are, however, mostly encountered from age 15 to 40, with a peak incidence at about age 25.

Clinical Presentation

Clinical Morphology

Several different morphologic forms of genital warts are recognized. The classical wart (and true condyloma accuminatum) is a skin-colored filiform papilloma approximately 3 to 10 mm high and 1 to 2 mm in diameter (Fig. 9-1). The terminal end on the larger lesions is brushlike and slightly whiter than the stalk itself. A larger variant of this type of wart can also occur. These larger lesions are less filiform and are made up of clustered closely set pink or red lobules that arise from a stalk (Fig. 9-2).

The most common morphologic presentation is that of flat warts appearing as barely elevated, smooth-surfaced, flat-topped papules 2 to 4 mm in diameter (Figs. 9-1 and 9-3). Warts that occur on the mucous membranes of the vagina and anus are almost always of this type. These lesions may be skin-colored, pink, brown, or, when on moist surfaces, white. Because of their small size, they may not be apparent until acetic acid soaks are applied (see below) (Fig. 9-4). These flat warts may cluster or may even become confluent, in which case they appear as a slightly elevated flat-topped plaques. When such plaques are on moist areas such as the vestibule they appear as white plaques and are thus easily confused with nonviral hyperkeratotic diseases (see Ch. 11).

Warts occurring on perigenital skin may have an appearance similar to hand warts (verruca vulgaris). These lesions are larger, flat-topped, square-shouldered papules 4 to 6 mm high and equally wide (Fig.

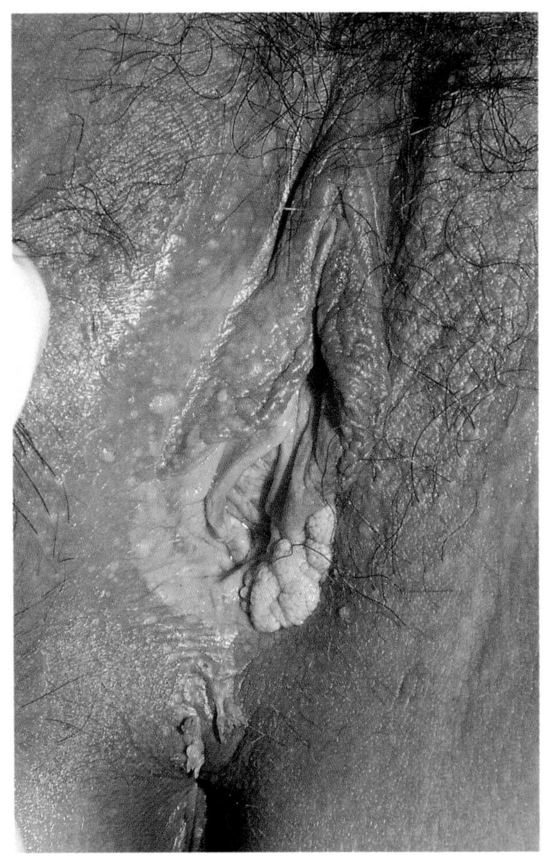

Fig. 9-1. Verrucous plaque of genital wart with several nearby flat warts. Small filiform warts are present on the perineal body.

9-5). The surface of such lesions is slightly rough because of the hyperkeratosis that is present. Color ranges from light brown to skin-colored.

Giant warts (sometimes called Buschke-Löwenstein tumors) are uncommonly encountered. Some are cauliflower-like in appearance (as if they were made up of several clusters) and others are smooth surfaced (Fig. 9-6). The largest lesions may be 5 to 10 cm in diameter. They may be pink, red, skin-colored, or somewhat pigmented.

Vestibular Papillomatosis

Special mention should be made of vestibular papillomatosis. This is a normal anatomic variant in which 10 to 100 small (1 to 2 mm) round papules stud the surface of the vulvar vestibule. In some cases, when the papillomas are especially numerous, the vestibule takes on a cobblestone-like appearance. Similar changes can occur within the vagina. These changes were originally thought to be caused by diffuse HPV infection, but hybridization studies are only positive for HPV DNA in about the same proportion of cases as in controls.[5,6] Clinical clues to the fact that these are anatomic variants rather than genital warts include the morphologic homogeneity (every papule is exactly the same size, color, and shape) and a distribution with almost perfect bilateral symmetry.

Symptoms

Anogenital warts of all types are mostly asymptomatic; mild itching is present in a minority of cases. Some of the larger warts, especially those that are pink or raspberry-like in appearance, are quite friable and bleed fairly easily. Pain is not usually associated with anogenital warts unless they are large enough to become mechanically irritated due to the binding of clothing or the trauma of coitus. Dyspareunia is not a feature of anogenital warts unless they are large enough to interfere mechanically with intromission. Some clinicians believe that HPV infection plays a role in vulvodynia/vestibulitis, but data to support this viewpoint are unimpressive[7] (see also Ch. 21).

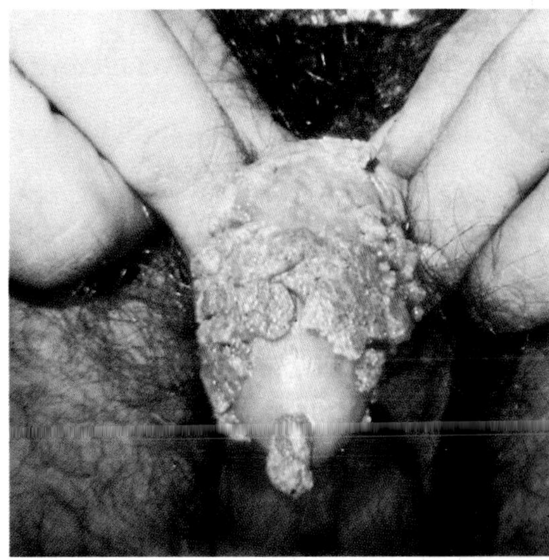

Fig. 9-2. Exuberant growth of penile and meatal genital warts.

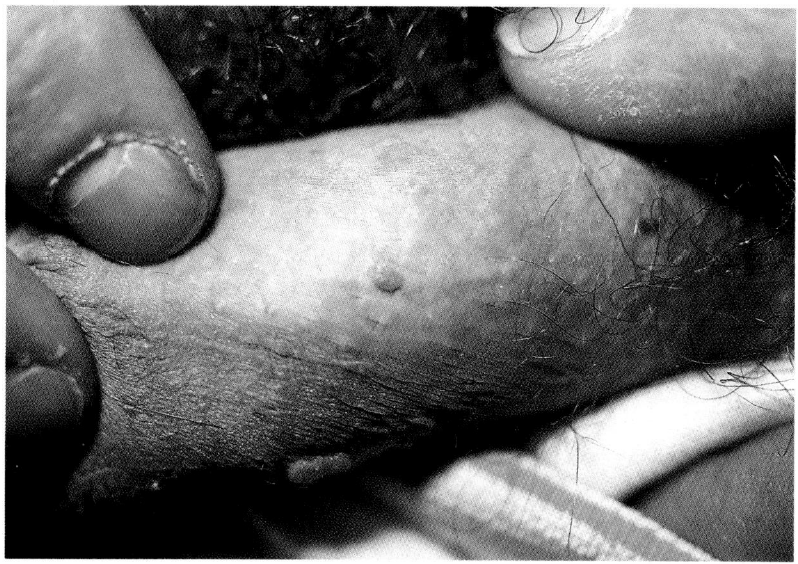

Fig. 9-3. Skin-colored, sharply demarcated, typical genital warts.

Distribution

HPV-induced anogenital lesions may occur anywhere on the skin and contiguous mucous membranes. In women, warts are most often found at the vaginal introitus, whereas in men they occur most frequently at the coronal sulcus and on the penile shaft. Other common locations include the vulvar vestibule in women, the glans penis in men, and the urethra,[8] anus, and perianal tissue in both sexes.[9] Approximately 50 percent of women with vulvar warts have evidence of cervical HPV infection,[10] and some of these women have cervical intraepithelial neoplasia (CIN) related to their cervical HPV infection.[11] Vaginal warts are encountered much less often. HPV DNA has also been recovered from urine[12] and semen.[13]

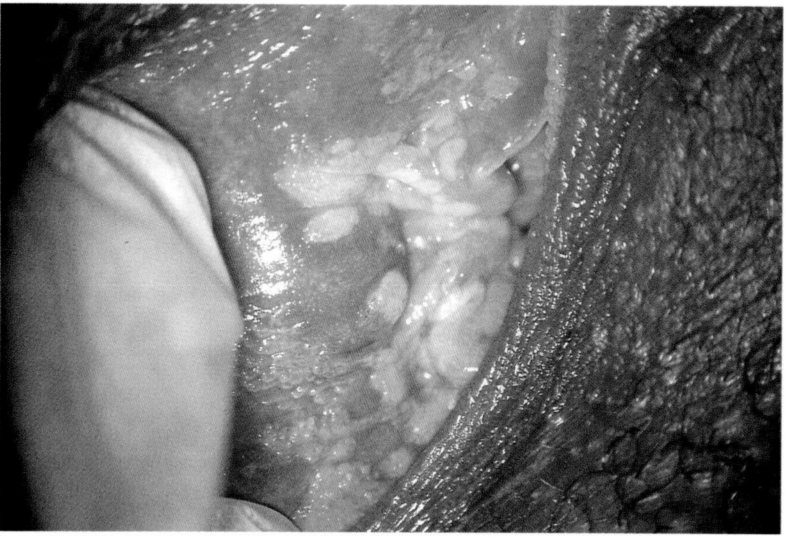

Fig. 9-4. Discrete, white papules of a subtle human papillomavirus infection following the application of acetic acid.

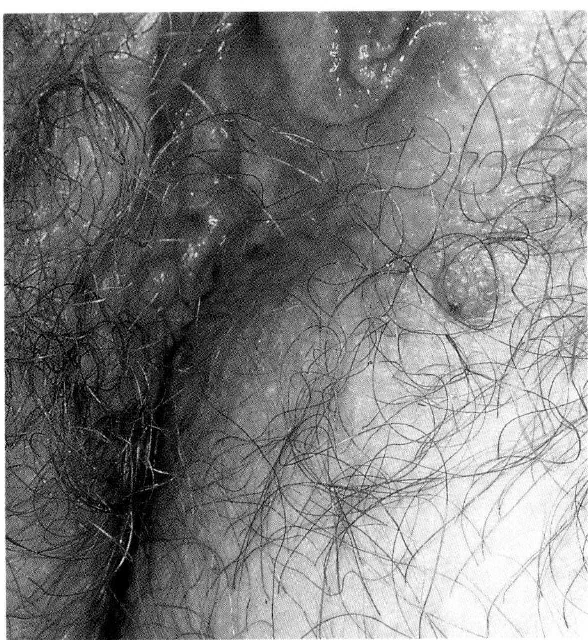

Fig. 9-5. Typical skin-colored wart with a papillomatous surface.

Diagnostic Approaches

Most warts can be recognized on the basis of clinical morphology, but biopsy is important in certain circumstances. Most importantly, varying degrees of dysplasia will be present in warts of two phenotypes: giant condylomata acuminata and flat-topped papules and plaques. This dysplasia cannot be recognized clinically, yet knowledge of its presence is critical in the determination of therapy and prognosis.

The application of 3 to 5 percent acetic acid (common white vinegar) soaks followed by examination with or without magnification[1] has been widely recommended as a means of increasing diagnostic sensitivity. This approach certainly allows for recognition of some lesions that might otherwise be missed, but questions remain as to the clinical usefulness of this technique.[14-16]

The controversy exists for three reasons. First, only about one half of the lesions so identified are true warts as judged by the presence of HPV DNA with molecular studies; the remainder are a hodgepodge of normal anatomic variants and benign, unimportant skin lesions. Second, viral replication is rarely occurring in these "subclinical" warts and thus they are probably low-risk lesions from a standpoint of contagion. Third, it is questionable what use there is in identifying these lesions if physicians are missing latent HPV in other unexamined sites such as the urethra, bladder, prostate, vagina, and rectum. We still use the acetic acid technique occasionally for purposes of contact tracing and for proof of cure post-therapy, but even in these settings it is of only minimal value.

Even more questions exist about the use of "molecular diagnosis" through DNA hybridization with or without PCR. This allows for exquisite sensitivity in determining whether or not HPV DNA is present

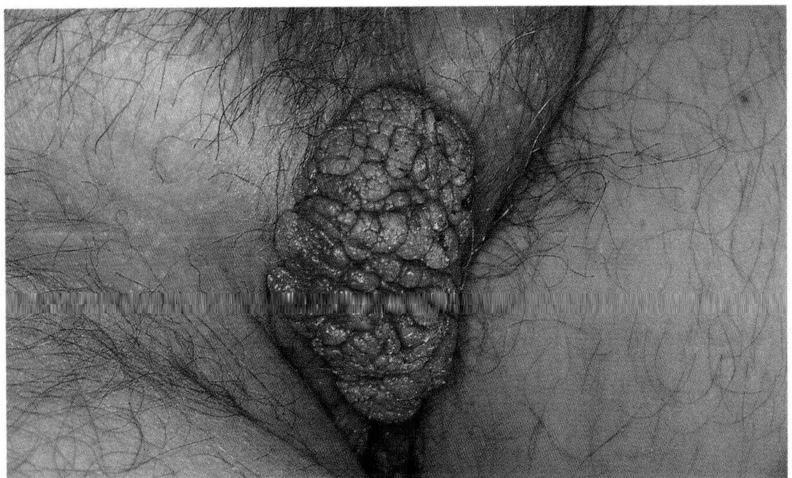

Fig. 9-6. Giant wart that deserves removal with histologic examination for the presence of verrucous squamous cell carcinoma (Buschke-Löwenstein tumor).

at a given site, but the usefulness of this information is not clear. Certainly we are not currently able to treat all of the 30 to 60 percent of patients who have laboratory evidence of HPV DNA nor can we treat, in any given patient, all of the rather large areas that can be identified by way of this approach. A commercial product, ViraPap, designed for use on the cervix, is available, but its use is probably best reserved for purposes of clinical research.

A commercial test, ViraType, is also available for purposes of typing the various strains of HPV DNA that might be present. The use of this test has some potential value in that it allows (theoretically at least) separation of "oncogenic" from "nononcogenic" HPV types. Unfortunately, the knowledge gained from typing is of limited usefulness[17] since only a small percent of infections with oncogenic types end in malignancy, and there are occasional reports of malignancy occurring with supposedly nononcogenic types. Basically, all patients with dysplasia in HPV-induced anogenital lesions need to be followed carefully regardless of which HPV type is responsible for the lesion.

Histology

Clinically evident warts due to HPV infection have equally apparent and characteristic microscopic changes. Epithelial thickening (acanthosis) with an overlying widened stratum corneum is present. In skin lesions, but not in mucous membrane lesions, there is papillomatosis, hypergranulosis, and focal, stacked parakeratosis. In all warts, koilocytosis is the single most important histologic feature. Koilocytosis is defined by the presence of numerous, usually clustered, vacuolar cells with darkly staining, round, or pyknotic nuclei surrounded by a clear halo. These cells are located in the upper portion of the epidermis and are never found below the midpoint of the epidermis. Koilocytosis is prominent in rapidly growing warts and is less apparent in older inactive lesions.

Unfortunately, many pathologists fail to recognize the phenomenon of "pseudokoilocytosis" and identify lesions as being of HPV origin on the presence of this feature alone. Pseudokoilocytosis is defined as the presence of infrequent, randomly scattered clear cells, located both above and below the epidermal midpoint. The nuclei are normal in appearance and stain at about the same density as those nuclei found in surrounding cells. Hybridization probes reveal HPV DNA no more often in these lesions than in anogenital control tissue.

Course and Prognosis

Proliferation of Warts

Clinical observation suggests that most HPV infections begin with inoculation of virus into a single site. A wart then develops at that site and in turn releases viral particles from the surface of the wart. These viral particles (from the "mother" wart) can then infect surrounding skin and mucous membranes, causing the development of many new, nearby "daughter" warts. The likelihood of spread to nearby areas of one's own skin and mucous membranes through this "seeding" effect depends in part on the health of surrounding tissue. Damage to the epithelium (from trauma, maceration, and so forth) appears to increase markedly the rate of spread.

It is also possible, but much less likely, to transfer the virus via the fingertip to some distant site on one's own body. Children with finger warts, for instance, sometimes develop genital warts as a result of this mechanism. The infrequency with which this occurs probably relates to the existence of a preferential body site for each of the numerous HPV types[18]; a given type will not grow well if it is transplanted to a nonpreferential location.

Spontaneous Resolution

Warts, like other viral lesions, activate an immunologic response on the part of the host.[18] Humoral immune response develops rapidly, but antibodies do not cause resolution; involution of warts depends on activation of cell-mediated immune (CMI) responsiveness. Humans reach an apogee of CMI responsiveness in late childhood. This is followed by a gradual dimunition with aging. Not surprisingly, then, warts of all types almost always spontaneously resolve in children and young adults but may persist indefinitely in older individuals.

Spontaneous resolution, when it does take place, requires months to years of infection. The reason for such slowness is not known, but it may relate to the intercellular (immunologically protected) location of HPV proteins in a cell type (keratinocyte) that has limited ability to process and present antigen to lymphocytes.

When warts resolve spontaneously, no trace of infection remains clinically visible. Nevertheless, in most cases, traces of HPV DNA probably remain at the lesional site in a latent phase. Reactivation of the latent DNA is apparently possible, and thus warts can recur. Put in another way, when viral particles are fully replicating (so-called productive infection) and virion assembly occurs, a visible wart is produced; resolution is accompanied by conversion to a nonproductive infection in which no virion assembly occurs and in which the HPV DNA remains in a latent state.

Contagion

Less is known about the spread of HPV than for most other viral diseases. This lack of knowledge stems from the fact that the virus cannot be cultured. Without evidence from cultures, there is no way to determine if warts are spread from person to person or if infection can be acquired from inanimate objects (fomites). Hybridization studies have demonstrated the presence of HPV DNA on underwear, on used vaginal specula, in the laser plume, and so forth,[19–21] but this does not really answer the question of acquisition from these sources. Epidemiologic studies of anogenital warts, however, suggest that person-to-person contact probably accounts for most transmission. Specifically, about 50 to 70 percent of the sexual contacts of individuals with anogenital warts are also infected.[14,15,22]

Nonsexual, person-to-person acquisition is, however, possible. A few infants, at the moment of birth, have been noted to have perianal warts; other infants have developed anogenital warts within weeks of birth (Fig. 9-7). These infants are presumed to have become infected on the basis of maternal birth canal infection.[23,24] This can be extended further. Laryngeal papillomatosis occurring secondary to HPV infection may not develop until midchildhood. Here, too, the infection seems to have remained latent (see below) for years before clinical expression develops. Based on these observations, it certainly seems possible that some anogenital warts in adults are also due to maternal infection (expression occurring after years of latency) rather than to recent sexual contact.[25]

Less often, anogenital warts in children develop as the result of autoinoculation from their own warts occurring elsewhere or from innocent exposure to care givers with hand warts.[23] The problem of sexual abuse as a cause of anogenital warts in children is discussed in the treatment section (see also Ch. 22).

Development of Anogenital Malignancy

Evidence strongly indicates that individuals with HPV infection are more likely than noninfected persons to develop squamous cell carcinoma.[26,27] This evidence is best developed for cervical infection, but vulvar, penile, and anal infections have the potential to induce malignant change as well. Clinically, this evolution occurs fairly rapidly for the cervix. Approximately 25 percent of patients with CIN I advance to CIN III in about 3 years of prospective follow-up.[28,29] On the other hand, progression appears to occur more slowly in the case of infection at other sites. For obvious ethical reasons one cannot follow patients beyond the point of in situ neoplasia, but plentiful evidence indicates that HPV infection is related to invasive and metastatic disease as well.

Clearly, infection with HPV alone does not explain this relationship: approximately 40 percent of adults are infected and yet appreciably fewer than 1 percent of adults develop the corresponding anogenital malignancy. The other factors important in HPV-related oncogenesis are discussed in the next section on pathogenesis.

Pathogenesis

Wart Biology

HPV is a double-stranded DNA virus that in humans has the capacity to infect only epithelial cells. As noted above, it cannot be routinely cultured, but molecular techniques allow for cloning of the virus and consequently for a reasonably good understanding of its pathophysiology. Approximately 70 HPV types are recognized; this is in dramatic contrast to herpes simplex virus, for which only two types have been described. For the purposes of this chapter, the 70 HPV types can be divided into those preferentially associated with anogenital infection and those that cause infection in other sites.

The anogenital types in turn can be divided into those with little or no oncogenic potential (HPV 6 and 11) and those with significant oncogenic potential (HPV 16, 18, 31, 33, 35, 51, and 52).[30] Fortunately, HPV 6 and 11 account for about 90 percent of all anogenital infections.

HPV resides within the nucleus of epithelial cells. The viral DNA of nononcogenic HPV types remains in an episomal location, whereas the viral DNA of oncogenic HPV types begins in an episomal location but subsequently becomes integrated into the host cell's chromosomal DNA as oncogenesis is initiated.

Incubation and Latency

Studies done on human volunteers many years ago revealed that warts developed, on average, 3 to 10 weeks after wart tissue was inoculated into the skin. These studies were not done with tissue from anogenital warts, but epidemiologic studies involving careful contact tracing indicate that a similar incubation period exists for anogenital infections as well.

The problem of determining incubation times is complicated by the existence of latency. HPV infection can be productive or nonproductive. Productive infection occurs when viral DNA is replicated, coating proteins are made, and the two are combined to form complete viral particles (virions). Nonproductive infection occurs when only viral DNA is present and no virions are assembled. Latency is characterized by nonproductive infection in which only HPV DNA is present. Cells can maintain the presence of HPV DNA for months and presumably even for years in this quiescent state. Then abruptly, and for reasons not understood, latency ends and productive infection begins, leading to the clinical development of warts.

Latency presumably explains the development of laryngeal papillomatosis in childhood and also probably explains the development of anogenital warts in the 50 to 75 percent of children in whom no evidence of sexual abuse can be identified. It may also explain the sudden appearance of anogenital warts in one member of a monogamous couple; the affected individual may have carried the virus in a latent state for years after either sexual or maternal acquisition.

Development of Visible Warts

HPV infection probably begins in those epithelial cells that lie at or just above the basal layer. Virion assembly, however, only occurs in the partially differentiated cells of the midlayers of the epithelium. Presumably one of the reasons the virus is so difficult to culture is because HPV replication cannot occur in the fully differentiated cells used in standard cell cultures. Once virions are assembled in the midepidermis, they are carried to the surface of the epithelium, where they are presumably shed along with the desquamating stratum corneum cells.

HPV virus needs a constant source of replicating cells to maintain a resident position within the midepidermis. Without a constant renewal of cells, all of the viruses would be carried to the surface and would be lost to the environment. To maintain a source of cell renewal, HPV DNA takes over a portion of the host cells' process which determines the rate of mitotic activity. In doing so it increases epithelial cell proliferation and creates the visible lesion clinically recognized as a wart. If the cell's proliferative process is appropriately controlled, the wart remains as a benign lesion. If regulation of mitotic control becomes seriously disturbed, a malignant process can be initiated (see below).

HPV-Induced Oncogenesis

Infection with HPV 16 and 18 (and less often HPV 31, 33, 35, 51, and 52) are associated with the potential development of malignancy.[30] This association has been most thoroughly studied with cervical infection, but all available knowledge indicates that the process is essentially identical for penile, vulvar, and anal disease.[27]

Current understanding suggests that the oncogenic property of HPV 16 and 18 occurs because their viral DNA becomes integrated into host cell chromosomal DNA, whereas the viral DNA of the nononcogenic types always remains in an episomal location. The first step in oncogenesis due to HPV 16 and 18 infection occurs when the circular viral DNA is nicked such that a strand of linear HPV DNA is formed; once the HPV DNA is in this linear form, integration into chromosomal DNA becomes mechanically possible. The nick in the viral DNA regularly occurs at a site (the E1 and E2 gene) that is responsible for regulatory control of the E6 and E7 viral genes. This integration of HPV DNA into chromosomal DNA represents the "initiation" step in an ongoing, multistep oncogenic process. The initation process is a permanent, mutational event producing abnormal host cell DNA that is then passed on to all future generations of the host cell.

Loss of regulatory control, related in part to disturbed function of the viral E1 and E2 genes, allows for excess production of the HPV E6 and E7 proteins; these proteins then bind to and inactivate the proteins p53 and p107, produced by the host cell tumor-suppressing genes. These tumor-suppressing genes represent the host cell's major mechanism for maintaining control of epithelial cell proliferation. Blocking their action appears to shut down programmed cell death (apoptosis) and allows for unchecked (i.e., cancerous) proliferation of these cells.

Of course, the process is not as simple as indicated here. The development of cancer is a multistep process and therefore many other factors in addition to HPV infection are required, including (1) impaired immune response; anogenital cancers occur at a very high rate in patients with the acquired immunodeficiency syndrome (AIDS)[31]; (2) the type of epithelial cell infected; cells at the cervical and anal transformation zones are more susceptible to malignant change than are keratinizing epithelial cells; (3) age at time of infection as measured by age at first intercourse[32]; cells infected at an early age seem more vulnerable than those infected later; and (4) the presence of tumor promotors or cocarcinogens; smokers are at appreciably higher risk than are nonsmokers.[33] A few other factors such as hormone use[34] and low erythrocyte folate levels[35] may also play a role in HPV-induced oncogenesis, but at this point the data are preliminary. In any event, the presence or absence of these additional factors (which determine whether or not HPV-initiated cells will eventually pursue a malignant course) may explain why only about 0.1 percent of the population develop anogenital malignancy even though 3 to 5 percent may be infected with HPV 16 and 18.

Treatment

Much controversy exists regarding the treatment for anogenital warts. In fact, some would argue that most warts could be left untreated. This position is based on the following data: (1) 40 percent of the sexually active population already has latent HPV infection, and no amount of treatment is going to reduce this prevalence; (2) HPV infection occurs in morphologic forms (latent infection) and in sites (urethra, bladder) that are not accessible for diagnosis and treatment—treatment of visible disease affects only the tip of the iceberg; (3) current methods of treatment are costly, uncomfortable, and do not even eradicate HPV DNA from treated sites; and (4) the course of anogenital warts is unpredictable—some, and maybe even most, will resolve spontaneously with sufficient passage of time.

In spite of these observations, treatment is probably warranted for equally good reasons: (1) visible warts represent the type of HPV infection with the greatest risk of contagion; treatment of these reduces most of the risk for sexual transmission; (2) HPV infection can be associated with the development of anogenital malignancy; anything done to reduce the risk of cancer will be worthwhile; and (3) patients are quite troubled by the presence of lesions that they recognize as abnormal[36,37]—they will insist on treatment.

Identification of Warts Requiring Treatment

Use of acetic acid soaks to identify lesions not otherwise visible originally seemed like a good idea[1] (see above). Now, some of the enthusiasm has waned. The high cost of testing (in terms of time spent), together with the troubling rate of false-positive and false-negative results, has increasingly limited our use of the test.

HPV infection is often not limited to a single site. For example, about 50 percent of the women with vulvar involvement have concomitant cervical infection.[10] Presumably, similar figures are true for other sites as well. Theoretically, then, when visible mucocutaneous lesions are encountered, all nearby mucosal sites (urethra, vagina, cervix, anal canal, and rectum) should be inspected. Clearly this is not possible as a public health policy. At the practical level the following approach might be considered. When perianal warts do not encroach on the anal verge, the likelihood of visible warts in the anal canal and rectum is low enough to warrant defering anoscopy. In both men and women, inspection of the urethra can be limited to the meatus. On the other hand, women with vulvar warts probably should have a cytologic smear taken from the cervix; colposcopy is indicated if either visible or cytologic abnormalities are found.

Treatment of Visible Warts

Additional material regarding the use of most of the treatment modalities discussed here can be found in Chapter 3 and in the review articles listed in the bibliography. Note that the term *clearance rate* is used rather than *cure rate;* HPV DNA is left at the site of some, maybe most, treated warts, resulting in ongoing latent infection.[38] The presence of HPV DNA at the treated sites probably accounts for the repeated observation that recurrence rates for warts treated with any modality average about 30 percent.

Podophyllin Resin

Historically podophyllin resin has been the most widely used treatment for anogenital warts. A 25 percent preparation in tincture of benzoin can be applied weekly or biweekly in the office. It is applied carefully with a small cotton swab to avoid getting other than minimal amounts on surrounding, normal skin. After drying for a few minutes the patient may dress and resume normal activities. Most authorities indicate that the podophyllin should be washed off 4 to 8 hours later, but we have found that there is little or no additional discomfort if it is simply left in place. This approach is inexpensive and efficient for the clinician. Unfortunately, patient acceptance is not terribly good partly because of the discomfort but mostly because the clearance rates are low enough to result in many return visits. Review of the literature suggests that a maximum cure rate of about 60 to 75 percent is possible with about six applications.

A new product, podofilox (Condylox), has recently been produced. It is much better standardized in terms of potency, and its use results in appreciably less discomfort. The product can be applied by the patient at home (see Ch. 3), which also enhances patient acceptability. In spite of these advantages, clearance rates are not appreciably better than those with the older preparation.[39]

Cryotherapy

Cryotherapy is replacing podophyllin as the most widely used therapeutic approach. Liquid nitrogen is preferred to carbon dioxide (dry ice) because of its colder temperature and greater efficacy. Liquid nitrogen can be used with a metal cryoprobe (particularly useful in treating the vagina and cervix) or can be applied directly to the lesion with a cotton-tipped applicator or in the form of a spray. A 15- to 30-second freeze is desirable with all techniques. Discomfort is moderately severe, but local anesthesia is not required. No special care is necessary following treatment. In 12 to 24 hours a blister forms under the wart, and 7 to 14 days later the wart (or at least most of it) sloughs off with the dead blister roof. Treatment efficacy is somewhat better than with podophyllin but this method still requires three to six treatments, 2 or 3 weeks apart, to obtain a 70 to 80 percent clearance rate.[40,41]

Trichloroacetic Acid

Trichloroacetic or dichloroacetic acid in a 50 to 85 percent solution is particularly effective for the treatment of the nonkeratotic, small, flat warts. It is applied in the office with a small cotton swab; care should be taken to avoid any application to perilesional normal skin. A significant burning sensation is felt within minutes, but thereafter little discomfort is noted. Here too, multiple applications at weekly or biweekly intervals are required to reach clearance rates of 70 to 80 percent.[40,41]

Fluorouracil

Topically applied 5 percent fluorouracil is used as both primary and adjuvant treatment after laser ablation. It is applied by the patient once or twice daily for 3 to 6 weeks. The resulting painful, inflammatory reaction is very troublesome to the patient, especially as it is so prolonged. Blinded studies are not possible because of the reaction it causes, and possibly for this reason there is a paucity of good studies objectively demonstrating its efficacy. Fluorouracil is considered by some as the treatment of choice for vaginal warts.[42] It is also thought to be useful in decreasing the recurrence rate in patients who have had primary treatment with destructive modalities.[42] Instructions regarding the use of fluorouracil are given in Chapter 3.

α-Interferon

Intralesionally injected α interferon was introduced with appreciable fanfare a few years ago, but enthusiasm for its use is not great today. The treatment is cumbersome, as only a very small area—in some cases each wart—must be separately injected multiple times. Moreover, the multiple needle sticks are painful, and a generalized toxic reaction is likely to occur at the initiation of therapy. Cure rates for individually treated warts are acceptably high, but complete clearance of multiple lesions is not often possible.[43] Systemic therapy in the form of subcutaneous or intramuscular injection seems to be ineffective in the primary treatment of anogenital warts; the effectiveness of α-interferon used as adjuvant therapy is controversial.[44,45]

Surgery

Surgical and destructive therapy of anogenital warts have increased in popularity primarily because the entire treatment can be carried out in one or two treatment sessions. Laser ablation, electrosurgical destruction, and surgical excision each have their proponents.[41,46,47] Choice among these modalities depends on one's particular skills and experience. Clearance rates are equally good with each and approach 90 to 95 percent in the short term; unfortunately, recurrences are such that the eventual clearance rates at the end of 6 months are only slightly higher than those listed above for cytotoxic therapy. Caution should be used when contemplating extended field treatment; long-term clearance rates are not better, and time to healing is prolonged and uncomfortable.[48] Additional material regarding the principles and practice of laser therapy for anogenital warts can be found in the review article by Reid.[47]

Treatment of Subclinical Disease

The term *subclinical* is used for lesions that are not visible until acetic acid soaks have been applied; magnification may be required to see the smallest lesions. As indicated above, only about one half of the lesions identified in this way prove to be caused by HPV infection. In spite of this high false-positive rate, some clinicians treat everything that is aceto-white as if it were HPV infection. This may be acceptable for small lesions, but is better avoided for larger lesions. Alternatively, one or more biopsies can be carried out to identify those aceto-white lesions that are warts, but care must be taken so that the histology is not overinterpreted. Specifically, true koilocytes must be differentiated from pseudokoilocytes (see above), which are regularly present in biopsies taken from genital mucocutaneous tissues.

Subclinical lesions are usually treated once they are identified. It could, however, be argued that these lesions do not require treatment since they presumably contain few, if any, fully formed viral particles and thus may be relatively noncontagious. If a decision to treat has been made, any of the treatments discussed above can be used; trichloracetic acid is particularly appropriate for the smaller lesions.

Treatment of Latent Disease

The term *latent* is used to indicate that no clinical lesions are present; by definition this type of HPV infection can only be identified with tests such as DNA hybridization.[1] HPV DNA can be present in a latent state for several centimeters around visible warts; thus large areas of genital tissue may be involved.[49] Moreover, latent lesions contain only fragments of HPV DNA without replicating virions and thus are presumably associated with little or no risk of contagion.

Latent infection presumably can convert to productive infection with consequent development of visible warts. For example, recurrence rates are higher when latency can be demonstrated in the normal tissue surrounding treated warts than when it is not present.[49] Nevertheless, the difficulty in identification, the low risk of contagion, and the large areas involved argue strongly against attempts to treat latent disease. In any event, it seems likely that no current form of treatment ever completely eradicates all traces of HPV DNA, anyway.[38]

Recurrences

Warts very frequently appear at the site of previously treated lesions. These are considered "recurrences" by both patient and clinician and their appearance carries the connotation that the treatment failed. This is not really true. As noted above, viral shedding from the original wart causes implantation into the surrounding tissue. This incubating or "latent" infection may then express itself as new wart formation weeks or months later. Thus the original wart may well have been successfully treated and the "recurrence" really represents the development of new lesions. For this reason, patients need to be aware that any treatment, no matter how complete and aggressive, is very likely to be followed by the appearance of additional warts. An understanding of this principle makes the patient less likely to be dissatisfied with treatment and more tolerant of the frequently necessary return visits and retreatment.

Warts appearing at a treated site, whether recurrent or new, can be treated with any of the modalities discussed above. Specifically, the appearance of these lesions does not imply that the original treatment was inadequate or represented a bad choice; in most instances it is quite appropriate to continue on with the original approach.

Warts in Pregnancy

Anogenital warts often increase in size and number during pregnancy. Infants born through an HPV-infected birth canal, whether warts are visible or not, are at appreciable risk of acquiring HPV infection.[24] Most often this exposure results in latent infection, but rarely anogenital warts or laryngeal papillomatosis will develop at a later date. For this reason, visible genital warts (presumably the type of HPV infection with greatest risk for transmission) in pregnant women should be treated. Large bulky warts should be treated for another reason as well; they increase the risk of tearing and bleeding at the time of parturition. Any of the conventional treatments except podophyllin, α-interferon, or flurouracil can be used. Podophyllin is easily absorbed through mucous membranes, and if large amounts are used there is significant risk of fetal neurotoxicity.

Anogenital Warts in Children

The presence of anogenital warts in infants and children requires, by statute, consideration of possible sexual abuse. If the clinicians involved are not skilled in carrying out this evaluation, they must find someone who is.

In acknowledging this responsibility, one should understand that only in a minority (probably less than 25 percent) of cases is evidence of sexual abuse found.[23] Also, typing of anogenital warts in children will not help to determine whether or not sexual abuse has occurred; most of the warts will be of the anogenital HPV type, but reasons other than sexual abuse can explain their presence (Fig. 9-7). These include acquisition from the mother at the time of birth, autoinoculation from warts elsewhere on the body, and nonsexual spread from family members who have warts.

As noted earlier, warts in children are almost certain to resolve spontaneously. This fact, coupled with the physical and possible pyschosexual trauma occasioned by repeated treatment, argues persuasively against treatment. If treatment is undertaken, use of podofilox (Condylox) at home by the parents offers a good, relatively nontraumatic option.

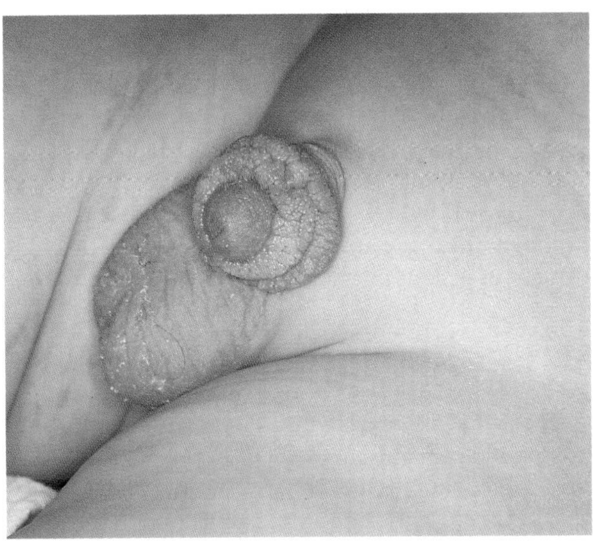

Fig. 9-7. Remarkable vegetative genital warts at the site of circumcision in an infant.

Analogies with Herpes Genitalis

Twenty years ago there was widespread publicity and outspoken concern about genital infection with herpes simplex virus (HSV). It was described as an extraordinarily contagious, dangerous, and incurable disease. Some of the same concerns are being voiced about HPV infection today. Physicians and patients have learned to cope with HSV infection and, because there are so many similarities between the two infections, we should learn to accept and cope with HPV infection as well.

A look at some of those similarities is instructive. First, they are about equally widespread, with 15 to 40 percent of the sexually active population being infected. Second, both are acquired mostly through sexual transmission, but both can also be acquired nonsexually as well. Third, they both have a latent phase: it occurs in the spinal ganglia for HSV and in the skin for HPV. Fourth, the active phase for both is treatable: acyclovir is administered for HSV and the various modalities discussed above can be used to clear visible warts. Fifth, the latent phase for both is incurable; latent infection lasts a lifetime for both diseases. Sixth, the latent phase for both may, from time to time, convert to the active phase, at which point visible lesions develop. Seventh, for both, contagion is high during the active phase and low, or absent, during the latent phase. Eighth, there are potential risks in pregnancy with both—more serious with HSV, less serious with HPV. Ninth, both have been linked with the development of malignancy—cervical only with HSV, more generalized with HPV.

Understanding these similarities should help us learn to deal with what is certainly a most difficult problem until we can prevent the infection through the use of a suitable vaccine.

MOLLUSCUM CONTAGIOSUM

This viral disease, as the name suggests, is quite contagious. As was once true for infection with HSV and HPV, molluscum contagiosum virus was primarily acquired through innocuous childhood transfer. Now all three infections occur most often in young adult life as a result of sexual transmission. The reason for this change is unknown but likely relates to smaller family size and less crowded sleeping conditions for children. Thus diseases previously transmitted through close personal contact in childhood (with consequent development of partial immunity) are now being passed at a later time in life when close personal contact, through sexual activity, once again occurs.

The prevalence of molluscum contagiosum in adults is low but rising[50]; a tenfold increase in genital infection was noted between 1966 and 1983. In spite of this rise, the prevalence in adults is lower than for HSV and HPV infection; it is probably less than 0.1 percent. Men and women are equally affected.

Clinical Presentation

The lesions of molluscum contagiosum occur as firm, smooth-surfaced, hemispherical papules 2 to 6 mm in diameter. These small papules are usually white or skin-colored but sometimes are so translucent as to simulate the presence of vesiculation (Fig. 9-8). The skin surrounding the lesions is usually normal in color, but sometimes a pink or red inflammatory halo is present. Less often the entire papule is inflamed and red; such lesions mimic folliculitis or furunculosis (Fig. 9-9). The inflammation develops when lesions are traumatized and virus proteins are consequently extruded into the dermis; the presence of these proteins incites a foreign body reaction.[51] A characteristic central umbilication is present at the summit of molluscum contagiosum papules about 25 percent of the time (Fig. 9-10). This umbilication, if present, is pathognomonic for the disease.

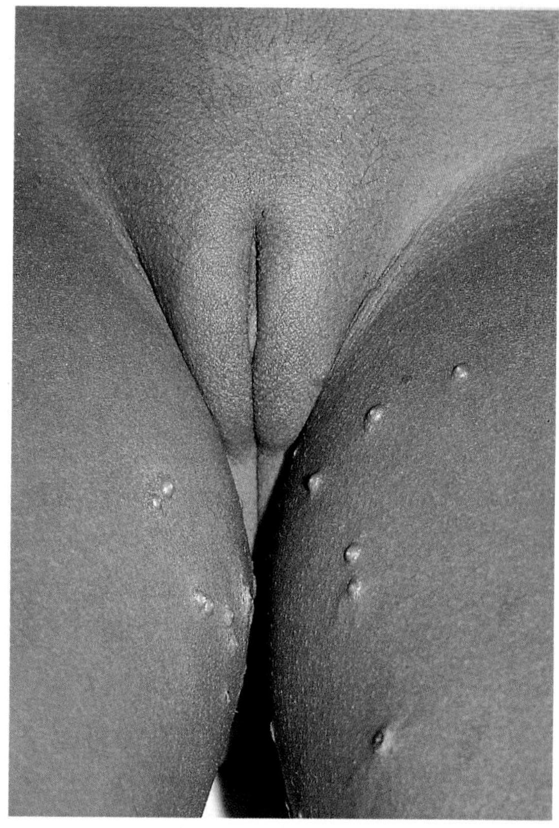

Fig. 9-8. Multiple white, shiny, dome-shaped papules of molluscum contagiosum.

Molluscum contagiosum can occur as a solitary lesion, but usually 5 to 30 lesions are present. Clustering of lesions can certainly occur but is less prominent than that seen with HPV-induced genital warts.

In men the lesions are found most often on the penile shaft, whereas in women the most common locations are the pubis, upper, inner thighs, and hair-bearing areas of the labia majora. Involvement of the mucous membranes of the genitalia can occur, but lesions in these sites are rarely encountered.

The lesions are asymptomatic and, for this reason, they are sometimes discovered incidentally in the course of genital examination for some other purpose.

A clinical diagnosis is usually possible especially if umbilicated lesions are present. However, sometimes

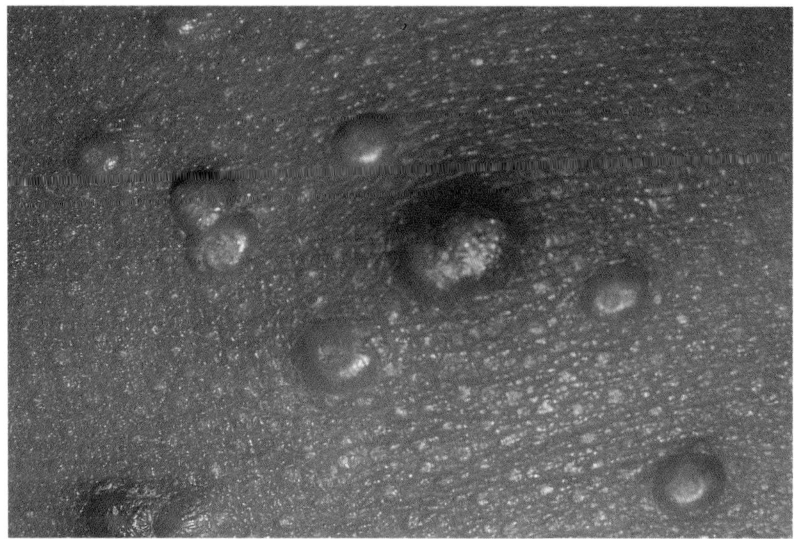

Fig. 9-9. An inflamed lesion of molluscum contagiosum surrounded by typical white and skin-colored shiny papules, some with a central dell.

in patients with AIDS, other infections (especially cryptococcosis) will mimic the lesions of molluscum contagiosum. Confirmation of a clinical diagnosis is easily obtained by way of biopsy or by extrusion of the molluscum bodies for cytologic (Tzanck) smears (see Ch. 2).

Course and Prognosis

In childhood, individual lesions of molluscum contagiosum resolve over 2 or 3 months, and the whole course of the disease is completed in a year or two. Data are not available regarding the course in adults, but probably all immunocompetent patients experience eventual spontaneous remission. On the other hand, those with depressed immune response, especially patients with AIDS, develop very large numbers of lesions and rarely experience spontaneous involution[52] (see also Molluscum Contagiosum in Ch. 24.) Resolution of an infection with molluscum contagiosum virus, as is true for other viral disease, seems to occur as a result of cell-mediated, rather than humoral, immune response.

Molluscum contagiosum is, with the exception of its contagiousness, a benign disease. Occasionally inflammation in one or more lesions occurs; these otherwise harmless lesions are quite tender and can heal with scarring. The molluscum contagiosum virus does not exist in a latent phase in ganglia or skin as do the herpes and wart viruses. For this reason, once an episode of molluscum contagiosum virus has ended, late recurrences are not encountered. However, the relatively long incubation period does result in the appearance of new lesions within weeks of what seemed to be complete eradication of the lesions. Reinfection is possible but does not seem to occur frequently.

Pathophysiology

Molluscum contagiosum is caused by a DNA virus of the poxvirus group. The virus is restricted to infection of mucocutaneous epithelial cells. The viral particles multiply in the cytoplasm of these cells, where they form inclusion granules (molluscum bodies, Henderson-Patterson bodies). These inclusion bodies are large enough to be easily visible with conventional light microscopy.

The virus has not been successfully cultured, but restriction endonuclease analysis demonstrates that two types of molluscum contagiosum virus (MCV I and II) exist. Most infections are with MCV I. These two types of virus do not appear to have the site specificity that occurs for HSV 1 and 2 infections.[53]

Viral particles are presumably shed from the surface of the lesions, where they are then spread to other areas or to other persons. Passage to other individuals seems to require fairly vigorous skin-to-skin contact. Development of genital lesions in adults occurs entirely by way of sexual activity. The virus is fairly easily transferred, but acquisition is enhanced by the presence of trauma to the skin. Most infections do not occur at the site of adnexal structures, but inoculation directly into the ostia of hair follicles occurs from time to time. The incubation period averages 1 to 2 months but is quite variable. This long incubation period makes contact tracing difficult.

Treatment

Although spontaneous resolution usually occurs, the lesions usually should be treated in order to reduce contagion, both to the host through autoinoculation, and to others through sexual contact. Treatment requires the removal of the centrally located molluscum body or destruction of the entire lesion. A skin curette can be used to "peel" the lesion away; this is most easily accomplished if the edge of the papule is first nicked with a blade. Alternatively, individual lesions can be treated with cryotherapy, cantharidin (Cantherone),[54] or trichloracetic acid.[55] Podophyllin resin or podofilox (Condylox)[56] and salicyclic acid preparations, as used for HPV-induced warts, are inconsistently effective. Electrosurgical destruction, laser ablation, and excision are not warranted because of potential scarring.[57]

Development of new lesions in and around the treated sites is quite common. This presumably occurs because of previously shed, incubating virus in nearby epithelial cells.[58] These new lesions are treated in the same manner as were the original lesions.

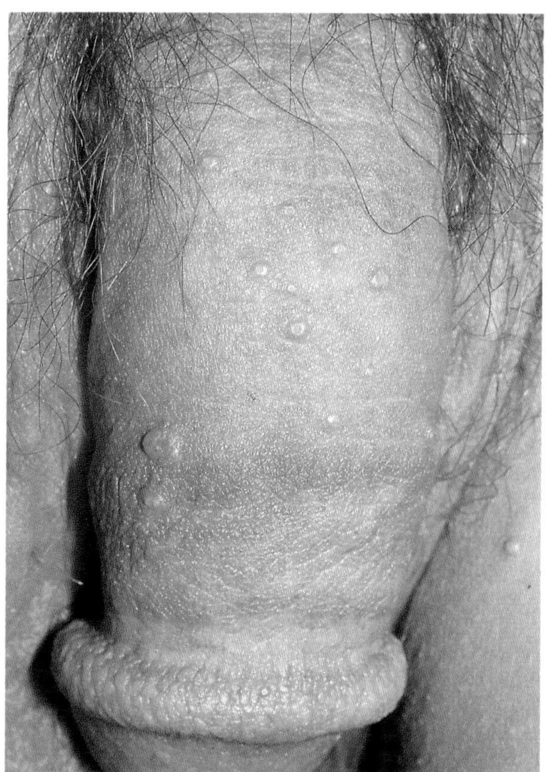

Fig. 9-10. Multiple lesions of molluscum contagiosum. Central umbilication is visible at the summit at this site of several lesions.

PEARLY PENILE PAPULES

Pearly penile papules are relatively common, distinctive tumors of the coronal sulcus that occur without racial predilection.

These asymptomatic, small papules usually develop during puberty and occur in up to 20 percent of young adult males.[59] More common in uncircumcised males, these are skin-colored or pink, monotonously regular, filiform, or digitate papules arranged in one or more rows around the coronal margin of the glans (Fig. 9-11). Their importance derives from frequent confusion clinically with condylomata acuminata, but there is no evidence that they are virally induced.[60]

Histologically, pearly penile papules are angiofibromas. They have no other associations or importance. Patients require no treatment other than reassurance.

VESTIBULAR PAPILLAE

Vestibular papillae are small papillomatous projections located in the vulvar vestibule. These are normal variants that are often mistaken for filiform genital warts (see also Vestibular Papillomatosis and Ch. 1).

Clinical Presentation

Although some physicians believe that vestibular papillae produce symptoms of burning, most feel that they are completely asymptomatic. Vestibular papillae are very monomorphous, smooth, and have a tubular appearance with a rounded tip (Fig. 9-12). The individual papillae are discrete, although closely set (Fig. 9-13). They may occur grouped in small patches, or may form symmetrical rows along skin lines through and around the edge of the vestibule.

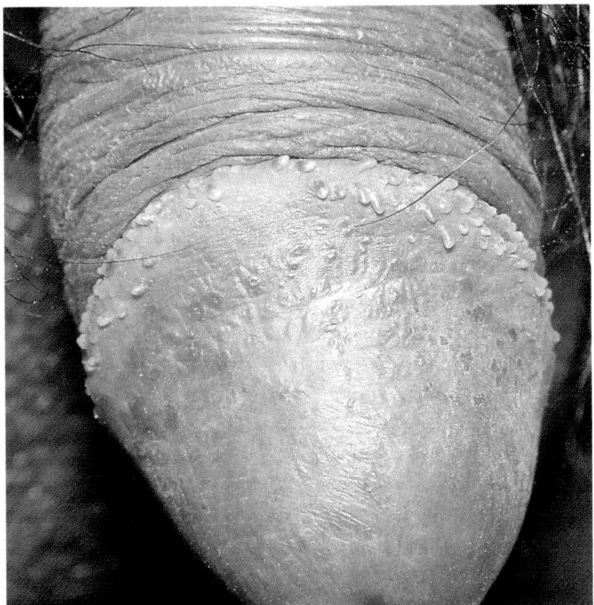

Fig. 9-11. Rows of uniform, digitate, skin-colored pearly penile papules around the corona.

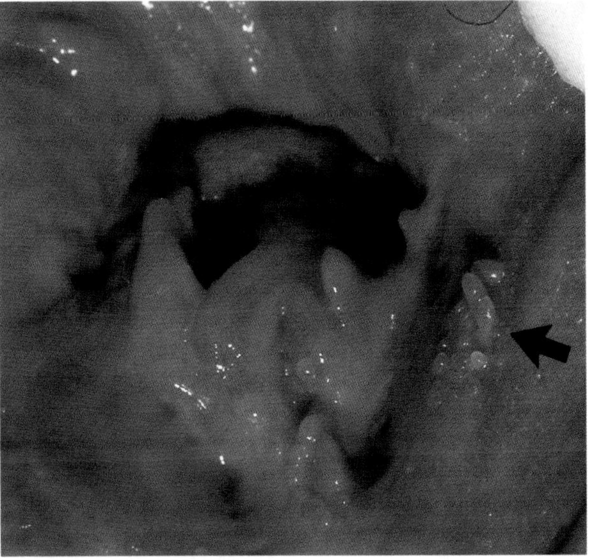

Fig. 9-12. Discrete, tubular, grouped vestibular papillae *(arrow)* with round tips.

Diagnosis

The differentiation of vestibular papillae from HPV infection can be made by differences in morphology and pattern. Those papillae that are HPV related tend to be irregular in height and shape with tapered tips, and individual papillae are often fused at the base. Often, there is a coarse, lobular texture to the papillae and surrounding skin, and nearby obvious genital warts heighten the clinician's suspicion of viral infection. Occasionally, nonspecific inflammation unassociated with HPV infection in the vestibule produces a reversible cobblestoned epithelial texture that can become accentuated into short papillae.

The diagnosis of vestibular papillae is made by the clinical appearance and, when necessary, by biopsy to rule out HPV infection. Histologically, HPV-related vestibular papillae show epithelial signs of wart infection, while physiologic papillae lack the vacuolated upper epidermal cells with hyperchromatic nuclei that are considered pathognomonic of HPV infection. Occasionally, glycogen-containing cells (pseudokollocytes) of the normal genital epithelium, which may appear vacuolated, is mistaken for these virus-containing cells, and an erroneous histologic diagnosis is made.

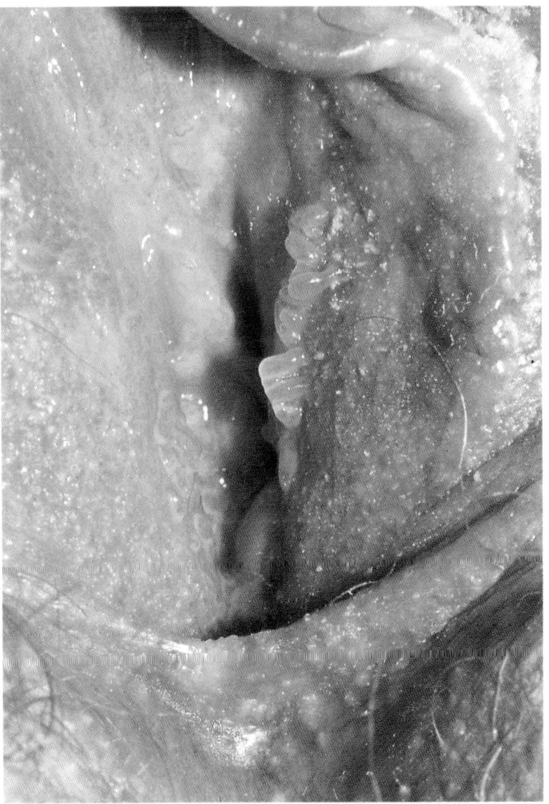

Fig. 9-13. Tubular, smooth, monomorphous, discrete vestibular papillae in a linear pattern.

Treatment

Vestibular papillae are asymptomatic and require no treatment other than reassurance.

HIDRADENOMA PAPILLIFERUM

Hidradenoma papilliferum is an uncommon benign tumor of apocrine sweat gland differentiation that occurs almost exclusively on the inner aspect of the labia majora or the interlabial fold of Caucasian women. This tumor appears as a skin-colored single nodule, although sometimes the color may be red or even bluish, and the surface may erode and exude papillomatous tissue or drain a serous fluid. The size is usually 1 cm or smaller. The diagnosis is often made on a biopsy performed to rule out a more significant tumor. Histologically, the tumor is filled with papillary projections covered by a single layer of cuboidal or columnar cells and a deeper layer of myoepithelial cells. Occasionally, these tumors may be mistaken histologically for an adenocarcinoma.

SYRINGOMAS

Syringomas are benign tumors derived from sweat glands. Isolated lesions can occur, but in the majority of patients they are numerous and found in clusters. Syringomas are most often encountered on the face, especially on the lower eyelids. Genital involvement, on the other hand, is thought to be rare; fewer than 20 cases have been reported. Personal experience, however, suggests that they occur much more frequently than this small number of reports suggest.

Genital lesions may represent the only site of involvement, or lesions in this location may occur as part of the condition termed diffuse eruptive syringomas. Women are affected appreciably more often than men; fewer than five cases of penile syringoma seem to have been reported in the English literature.[61,62] The onset of genital lesions is usually around puberty, but late-onset and childhood cases have been reported.[63]

Clinical Presentation

Individual lesions are smooth-surfaced, skin-colored, dome-shaped papules 2 to 5 mm in diameter. Twenty to 100 or more papules may be present. These multiple lesions are usually found in clusters that are located bilaterally. Within the clusters, the lesions are very closely set, but total confluence does not occur. The distribution of syringomas is restricted to the nonmucosal aspects of the genitalia. Most lesions are asymptomatic, although pruritus can occur and may lead to the diagnosis of the previously unrecognized syringomas.[64]

Syringomas clinically resemble the papules of Fox-Fordyce disease, but the latter are darker and much more pruritic. Syringomas, especially those occurring on the penis, may be mistaken for genital warts.[65]

Diagnosis, Pathogenesis, and Treatment

Histologically, clusters of malformed sweat glands are found in the connective tissue. Most authorities believe that the tumors arise from eccrine, rather than apocrine, sweat glands. Data currently available suggest that they derive from the ductal, rather than the secretory, portion of the eccrine structures.

Once present the lesions remain in place indefinitely. They have a benign course; malignant counterparts have not been described. Treatment is not necessary, although individual lesions can be eradicated with laser ablation[66] or light electrosurgery. Alternatively, clusters of lesions can be surgically excised.

SKIN TAGS AND FIBROEPITHELIAL POLYPS

Skin tags (acrochordons) and fibroepithelial polyps are extraordinarily common benign lesions and may be found in 5 percent or so of the population. They represent similar pathologic processes, but by convention the former term is used for small lesions (which are usually multiple) and the latter for solitary large lesions.

Clinical Presentation

Skin tags occurring in the axillae and around the neck (the most common sites) are small, soft, filiform papules 1 mm in diameter and 1 to 3 mm in length. Those occurring in the anogenital region are fewer in number and larger in size. Thus they are soft and filiform but are 1 to 2 mm in diameter and 3 to 5 mm in length.

Fibroepithelial polyps (soft fibromas), on the other

hand, occur more often in the anogenital region than in the axillae. These polyps are baglike outpouchings of normal-appearing skin. They are 5 to 15 mm at their widest diameter but are usually attached by a thin stalk, which may be only 1 to 2 mm in diameter (Fig. 9-14). These large lesions may have a wrinkled surface. Clinically, fibroepithelial polyps are almost indistinguishable from neurofibromas.

Skin tags and fibroepithelial polyps are usually skin-colored, but especially in dark-skinned individuals, they may be more darkly pigmented than the surrounding skin. These lesions are most often found on the upper inner thighs but are also seen in the crural folds and in the infragluteal creases.

Skin tags and polyps are asymptomatic unless they become inflamed secondary to trauma. Occasionally the larger, polypoid lesions suddenly enlarge and turn black; this spontaneous necrosis probably occurs as result of torsion of the stalk.

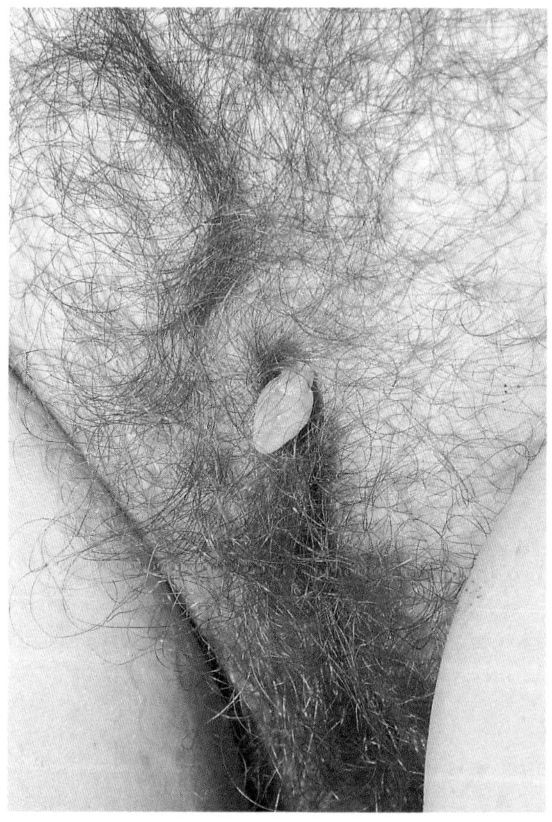

Fig. 9-14. A typical fleshy, skin-colored, pedunculated fibroepithelial polyp.

Histology and Diagnosis

Histologically the lesions appear as an outpouching of normal skin with some increase in the number of small capillaries and flattening of the epithelium. The smaller lesions sometimes show a few benign nevus cells or changes similar to those found in seborrheic keratoses. Lesions identical in clinical appearance to skin tags and fibroepithelial polyps are sometimes found to be intradermal nevi, neural nevi, seborrheic keratoses, and neurofibromas when microscopic examination is carried out.

Pathogenesis

The pathogenesis of these lesions is unknown. The tendency for skin tags located on the neck, chest, and axillae to occur more frequently in women suggests that a hormonal influence may be important. These same lesions occur in larger numbers in individuals who are obese. The meaning of this observation is unknown, but possibly it relates to estrogen metabolism in fat stores.

Treatment

Skin tags and fibroepithelial polyps follow a benign course. Treatment is not necessary unless they are in a location that might lead to irritation and inflammation. Larger lesions can be snipped at the base with or without local anesthesia. Smaller lesions can also be clipped or can be destroyed with cryotherapy or light electrosurgery.

LICHEN NITIDUS

Lichen nitidus is an uncommon inflammatory skin disorder found primarily over the penis, lower trunk, and arms.

Clinical Presentation

Occurring at any age and in any race, there is no gender predominance, although the penis is preferentially affected, whereas the vulva is not (Fig. 9-15). Lichen nitidus is generally asymptomatic, but mild pruritus may be present. Lesions consist of tiny, skin-colored to pink, shiny papules less than 1 mm in size. These monomorphous papules are dome-shaped to flat-topped and are distributed in a regular, follicular-appearing (although not truly follicular) pattern

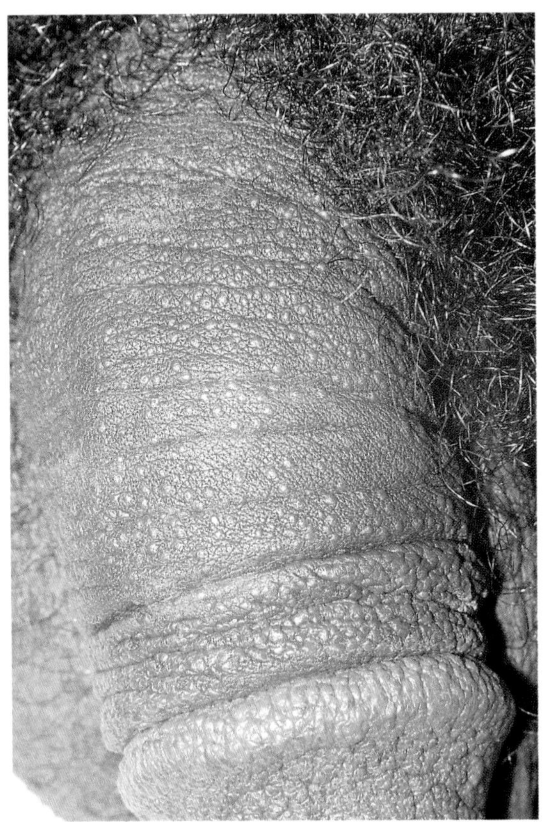

Fig. 9-15. Monotonous, shiny, pinpoint-sized papules of lichen nitidus.

over the shaft and glans of the penis as well as the lower abdomen, buttocks, and arms. Lichen nitidus exhibits the Köbner phenomenon, in which papules occur in areas of injury. Usually a careful examination reveals a line of tiny papules, somewhere, produced by a scratch. Generalized and confluent disease occurs occasionally, and fine scale is sometimes present in this variant.

Histology

Histologically, lichen nitidus consists of sharply circumscribed, small granulomatous nodules. These are located in the superficial dermis, partially encased by a rim of epidermis that has proliferated downward.

Pathogenesis

The etiology of lichen nitidus is unknown. It has been believed to be associated with tuberculosis or another unidentified organism, and some have felt that lichen nitidus represents a variant or close relative of lichen planus.

Treatment

Some patients experience a remission soon after onset, whereas others have resolution only after many years or never. A topical corticosteroid cream may improve pruritus in those who itch, especially if secondary eczema has developed, and a high-potency topical steroid or oral prednisone may improve lesions. Oral psoralens followed by exposure to ultraviolet A light (PUVA) have been reported to be useful,[67] as has oral etretinate.[68]

VERRUCIFORM XANTHOMA

Verruciform xanthoma was originally reported as a lesion arising only on the oral mucous membranes. Subsequently, a few lesions have been identified on the vulva, penis, and scrotum. Single lesions, in the form of a papule or plaque, can occur but clustered papules have also been reported. The surface of the lesion may be smooth but more often it is papillomatous or verrucous. Verruciform xanthomas occurring in the genital area are almost always clinically misidentified as warts. Histologically, foam cells filled with lipid are densely packed under an acanthotic epithelium that demonstrates hyperkeratosis and parakeratosis. The source of the lipid and the reason for its deposition are unknown. The lesions appear to be benign.

PSEUDOEPITHELIOMATOUS, MICACEOUS, AND KERATOTIC BALANITIS

Pseudoepitheliomatous, micaceous, and keratotic balanitis was first recognized and reported by Lortat-Jacob and Civatte in 1961. Since then only a few additional cases have been reported.[69] The term *balanitis* was used in the title as the original authors believed that the process was benign. This disease appears to occur only in men over the age of 50.

Clinical Appearance

The clinical appearance is described as a thick white laminated scale encasing the glans penis. The descriptive term *armorlike keratosis* has been used to emphasize the solid, thick nature of the process. Sometimes crusting, in addition to scale, is found.

Histology and Diagnosis

Biopsy reveals hyperkeratosis, acanthosis, and varying degrees of dysplasia. Generally, the lesions have a prolonged course of many years, but eventual development of squamous cell carcinoma has been reported several times.[70,71] The authors of these two reports felt that the process was a form of verrucous carcinoma. In one instance, a sarcoma developed at a treated site.[72]

Treatment

Partial improvement has been reported with the use of cryotherapy and topically applied fluorouracil (Efudex, Fluroplex). However, given the tendency to form true squamous cell carcinoma, excisional surgery is preferred.

REFERENCES

Anogenital Warts

1. Sawchuk WS: Ancillary diagnostic tests for detection of human papillomavirus infection. Dermatol Clin 9:277, 1991
2. Chuang T, Perry HU, Kurland LT et al: Condyloma accuminata in Rochester, Minnesota, 1950–1978: epidemiology and clinical features. Arch Dermatol 120:469, 1984
3. Bauer HM, Ting Y, Greer CE et al: Genital human papillomavirus infection in female university students as determined by a PCR-based method. JAMA 265:472, 1991
4. Kemp EA, Hakenwerth AM, Laurent SL et al: Human papillomavirus prevalence in pregnancy. Obstet Gynecol 79:649, 1992
5. Bergeron C, Ferenczy A, Richart RM et al: Micropapillomatosis labialis appears unrelated to human papillomavirus. Obstet Gynecol 76:281, 1990
6. Moyal-Barracco M, Leibowitch M, Orth G: Vestibular papillae of the vulva. Arch Dermatol 126:1594, 1990
7. Furlonge B et al: Vulvar vestibulitis syndrome: a clinicopathologic study. Br J Obstet Gynaecol 98:73, 1991
8. Hillman RJ, Botcherby M, Ryait BK et al: Detection of human papillomavirus DNA in the urogenital tracts of men with anogenital warts. Sex Trans Dis 20:21, 1993
9. Sonnex C et al: Anal human papillomavirus infection in heterosexuals with genital warts: prevalence and relation with sexual behavior. Br Med J 303:1243, 1991
10. Kulski JK, Demeter T, Rakoczy GF et al: Human papillomavirus coinfections of the vulva and uterine cervix. J Med Virol 27:244, 1989
11. Rowen D, Carne CA, Sonnex C, Cooper P: Increased incidence of cervical cytological abnormalities in women with genital warts or contact with genital warts: a need for increased vigilance? Genitourin Med 67:460, 1991
12. Das BC, Gopalkrishna V, Sharma JK et al: Human papillomavirus DNA in the urine of women with preneoplastic cervical lesions. Lancet 340:1417, 1992
13. Green J, Monteiro E, Bolton VN et al: Detection of human papillomavirus DNA by PCR in semen from patients with and without penile warts. Genitourin Med 67:207, 1991
14. Schultz RE, Miller JW, MacDonald GR et al: Clinical and molecular evaluation of acetowhite genital lesions in men. J Urol 143:920, 1990
15. Hippelainen M, Yliskoski M, Saarikoski S et al: Genital human papillomavirus lesions of the male sexual partners: the diagnostic accuracy of peniscopy. Genitourin Med 67:291, 1991
16. Mazzatenta C, Andrassi L, Biagioli M et al: Detection and typing of genital papillomaviruses in men with a single polymerase chain reaction and type-specific DNA probes. J Am Acad Dermatol 28:704, 1993
17. Sedlacek TV, Sedlacek AE, Neff D, Rando RF: The clinical role of human papillomavirus typing. Gynecol Oncol 42:222, 1991
18. Jenson AB, Kurman RJ, Lancaster WD: Tissue effects of and host response to human papillomavirus infection. Dermatol Clinics 9:203, 1991
19. Ferenczy A, Bergeron C, Richart RM: Human papillomavirus DNA in fomites on objects used for the management of patients with genital human papillomavirus infections. Obstet Gynecol 74:950, 1989
20. Bergeron C, Ferenczy A, Richart: Underwear: contamination by human papillomaviruses. Am J Obstet Gynecol 162:25, 1990
21. Wisniewski PM, Warhol MJ, Rando RF et al: Studies on the transmission of viral disease via the CO_2 laser plume and ejecta. J Reprod Med 35:1117, 1990
22. Selvey L, Buntin DW, Kennedy L, Frazer IH: Male partners of women with genital human papillomavirus infection. Med J Aust 150:479, 1989
23. Obalek S, Misiewicz, Jablonska S et al: Childhood condyloma acuminatum: association with genital and cutaneous human papillomaviruses. Pediatr Dermatol 10:101, 1993
24. Sedlacek TV, Lindheim S, Eder C et al: Mechanism for human papillomavirus transmission at birth. Am J Obstet Gynecol 161:55, 1989
25. Pao CC, Tsai PL, Chang YL, Hsieh TT: Non-sexual papillomavirus transmission routes. Lancet 339:1479, 1992
26. Quan MB, Moy L: The role of human papillomavirus in carcinoma. J Am Acad Dermatol 25:698, 1991
27. Pfister H, Fuchs PG: Relation of papillomaviruses to anogenital cancer. Dermatol Clin 9:267, 1991
28. Kirby AJ, Spiegelhalter DJ, Day NE et al: Conservative treatment of mild/moderate cervical dyskeratosis: long-term outcome. Lancet 339:828, 1992
29. Koutsky LA, Holmes KK, Critchlow CW et al: A cohort study of the risk of cervical intraepithelial neoplasia grade 2 or 3 in relation to papillomavirus infection. N Engl J Med 327:1272, 1992
30. Lorincz AT, Reid R, Jenson AB et al: Human papillomavirus infection of the cervix: relative risk associations of 15 common anogenital types. Obstet Gynecol 79:328, 1992

31. Palefsky JM, Gonzales J, Greenblatt RM et al: Anal intraepithelial neoplasia and anal papillomavirus infection among homosexual males with group IV HIV disease. JAMA 263:2911, 1990
32. Parazzini F, La Vecchia C, Negri E et al: Risk factors for cervical intraepithelial neoplasia. Cancer 69:2276, 1992
33. Daling R et al: Cigarette smoking and the risk of anogenital cancer. Am J Epidemiol 135:180, 1992
34. Vandenvelde C, Van Beers D: Oral contraceptives and papillomavirus persistence in normal cervix. Lancet 339:1294, 1992
35. Butterworth CE, Hatch KD, Macaluso M et al: Folate deficiency and cervical dysplasia. JAMA 267:528, 1992
36. Voog E, Lowhagen GB: Follow-up of men with genital papilloma virus infection. Acta Derm Venereol (Stockh) 72:185, 1992
37. Persson G, Dahlof LG, Krantz I: Physical and psychological effects of anogenital warts on female patients. Sex Trans Dis 20:10, 1993
38. Zhu WY, Blauvelt A, Goldstein BA et al: Detection with the polymerase chain reaction of human papillomavirus DNA in condylomata acuminata treated in vitro with liquid nitrogen, trichloracetic acid, and podophyllin. J Am Acad Dermatol 26:710, 1992
39. Greenberg MD, Rutledge LH, Reid R et al: A double-blind, randomized trial of 0.5% podofilox and placebo for the treatment of genital warts in women. Obstet Gynecol 77:735, 1991
40. Godley M, Bradbeer C, Gellan M et al: Cryotherapy compared with trichloroacetic acid in treating genital warts. Genitourin Med 63:390, 1987
41. Stone K, Becker T, Hadgu A et al: Treatment of external genital warts: a randomised clinical trial comparing podophyllin, cryotherapy, and electrodesiccation. Genitourin Med 66:16, 1990
42. Krebs HB: Treatment of genital condylomata with topical 5-fluorouracil. Dermatol Clin 9:333, 1991
43. Trofatter KF Jr: Interferon treatment of anogenital human papillomavirus-related diseases. Dermatol Clin 9:343, 1991
44. Petersen CS, Bjerring P, Larsen J et al: Systemic INFalpha2b increases the cure rate in laser treated patients with multiple persistent genital warts; a placebo-controlled study. Genitourin Med 67:99, 1991
45. Hopfl RM, Sandbichler M, Zelger BWH et al: Adjuvant treatment of recalcitrant genitoanal warts with systemic recombinant interferon-alpha-2c. Acta Derm Venereol (Stockh) 72:383, 1992
46. McMillan A, Scott G: Outpatient treatment of perianal warts by scissor excision. Genitourin Med 63:114, 1987
47. Reid R: Physical and surgical principles governing carbon dioxide laser surgery on the skin. Dermatol Clin 9:297, 1991
48. Riva JM, Sedlacek TV, Cunnane MF, Mangan CE: Extended carbon dioxide laser vaporization in the treatment of subclinical papillomavirus infection of the lower genital tract. Obstet Gynecol 73:25, 1989
49. Ferenczy A, Mitao M, Nagai N et al: Latent papillomavirus and recurring genital warts. N Engl J Med 313:784, 1985

Molluscum Contagiosum

50. Oriel JD: The increase in molluscum contagiosum. Br Med J 294:74, 1987
51. Brandrup F, Asshenfeldt P: Molluscum contagiosum-induced comedo and secondary abscess formation. Pediatr Dermatol 6:118, 1989
52. Schwartz JJ, Myskowski PL: Molluscum contagiosum in patients with human immunodeficiency virus infection. A review of twenty-seven patients. J Am Acad Dermatol 27:583, 1992
53. Porter CD, Blake NW, Archard LC et al: Molluscum contagiosum virus types in genital and non-genital lesions. Br J Dermatol 120:37, 1989
54. Epstein E: Cantharidin treatment of molluscum contagiosum. Acta Derm Venereol (Stockh) 69:91, 1989
55. Garrett SJ, Robinson JK, Roenigk HH: Trichloroacetic acid peel of molluscum contagiosum in immunocompromised patients. J Dermatol Surg Oncol 18:855, 1992
56. Deleixhe-Mauhin F, Pierard-Franchimont C, Pierard GE: Podophyllotoxin in the treatment of molluscum contagiosum. J Dermatol Treat 2:99, 1991
57. Friedman M, Gal D: Keloid scars as a result of CO_2 laser for molluscum contagiosum. Obstet Gynecol 70:394, 1987
58. Smith KJ, Skelton HG, Yeager J et al: Molluscum contagiosum. Ultrastructural evidence for its presence in skin adjacent to clinical lesions in patients infected with human immunodeficiency virus type 1. Arch Dermatol 128:223, 1992

Pearly Penile Papules

59. Neinstein LS, Goldenring J: Pink pearly papules: an epidemiologic study. J Pediatr 105:594, 1984
60. Ferenczy A, Richart RM, Wright TC: Pearly penile papules: absence of human papillomavirus DNA by the polymerase chain reaction. Obstet Gynecol 78:118, 1991

Syringomas

61. Lo JS, Dijkstra JWE, Bergfeld WF: Syringomas on the penis. Int J Dermatol 29:309, 1990
62. Sola Casas MA, Soto De Delas J, Redondo Bellon P, Quintanilla Gutierrez E: Syringomas localized to the penis. Clin Exp Dermatol 18:384, 1993
63. Scherbenske JM, Luptou GP, James WD, Kirkle DB: Vulvar syringomas occurring in a 9-year-old child. J Am Acad Dermatol 19:575, 1988
64. Carter J, Elliot P: Syringoma—an unusual cause of pruritus vulvae. Aust NZ Obstet Gynaecol 4:382, 1990
65. Lipshutz RL, Kantor GR, Vonderheid EC: Multiple penile syringomas mimicking verrucae. Int J Dermatol 30:69, 1991
66. Martin F, Escallier F, Collet E et al: Traitement par le laser CO_2 des syringomes vulvaires multiples. Nouv Dermatol 12:149, 1993

Lichen Nitidus

67. Randle HWl, Sander HM: Treatment of generalized lichen nitidus with PUVA. Int J Dermatol 25:330, 1986
68. Aram H: Association of lichen planus and lichen nitidus. Treatment with etretinate. Int J Dermatol 27:117, 1988

Pseudoepitheliomatous, Micaceous, and Keratotic Balanitis

69. Tio TT, Blindeman L, van Ulsen J: Pseudoepitheliomatous, keratotic and micaceous balanitis of Lortat-Jacob and Civatte. Br J Dermatol 123:265, 1990

70. Bargman H: Pseudoepitheliomatous, keratotic, and micaceous balanitis. Cutis 35:77, 1985
71. Beljaards RC, Van Dijk E, Hausman R: Is pseudoepitheliomatous, micaceous and keratotic balanitis synonymous with verrucous carcinoma? Br J Dermatol 117:641, 1987
72. Irvine C, Anderson JR, Pye RJ: Micaceous and keratotic pseudoepitheliomatous balanitis and rapidly fatal fibrosarcoma of the penis occurring in the same patient. Br J Dermatol 116:719, 1987

SUGGESTED READINGS

Anogenital Warts

Cobb MW: Human papillomavirus infection. J Am Acad Dermatol 22:547, 1990

This 20-page review covers all of the general aspects of HPV infection, but there is little in it specifically about anogenital infection.

Ling MR: Therapy of genital human papillomavirus infections. Part I: Indications for and justification of therapy. Int J Dermatol 31:682, 1992

Ling MR: Therapy of genital human papillomavirus infections. Part II: Methods of treatment. Int J Dermatol 31:769, 1992

These two articles contain a very complete and authoritative review regarding treatment of anogenital HPV infections.

Quan MB, Moy RL: The role of human papillomavirus in carcinoma. J Am Acad Dermatol 25:698, 1991

This is a reasonably up-to-date review of the fast-moving story on HPV-induced oncogenesis.

Reid R, Campion MJ: The biology and significance of human papillomavirus infections in the genital tract. Yale J Biol Med 61:307, 1988

This remarkably complete review is written from a gynecologic perspective.

Sehgal VN, Koranne RV, Srivastava: Genital warts. Current status. Int J Dermatol 28:75, 1989

This short review is written from a dermatologic perspective.

Molluscum Contagiosum

Brown ST, Nalley JF, Kraus SJ: Molluscum contagiosum. Sex Trans Dis 8:227, 1981

Although this article is more than ten years old, it provides an excellent summary of the disease.

Vestibular Papillae

Moyal-Barracco M, Leibowitch M, Orth: Vestibular papillae of the vulva. Lack of evidence for human papillomavirus etiology. Arch Dermatol 126:1594, 1990

This article reports on examination of papillomatous lesions of the vulvar vestibule for human papillomavirus by the Southern blot technique and then contrasts the clinical appearance of lesions associated with the presence of virus with those unassociated with this positive finding.

Lichen Nitidus

Arndt K: Lichen nitidus. p. 1144. In Fitzpatrick TB, Eisen AZ, Wolff K et al (eds): Dermatology in General Medicine. McGraw-Hill, New York, 1993

This chapter is a succinct review of the disease, with color photographs.

Verruciform Xanthoma

De Rosa G, Barra E, Gentile R et al: Verruciform xanthoma of the vulva: case report. Genitourin Med 65:252, 1989

Geiss DF, Del Rosso JQ, Murphy J: Verruciform xanthoma of the glans penis: a benign clinical simulant of genital malignancy. Cutis 51:369, 1993

George WM, Azadeh B: Verruciform xanthoma of the penis. Cutis 44:167, 1989

10 Skin-Colored Nodules

SECONDARY SYPHILIS

Lesions of secondary syphilis occurring on dry glabrous skin consist of erythematous, sharply marginated slightly scaling papules, whereas those occurring on moist skin or mucous membranes (condylomata lata) are skin-colored or white. In spite of these morphologic distinctions, all forms of secondary syphilis are covered in this chapter.

Clinical Presentation

The lesions of secondary syphilis that occur on the trunk, pubic area, buttocks, and thighs are small, fairly sharply marginated, red papules 3 to 10 mm in diameter (Fig. 10-1). The papules are bright red at first and become more dusky as they age. In dark-skinned individuals, the red color is masked and the lesions appear pigmented. The papules may or may not have discernible overlying scale. Individual lesions remain discrete; coalescence to form plaques rarely occurs.

Those lesions that occur on the penis and scrotum are often slightly larger and may be less sharply marginated. In blacks and other dark-skinned individuals, ringlike (annular) lesions up to 2 cm in diameter may be present (Fig. 10-2). The surface of the lesions on the male genitalia may be moist or slightly scaly.

Condylomata lata are larger (1 to 2 cm), more elevated, flat-topped papules and small plaques (Fig. 10-3). The lesions are quite variable in color; skin-colored, pink or dusky hues may be found. In moist areas, surface scale becomes hydrated, and consequently the surface may appear white. Condylomata lata are typically found on the female genitalia and in the perianal area in both sexes. Here, too, the surface may be either moist (and even visibly eroded) or dry and slightly scaly.

When a suspicion of secondary syphilis is raised, a general examination should be carried out. Red papules similar to those seen on the trunk are often present on the face; flat-topped firm papules are usually present on the palms and soles. White patches and erosions may occur on the mucous membranes of the mouth; patchy alopecia can often be found on the scalp. Generalized lymphadenopathy is regularly encountered, and sometimes hepatosplenomegaly is present. Keep in mind that the lesions of secondary syphilis, especially those that are moist, are quite contagious; gloves should be worn for the entire examination.

Diagnosis

Dark-field examination of serum recovered when moist lesions are scraped will reveal the causative spirochete, *Treponema pallidum.* For practical purposes, however, the diagnosis is usually confirmed through serologic testing (see under Primary Syphilis, Ch. 17).

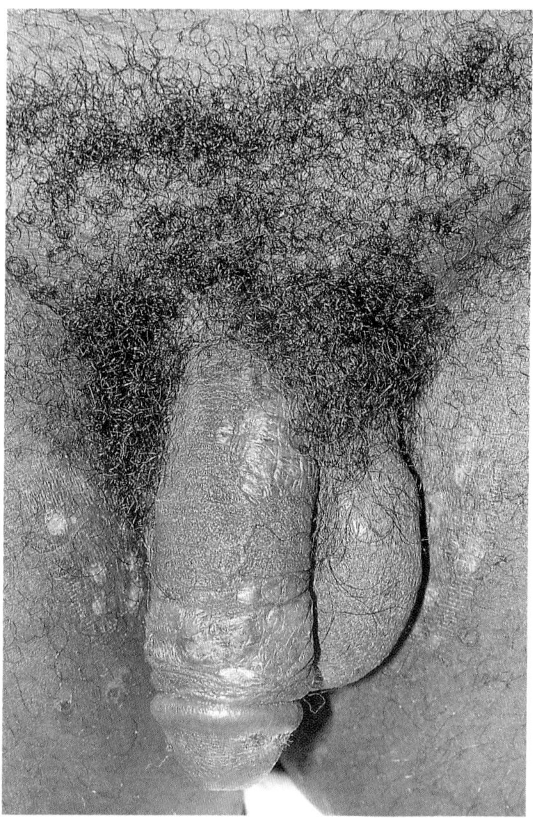

Fig. 10-1. Hypopigmented and pink, scaling papules of secondary syphilis in a black patient who exhibits less visible erythema than would most lighter-complexioned people.

Course and Prognosis, Pathogenesis, and Treatment

Discussion of the course, prognosis, pathogenesis, and therapy of syphilis can be found in Chapter 17 in the section on primary syphilis.

SCLEROSING LYMPHANGITIS

Clinical Presentation

Sclerosing lymphangitis occurs only in men. It begins with the sudden onset of a cordlike thickening of tissue that develops circumferentially at the corona or just posterior to the coronal sulcus (Figs. 10-4 and 10-5). The lesion is usually skin-colored, firm, and painless. In some instances slight inflammation will be present, in which case some redness and tenderness may be noted. No lymphadenopathy is found.

Histology

Histologically, a thrombosed vessel with some surrounding chronic inflammatory reaction is noted. Older lesions may show evidence of recanalization. Controversy exists as to the nature of the vessel involved[1]; a recent study presented data suggesting that the occluded vessels were lymphatic in origin.[2]

Pathogenesis

The etiology of the problem is unknown. Since it tends to develop in men who are hyperactive sexually, it is likely that trauma plays an important role. Infection does not seem to cause the problem, although nonrelated sexually transmitted diseases are often present.

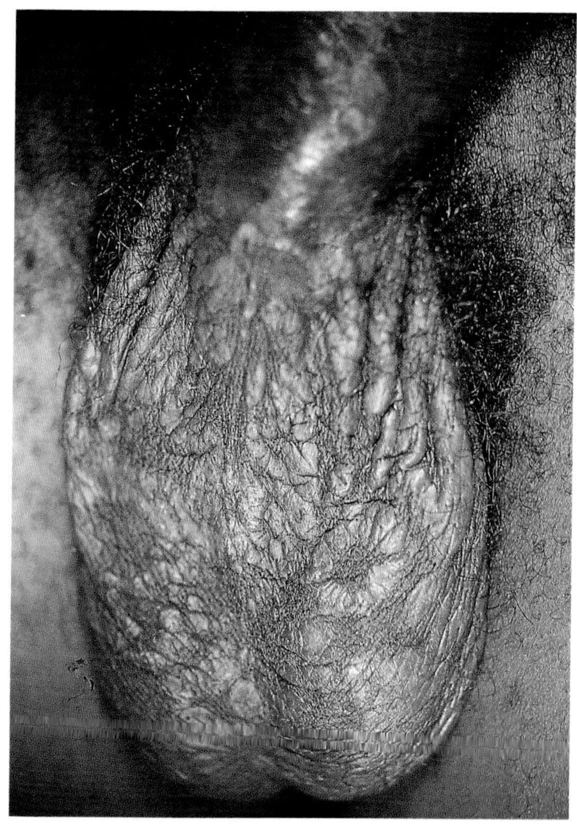

Fig. 10-2. Small, annular, well-demarcated, scaling plaques of secondary syphilis over the scrotum.

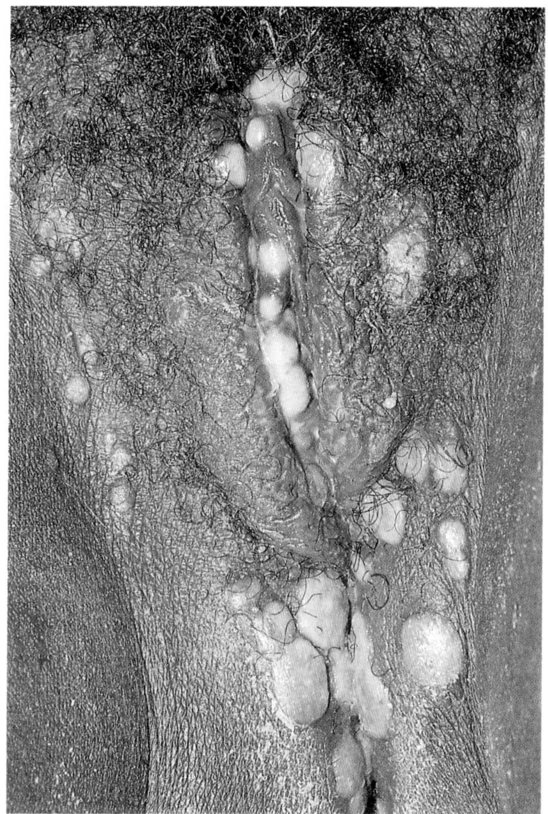

Fig. 10-3. Flat-topped, moist, white papules of condylomata lata over the modified mucous membranes, and skin-colored, pink, and scaling lesions over keratinized skin in a patient with secondary syphilis.

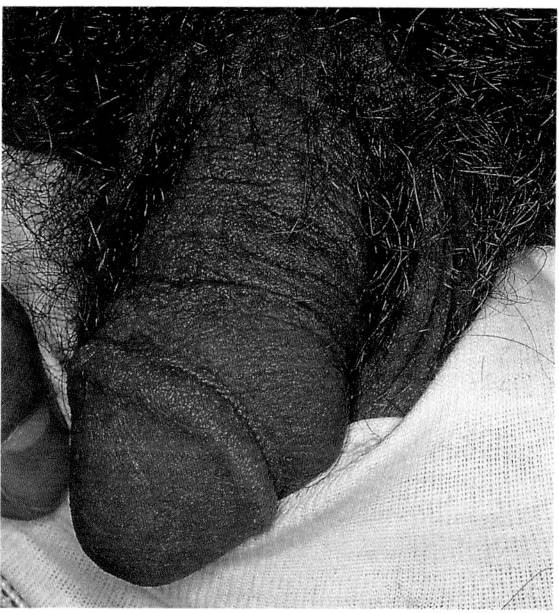

Fig. 10-4. Firm nodule of sclerosing lymphangitis.

Treatment

Cessation or reduction in sexual activity is recommended, and the lesion resolves spontaneously over a period of 1 or 2 months. Surgical removal of the indurated tissue can be carried out in the rare instance in which tenderness is troublesome and persistent.[3]

CYSTS

Cysts are benign nonsolid tumors or dilations of normal components of the skin or its appendages or of glandular ducts. Genital cysts are common and are usually asymptomatic unless inflamed (see also Inflamed Cysts in Ch. 8).

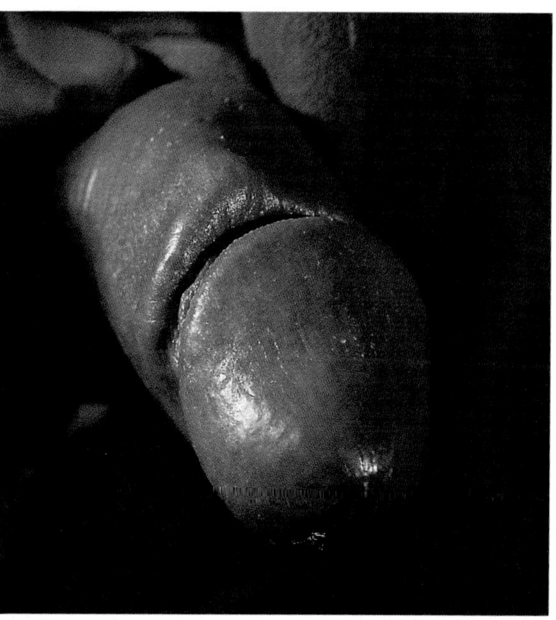

Fig. 10-5. Cord of sclerosing lymphangitis in a typical location on the penis.

EPIDERMAL CYSTS

The most common cysts are epidermal, sometimes referred to by the misnomer sebaceous cysts. These occur when squamous epithelium is present in the dermis without an adequate surface outlet, so that desquamated epithelial cells and keratin debris collect within this dermal sphere of epithelium. These cysts usually arise from hair follicles that become obstructed and then are distended by keratin from the stratum corneum of the follicular epithelium deep to the obstruction (Fig. 10-6). Less often, epithelium can be displaced into the dermis by trauma, such as an episiotomy. The hydrated keratin within the cyst gives the lesion a white or yellowish color, although deeper lesions may be skin-colored (Figs. 10-7 and 10-8). An epidermal cyst is firm and, unless inflamed, nontender; it varies in size from about 1 mm to several centimeters. They are especially common on the scrotum and labia majora, although the penile shaft, labia minora, and vagina can be affected. They may be single or multiple. Occasionally and most often as a result of trauma or manipulation, the cyst may rupture; the contents induce a brisk and painful foreign-body inflammatory response.

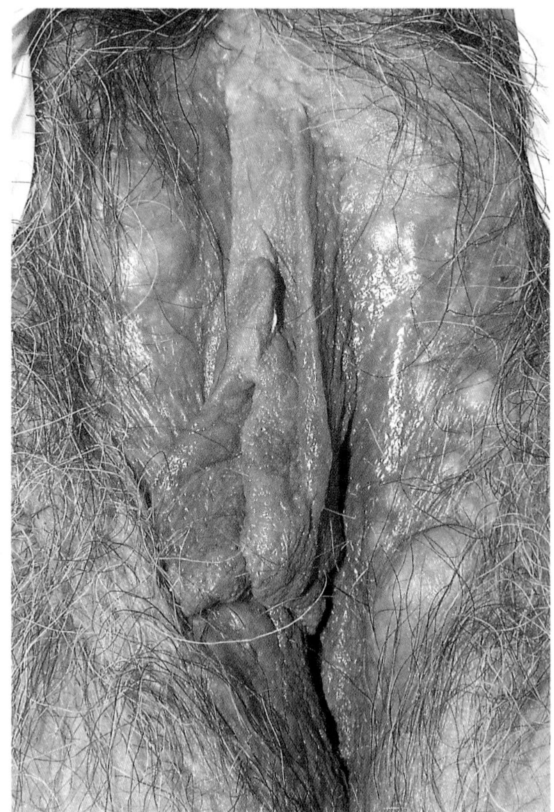

Fig. 10-7. Multiple skin-colored and yellow epidermal cysts.

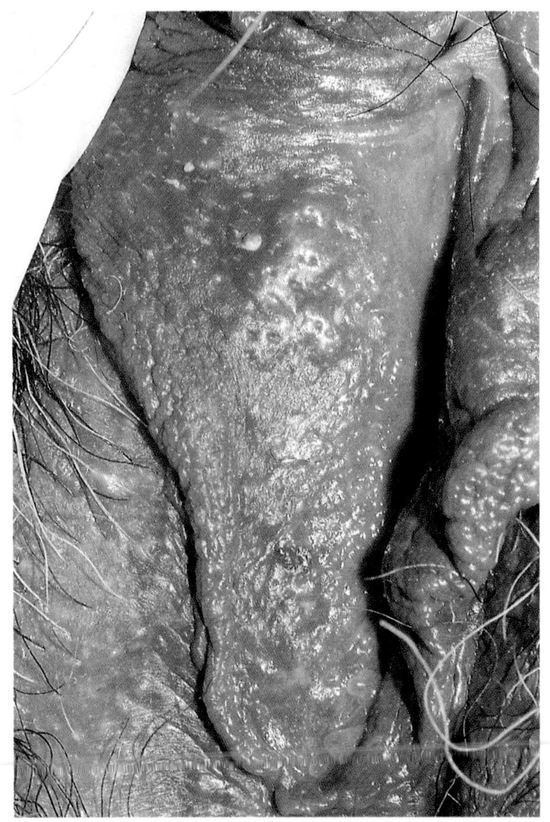

Fig. 10-6. Comedones and small epidermal cysts over the inner labia minora, a manifestation of the hair follicles that are present in some patients in this area. A pigmented nevus is also present.

Histologically, the cysts consist of squamous epithelium with contents of keratinous material. Epidermal cysts do not require therapy except for cosmetic reasons or if inflamed. The treatment of epidermal cysts is surgical. Although a cyst can be incised and drained of its cheesy, often malodorous contents with good short-term results, this usually results in recurrence. For definitive treatment, the epithelial sac should be removed at a time when the cyst is not inflamed so that scarring and discomfort are minimized.

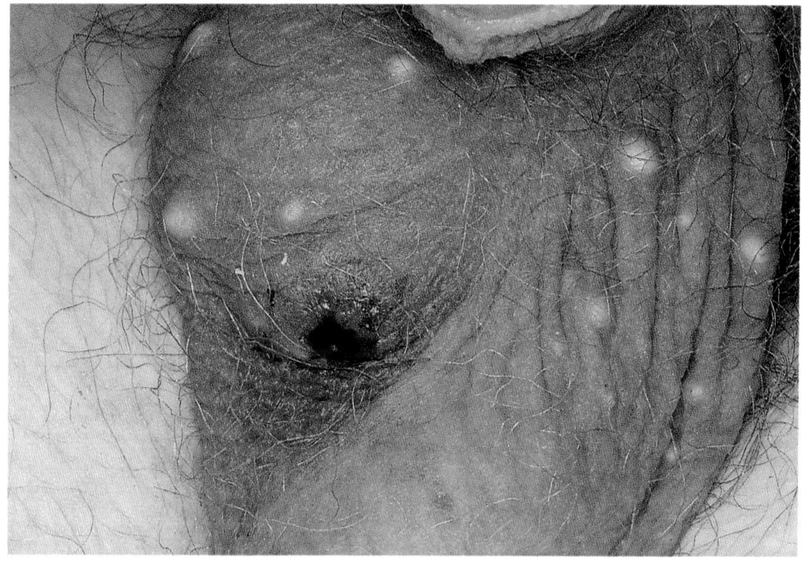

Fig. 10-8. These small, white firm nodules are distinctive for scrotal epidermal cysts. Inflammation is present at the site of an incision and drainage.

BARTHOLIN'S GLAND DUCT CYSTS

Bartholin's gland duct cysts are common genital cysts, occurring in about 2 percent of women. These cysts result from obstruction of this major vulvar vestibular mucous-secreting gland with subsequent distention of the duct. The Bartholin's gland is deeper than the minor vestibular glands, so that the resulting cyst often presents as a less discrete, skin-colored swelling of the inner, posterior portion of the labium majus (Fig. 10-9), although a well-demarcated nodule similar to mucoid vestibular cysts occasionally occurs. Smaller cysts may be palpable but not visible. Histologically, a Bartholin's gland duct cyst is lined by transitional or squamous epithelium if the obstruction is within the main duct, but tall columnar cells may line the cyst if it originates in an acinus.

Obstruction of the duct may occur as a result of infection, inspissated mucous, or trauma. In the past, inflamed Bartholin's gland duct cysts were nearly always felt to be infected, but it is now recognized that cysts and abscesses are often sterile on culture.

Although asymptomatic unless inflamed or very large, Bartholin's gland cysts are sometimes predisposed to recurrent inflammation. Gonorrhea is an important cause of inflamed Bartholin's cysts and abscesses and should be ruled out. Incision and drainage or aspiration are useful short-term therapies

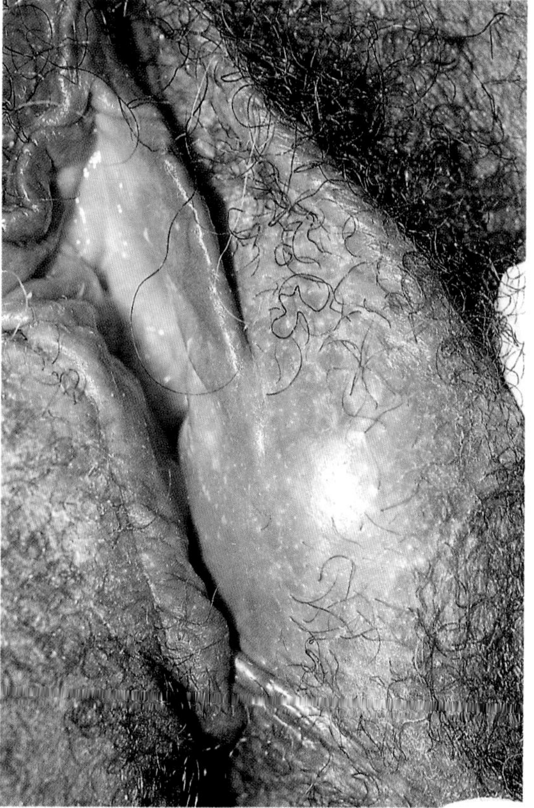

Fig. 10-9. Diffuse swelling of an uninflamed Bartholin's gland duct cyst in the posterior vulva.

but often are associated with recurrence. However, removal of the gland and cyst may result in unacceptable morbidity. In addition to oral antibiotics for infected cysts, marsupialization or the use of a Word catheter as discussed previously (Ch. 8) may be indicated for definitive treatment. The new appearance of a Bartholin's duct cyst in a postmenopausal woman should raise the suspicion of malignancy.

PILONIDAL CYSTS

Pilonidal cysts are abscesses that develop as a foreign-body inflammatory response to hair within the dermis. The hair may simply be ingrown or the abscess may occur in response to a ruptured dermoid cyst. Although most pilonidal cysts and sinuses are in the lower sacrococcygeal area, some may occur in the genital, primarily vulvar, area. The most common genital location is periclitoral, but other areas include the mons pubis and the perineum. These cysts appear as an erythematous papule or nodule that may become eroded and drain, forming a chronic sinus tract. Treatment is by complete surgical removal when the inflammation has subsided. Removal of the entire sinus tract is essential to prevent recurrence.

DERMOID CYSTS

Dermoid cysts are cystic tumors containing multiple structures of ectodermal origin, including keratin, hair, and sometimes teeth. These cysts may be asymptomatic or they may cause symptoms from size and pressure on surrounding structures, from rupture with resulting foreign body reaction such as a pilonidal sinus, or from malignant degeneration. Treatment is surgical excision.

INGUINAL HERNIAS

Inguinal hernias, occurring almost exclusively in men, result from extrusion of bowel through the inguinal ring following the same pathway through which testes descend from their original position in the abdomen. This presents as a boggy scrotal swelling that can usually be reduced by gentle pressure back through the inguinal ring. Even when asymptomatic, surgery to reinforce the peritoneum is indicated to prevent incarceration of the hernia and ischemia of the trapped bowel.

CYSTS OF THE CANAL OF NUCK AND HYDROCELES

Cysts of the canal of Nuck (in women) and hydroceles (in men) are cystic, serous fluid-containing swellings in the inguinal crease, the anterior labia majora, or scrotum. These cysts arise from remnants of peritoneum as it passes through the inguinal canal, called the processus vaginalis peritonei or canal of Nuck. If this embryonic structure is incompletely obliterated during fetal life, occlusion of the outlet of this peritoneal diverticulum produces a cyst, and multiple sites of occlusion produce multiple cysts. These cysts may occur anywhere along the path of the inguinal canal, or within the labia majora or scrotum. These cysts are lined with flattened cuboidal cells and generally are asymptomatic, requiring no treatment. When large or uncomfortable, they may be excised surgically, although they may recur.

MUCOUS CYSTS OF THE VULVA AND VAGINA

Mucous cysts of the vulva and vagina are common and may arise from any of several different structures. Cysts of Skene's (paraurethral) duct lie in the distal urethra and open within or just outside the urethral orifice. Occlusion of these ducts results in a cystic swelling at the urethral opening. These cysts may reach 2 cm in size. Many are asymptomatic, but others produce dyspareunia or urinary outlet obstruction and require surgical removal.

Other mucous cysts of the vulva and vagina are generally developmental, occurring from vestigeal embryonic structures including the mesonephric (Gartner's) duct, paramesonephric (müllerian) duct, and urogenital sinus. Cysts of the vulvar vestibule are believed to derive primarily from the urogenital sinus, whereas vaginal cysts develop from the mesonephric ducts and the paramesonephric ducts. Clinically, these cysts are often indistinguishable, and for practical purposes differentiation is unimportant. It is important, if treatment is contemplated, to differentiate vaginal cysts from a urethral diverticulum.

MUCOUS CYSTS OF THE VULVAR VESTIBULE

Mucous cysts of the vulvar vestibule are relatively common. Although many are believed to be developmental cysts that arise from persistent urogenital sinus epithelium, others probably develop as a result of obstruction of the minor vestibular glands, which are small invaginations of glandular tissue of the vulvar vestibule. Vestibular cysts are usually under 2 cm in size and may be yellow, bluish, or skin-colored, often with a translucent quality (Figs. 10-10 and 10-11). Histologically, these cysts show a lining of columnar epithelium, sometimes with squamous metaplasia. These cysts are filled with mucous secretions and are usually asymptomatic, requiring no therapy.

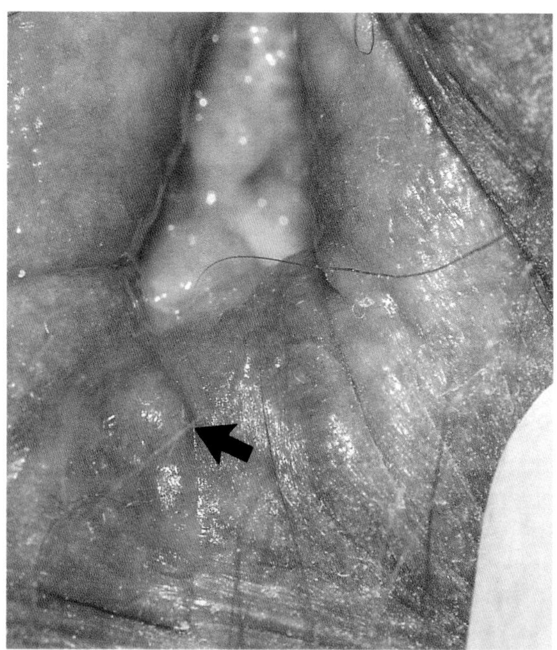

Fig. 10-11. A skin-colored, translucent vestibular cyst *(arrow).*

GARTNER'S CYSTS

Gartner's cysts are cystic dilations of remnants of the wolffian (mesonephric) ducts. These embryonal structures largely degenerate in fetal life, except for fragments at the lateral vagina. They are most often multiple and small, occurring as small surface irregularities arranged in a linear pattern along the anterolateral vagina or hymeneal ring. Larger cysts may also occur anteriorly in the vagina, occasionally producing dyspareunia or symptoms from pressure on urinary structures. The cysts are lined with mucus-secreting cuboidal or columnar epithelium on a basement membrane and exhibit smooth muscle within the wall. Because these cysts are usually asymptomatic and are discovered only incidentally on physical examination, removal is usually unnecessary.

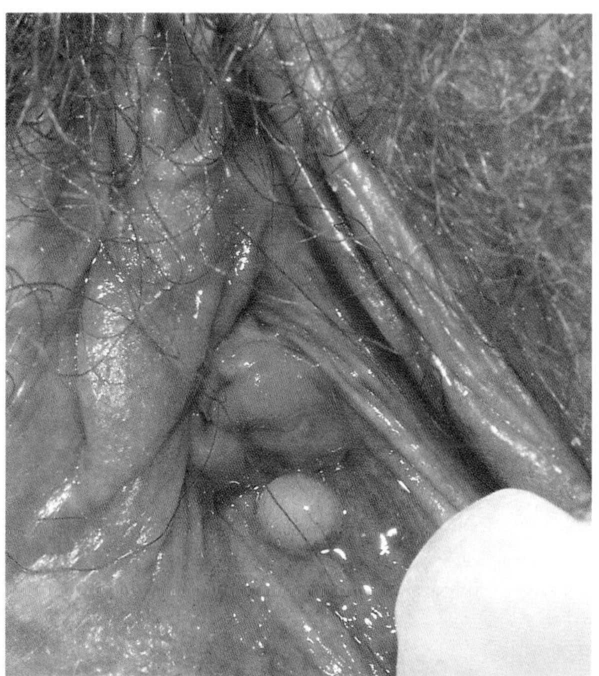

Fig. 10-10. This vestibular cyst is yellow, although some are skin-colored or blue.

PARAMESONEPHRIC (MÜLLERIAN) DUCT CYSTS

Paramesonephric (müllerian) duct cysts are vaginal cysts that arise from remaining fragments of the glandular epithelium that lines the vagina during fetal life, before the upward migration of squamous epithelium that ultimately constitutes the vaginal epithelial layer. These cysts may occur anywhere in the vagina, but most often are found anteriorly. They are usually less than 2 cm, but may sometimes be larger, occasionally causing dyspareunia or urinary symptoms. Because the paramesonephric ducts eventually create the final columnar epithelium of the endocervix, endometrium, and endosalpinx, the cyst lining may be any or all of these three different types. Most common is the tall columnar cells typical of the endocervix. Paramesonephric duct cysts usually require no treatment.

NEUROFIBROMAS

Neurofibromas of the anogenital region have been reported primarily in a vulvar location. Some of these occurred as isolated lesions,[4] but most have developed in the setting of generalized neurofibromatosis (von Recklinghausen's disease). The prevalence of vulvar involvement in von Recklinghausen's disease is not known but may be as high as 20 percent. The lesions are clinically and histologically similar regardless of the setting in which they occur.

Two morphologic forms of neurofibromas occur. The first is a pedunculated lesion that appears as an outpouching of the skin. Some of these lesions are nodular, whereas other are polypoid and are attached to the skin with a stalk (Fig. 10-12). Both are skin-colored, soft, and sometimes wrinkled in appearance; their size is usually less than 3 cm in diameter. The second is a deep "plexiform" lesion. These larger lesions usually appear as a deeper, slope-shouldered enlargement of the labia majora or the clitoris, or both.[5] They, too, are skin-colored and soft but may have the characteristic "bag of worms" consistency of plexiform neurofibromas elsewhere. This second type arises from deeper nerves in the subcutaneous tissue.

Small pedunculated lesions, whether solitary or associated with generalized neurofibromatosis, are benign lesions. These small lesions do not require treatment unless they are in a location or of a size that is troublesome to the patient, in which case they can be surgically removed. Plexiform neurofibromas arise in the setting of von Recklinghausen's disease, and they have approximately a 5 percent risk of evolving into a malignant sarcoma. Surgical excision of these lesions is generally warranted, but more often than not they cannot be completely excised because of their depth and interrelationship with other deep structures.

NEUROMAS

Neuromas are not usually clinically recognized and instead are found incidentally at the time of surgery carried out for other reasons. There is almost no description of this condition in the literature, but anecdotally they are found with some frequency in women who are undergoing excisional surgery for vulvodynia or other forms of vulvar pain.[6] It is not clear if the neuromas identified in this setting are

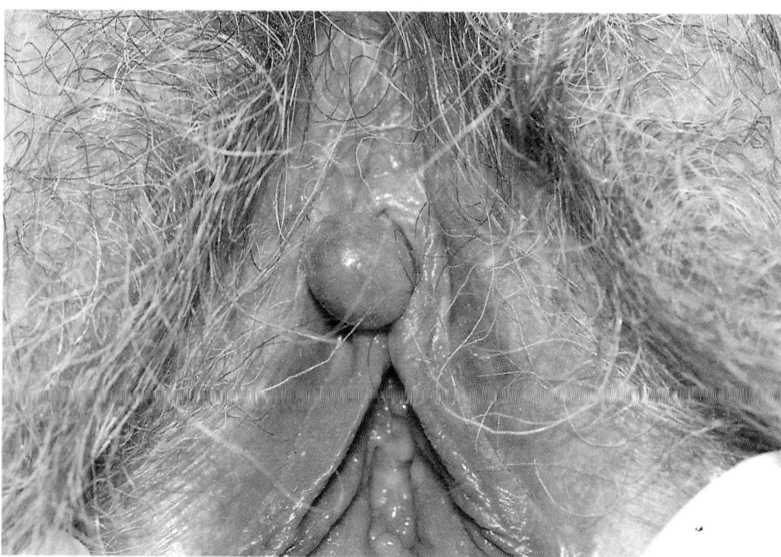

Fig. 10-12. Skin-colored, soft nodule of a clitoral neurofibroma in a patient without neurofibromatosis.

responsible for the pain or whether they represent incidental lesions.

FIBROMAS AND FIBROSARCOMAS

Fibromas and fibrosarcomas are uncommon tumors primarily reported in women. They usually arise in the labia majora, but lesions have been found at the perineal body and vaginal introitus. Two clinical types occur. The first type is a pedunculated lesion similar in appearance to the fibroepithelial polyp; however, on palpation a fibroma is firm whereas a fibroepithelial polyp is soft. The second type is a slope-shouldered firm nodule that is not pedunculated. Both types of lesions are asymptomatic, slow-growing, skin-colored, and smooth-surfaced. Lesions are usually several centimeters in diameter, but a few giant lesions have been reported. Fibromas and fibrosarcomas may develop at any age.

On biopsy the tumors consist of densely packed, parallel, and intertwining bundles of collagen fibers. A few lesions showing the malignant changes of dermatofibrosarcoma have been reported. Lesions with a benign histology rarely recur after excision; those with a malignant histology are very likely to recur and eventually lead to death.

LIPOMAS AND LIPOSARCOMAS

Lipomas are common fatty hamartomas of the subcutaneous tissue. They are frequently encountered on the lower abdomen and thighs. They also develop specifically within the labia majora and around the clitoris. Lipomas usually occur as a skin-colored, soft, rounded mass; most are only a few centimeters in diameter, but larger lesions have been reported. They are asymptomatic except in the rare setting of Dercum's disease (adiposis dolorosa), in which pain may be present. Lipomas develop so insidiously that most patients are not aware of any growth or enlargement. If a patient should describe a rapid growth pattern, biopsy should be considered to rule out the presence of a liposarcoma. Histologically lipomas demonstrate a proliferation of mature fat cells with intermingled fibrous strands. Treatment is not medically necessary, but lipomas can be removed with liposuction or they can be surgically excised.

Liposarcomas are fairly common soft tissue malignancies but are rarely reported to occur in the anogenital region.[7] This rarity can be explained by the fact that liposarcomas, in contradistinction to lipomas, arise from intermuscular fascial planes rather than from lipocytes in the subcutaneous tissue. Also, for this reason, liposarcomas arise de novo and do not evolve from lipomas. Clinically, liposarcomas present skin-colored nodules that are much more firm on palpation than are lipomas. Metastases occur commonly. Histologically, the tumor is composed of lipocytes with spindle-shaped nuclei; the degree of nuclear atypicality is highly variable.

LANGERHANS CELL HISTIOCYTOSIS

Fewer than 50 cases of Langerhans cell histiocytosis (LCH) (histiocytosis X) occurring in the anogenital area have been reported.[8] Genital LCH occurs mostly in children and young adults, but development in older individuals has been documented.[9] Nearly all of the patients have been female, but a few males have been reported.[10]

LCH may be confined to the anogenital area, or anogenital lesions may occur as part of disseminated disease. In either case, systemic involvement may or may not be present. The most common lesions encountered in the localized form of the disease occur on the vulva and consist of skin-colored nodules and plaques that are usually ulcerated. In the disseminated (Letterer-Siwe) form of the disease, an inflammatory eruption simulating that of seborrheic dermatitis may be found in the intertriginous folds. Some of them may be purpuric.

The histologic appearance of the lesions is distinctive and consists of a granulomatous reaction with prominent histiocytes (some of which may be foamy) with accompanying giant cells, eosinophils, neutrophils, and plasma cells. Treatment of LCH lies outside the scope of this book.

GRANULAR CELL TUMORS

Granular cell tumors are rare neoplasms. They are more common in women than in men, and blacks seem to be particularly predisposed. The tongue is the most common site, but about 5 percent occur on the vulva. Lesions are most often solitary, but in about 10 to 15 percent of the cases multiple lesions are found. Onset is usually in early adult life, but a few cases have occurred in children.[11]

Vulvar lesions account for almost all of the granular cell tumors involving the genitalia; fewer than 100 women with these tumors have been reported. The neoplasms are primarily situated on the labia majora and present as rounded, firm lesions with somewhat indistinct margins (Fig. 10-13). Most are skin-colored and smooth-surfaced, but some display hyperkeratosis or even a verrucous surface. The average size is 2 to 4 cm, but larger lesions can occur. Nearly all of the vulvar lesions have been solitary. These tumors are slow-growing and asymptomatic.

The histology of granular cell tumors is distinctive. The tumor is made up of large cells containing granule-filled, pale cytoplasm. The granules, which are period acid-Schiff (PAS) positive, appear to be phagolysosomes. The cells are morphologically benign in most cases, but a few instances showing cellular atypicality have been reported. Those demonstrating histologic atypicality may metastasize and, surprisingly, so do some of those that are microscopically benign.[12] Excision is the treatment of choice; margins should be checked to minimize the possibility of recurrence.

GENITAL EDEMA

Noninflammatory swelling of the genitalia generally occurs in four settings. The first is that of congenital abnormalities of lymphatic vessels.[13] Edema can develop as a component of congenital lymphedema (Milroy's disease); diagnosis is based on the history of presence since infancy and on the occurrence of accompanying lymphedema of either or both lower extremities. Alternatively, the edema can develop as part of the condition known as lymphangioma circumscriptum, in which case surface changes consisting of clustered thick-walled "vesicles" (lymphangiectasias) will be noted. Lymphangiectasia, with or without associated edema, can also occur as an acquired condition secondary to lymphatic damage occurring in association with various types of inflammatory disease[14] (see also below).

The second setting is that of angioedema occurring as a result of a localized allergic reaction (Fig. 10-14), most commonly seen in men and women who have contact allergies to latex. It therefore occurs in those who are using latex condoms or latex diaphrams. Genital edema can also be seen postcoitally in women who have the rare condition of allergy to components of their sexual partner's ejaculate.[15] In both instances the reaction appears to be mediated by an IgE mechanism and for this reason generalized anaphylaxis is possible. Genital edema due to angioedema is recognized by the rapid development of swelling and by the repetitive pattern of occurrence (see also under Contact Urticaria in Ch. 5).

The third setting is that of infectious or postinfectious lymphatic damage. The most common infec-

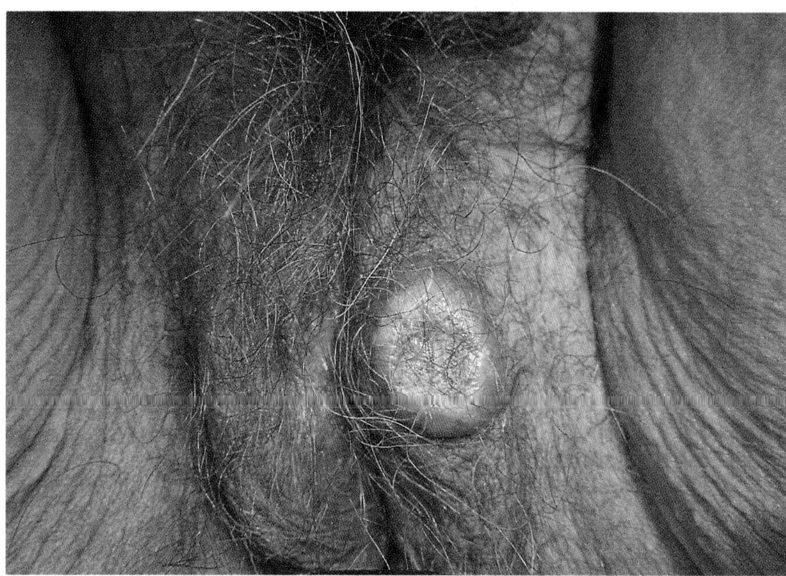

Fig. 10-13. Firm, pink granular cell tumor of the vulva. (Courtesy of David N. Flieger, M.D.)

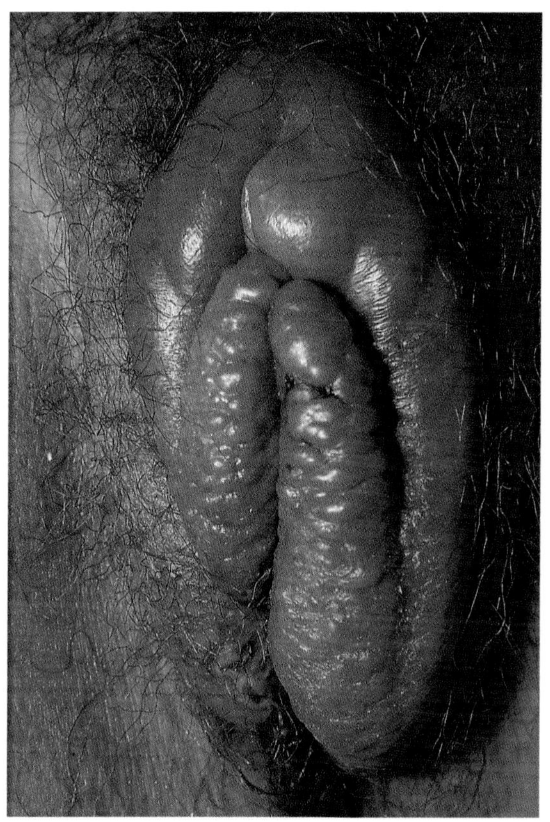

Fig. 10-14. Gross edema of the labia minora. Resolution occurred spontaneously, in 2 weeks.

tion (but probably the one most often missed) is episodic cellulitis due to streptococcal or staphylococcal infection. These infections are often quite subtle, with only slight redness and tenderness occurring at the time of the infection; mild fever may or may not be present. The episodes of cellulitis due to these organisms tend to be recurrent. As a result of repetitive lymphatic damage, lymphedema, which is mild and transient at first, gradually increases, and then becomes more permanent.

Some of the less common infections that cause persistent genital edema include lymphogranuloma venereum, granuloma inguinale, filariasis, leishmaniasis, and Bartholin's gland duct abscess with rupture. Other inflammatory disease should be mentioned even though they are not, strictly speaking, infections: hidradenitis suppurativa, Crohn's disease, and (rarely) severe atopic/neurodermatitis. Since all of these are substantive and symptomatic processes, patient history should allow for proper identification.

The fourth setting is the development of granulomatous genital lymphedema, similar to that occurring on the lips (Melkersson-Rosenthal syndrome).[16] This edema is typically episodic and soft at first but gradually becomes firm and more persistent. Identification requires biopsy, sometimes on several occasions. The histologic changes are nonspecific in the beginning, but the typical granulomatous pattern develops with the passage of time. Speculation suggests that a relationship might exist between this process and both sarcoidosis and Crohn's disease. Intralesionally injected or systemically administered steroids may be helpful for this condition.

Treatment for noninflammatory edema depends on which of these conditions are identified, but in any case, long-term antibiotic treatment is well worth trying since there is little to lose and, potentially, much to gain.

REFERENCES

Sclerosing Lymphangitis

1. Leventhal LC, Jaworsky C, Werth V: An asymptomatic penile lesion. Arch Dermatol 129:365, 1993
2. Tanii T, Hamada T, Asai Y et al: Mondor's phlebitis of the penis: a study with factor VIII related antigen. Acta Derm Venereol (Stockh) 64:337, 1984
3. Broaddus SB, Leadbetter GW: Surgical management of persistent symptomatic nonvenereal sclerosing lymphangitis of the penis. J Urol 127:987, 1982

Neurofibromas

4. Venter PF, Rohm GF, Slabber CF: Giant neurofibromas of the labia. Obstet Gynecol 57:128, 1981
5. Nogita T, Kawabata Y, Tsuchida T et al: Clitoral and labial involvement of neurofibromatosis. J Am Acad Dermatol 23:937, 1990

Neuromas

6. Sonnendecker EWW, Cohen RJ, Dreyer L et al: Neuroma of the vulva. A case report. J Reprod Med 38:33, 1993

Lipomas and Liposarcomas

7. Brooks JJ, LiVolsi VA: Liposarcoma presenting on the vulva. Am J Obstet Gynecol 156:73, 1987

Langerhans Cell Histiocytosis

8. Axiotis CA, Merino MJ, Duray PH: Langerhans cell histiocytosis of the female genital tract. Cancer 67:1650, 1991
9. Modi D, Schulz EJ: Skin ulceration as sole manifestation of Langerhans-cell histiocytosis. Clin Exp Dermatol 16:212, 1991
10. Cavender PA, Bennett RG: Perianal eosinophilic granuloma resembling condyloma latum. Pediatr Dermatol 5:50, 1988

Granular Cell Tumors

11. Guenther L, Shum D: Granular cell tumor of the vulva. Pediatr Dermatol 10:153, 1993
12. Majmudar B, Castellano PZ, Wilson RW, Siegel RJ: Granular cell tumors of the vulva. J Reprod Med 35:90, 1990

Genital Edema

13. Dijkstra JWE, Bergfeld, Kay R: Congenital lymphedema of genitalia and extremities. Cleve Clin Q 51:553, 1984
14. Handfield-Jones SE, Prendiville WJ, Norman S: Vulval lymphangiectasia. Genitourin Med 65:335, 1989
15. Freeman S: Woman allergic to husband's sweat and semen. Contact Dermatitis. 14:110, 1986
16. Larsson E, Weatermark P: Chronic hypertrophic vulvitis—a condition with similarities to cheilitis granulomatosa (Melkersson-Rosenthal syndrome). Acta Derm Venereol (Stockh) 58:92, 1978

SUGGESTED READINGS

Secondary Syphilis

Chapel TA: Primary and secondary syphilis. Cutis 33:47, 1984

Hira SK, Patel JS, Bhat SG et al: Clinical manifestations of secondary syphilis. Int J Dermatol 26:103, 1987

Hook EW III, Marra CM: Acquired syphilis in adults. N Engl J Med 326:1060, 1992

Mindel A, Tovey SJ, Timmins DJ, Williams P: Primary and secondary syphilis, 20 years' experience. 2. Clinical features. Genitourin Med 65:1, 1989

Sclerosing Lymphangitis

Wright RA, Judson FN: Penile venereal edema. JAMA 241:157, 1979

This paper reviews 24 cases of the disease and, among other points, describes the high frequency of concomitant sexually transmitted diseases. A color photograph of a typical lesion is presented.

11 White Patches and Plaques

LICHEN SCLEROSUS

Lichen sclerosus (Lichen sclerosus et atrophicus, hypoplastic dystrophy, kraurosis vulvae, balanitis xerotica obliterans) is a relatively common hypopigmented skin disorder that exhibits a strong predilection for genital skin, usually without affecting other areas. The International Society for the Study of Vulvovaginal Disease (ISSVD) has determined that the proper terminology for this disease is *lichen sclerosus.* This addresses the issue that affected skin is not literally *atrophic,* a term derived from the Greek "for lack of nourishment." However, *atrophic* has a dermatologic definition as well, referring to thinning and flattening of the skin, a characteristic of lichen sclerosus. Therefore, this disease retains its full name in many nongynecology settings.

Until recently, gynecologic terminology classified lichen sclerosus as hypoplastic dystrophy, as compared with hyperplastic dystrophy (neurodermatitis and other causes of epithelial hyperplasia) or mixed dystrophy (lichen sclerosus with superimposed neurodermatitis). Whereas both lichen sclerosus and lichen sclerosus et atrophicus are acceptable terminology, the term *dystrophy* should be avoided, since it confuses by referring to totally unrelated diseases.

Clinical Presentation

Although by far most common on the vulva and perianal skin of adult women, lichen sclerosus occurs in both sexes and at any age. This disease is uncommon in infancy, but it has been reported in children as young as 4 weeks. Lichen sclerosus is well known to occur in prepubertal girls, and despite its reported rarity in young boys, several reviews of the histology of foreskins removed during circumcision for phimosis in boys have shown the presence of lichen sclerosus in many[1,2] (Fig. 11-1). Lichen sclerosus is most common in white and Hispanic patients and is rare in blacks.

Pruritus is a common presenting complaint, especially in women. Itching may be excruciating and life-ruining. Pain also occurs, especially as a consequence of scratching fragile skin or in association with coitus. Some patients describe frequent sores or bleeding. However, some patients are totally asymptomatic, and skin changes are discovered only on a routine examination. Patients are often well until an intermittent event such as vulvovaginal candidiasis precipitates symptoms that continue after appropriate therapy for the precipitating event (Fig. 11-2).

Clinically, classic lichen sclerosus presents as well-demarcated white plaques of thin, fragile skin. These

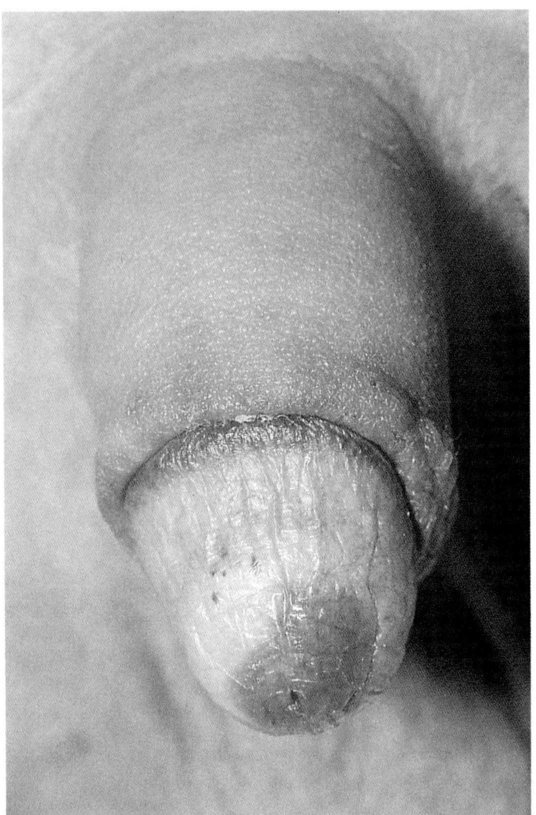

Fig. 11-1. Typical white, crinkled skin of the glans of a small boy diagnosed with lichen sclerosus at circumcision for "idiopathic" phimosis.

plaques usually occur first on the modified mucous membranes of the vulva or perianal area of women, or under the foreskin of uncircumcised males. Some believe that this distribution occurs partly because lichen sclerosus seems to exhibit Köbner's phenomenon: the disease appears at a site of injury or irritation, such as occurs in these areas from warmth, friction, and accumulation of sweat and keratin debris. Characteristic, fine surface crinkling is common (Fig. 11-3), but surface appearance and texture vary depending upon the location, degree of dampness, and extent of scratching. Atrophic modified mucous membrane skin often appears smooth, without the normal surface irregularities produced by sebaceous glands and skin lines. Because of the atrophic changes, fragility manifested by erosions and purpura are common (Figs. 11-4 and 11-5). A less common consequence of fragility is blistering that may be hemorrhagic. More marked disease is characterized by hyperkeratosis often produced by rubbing or scratching (Fig. 11-6). This may appear as scale or as irregular keratotic papules or plaques that are white as a result of hydration.

As the disease progresses, scarring obliterates the typical skin texture, and normal genital structures are resorbed. The labia minora scar (agglutinate) to the inner aspect of the labia majora and eventually are resorbed without a trace (Fig. 11-7). This process also occurs when the clitoral prepuce scars over the clitoris and to surrounding skin, until the clitoris is completely buried (Figs. 11-7 and 11-8). With severe disease, the vaginal introitus narrows abnormally until the associated fragility and inelasticity render intercourse painful or impossible, even though lichen

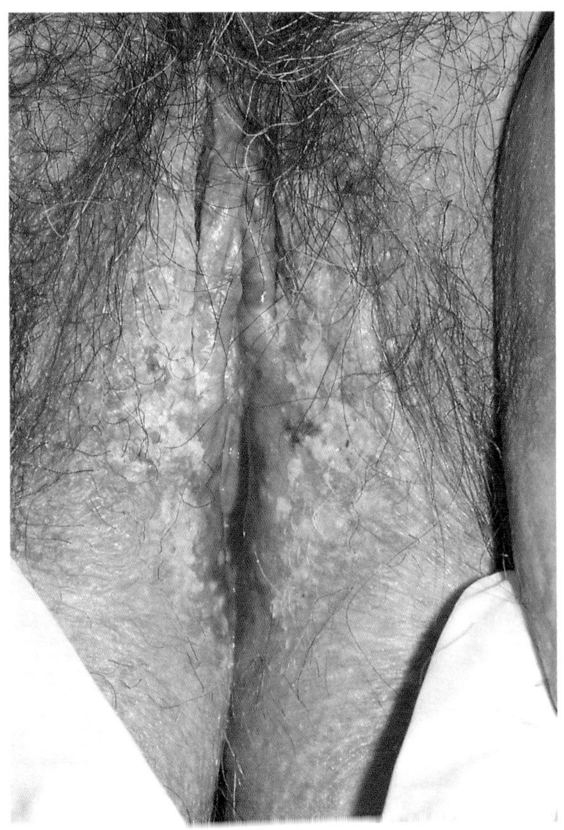

Fig. 11-2. The delicate skin of lichen sclerosus is at an increased risk of secondary infection, as in this patient with a superimposed candidal and streptococcal infection. The secondary processes sometimes initially obscure the underlying skin changes of lichen sclerosus, especially in children and postmenopausal women.

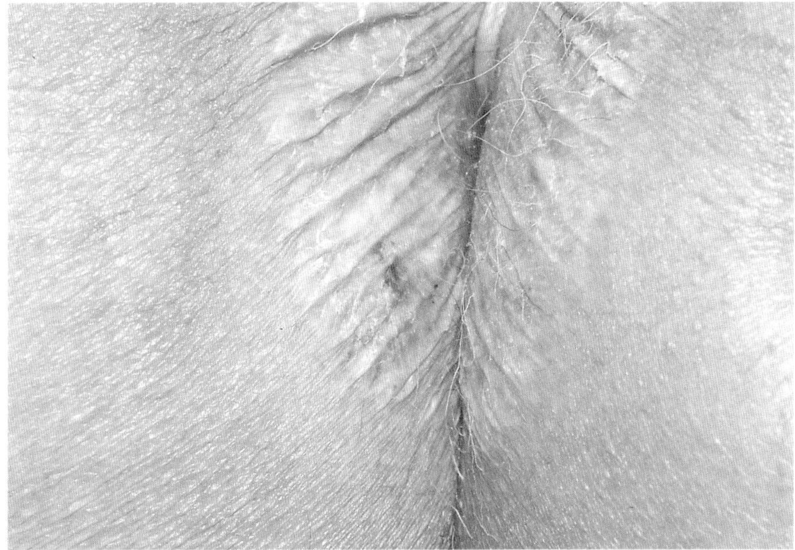

Fig. 11-3. Sharply marginated, white plaque of lichen sclerosus with classic fine crinkling and fragility as evidenced by purpura.

sclerosus never extends to the vagina or cervix. These late and severe changes are nonspecific and are referred to as kraurosis vulvae. Patchy hyperpigmentation occurs in some with lichen sclerosus (Fig. 11-7). In the absence of the most specific findings of fine crinkling, thinning, and purpura, other scarring diseases, especially cicatrical pemphigoid and late erosive lichen planus, should be considered in the diagnosis (see Desquamative Vaginitis in Ch. 7, and these specific diseases).

Similar changes occur on the penis (Figs. 11-9 and 11-10). Lesions are generally found on the glans and inner aspect of the foreskin, sometimes extending to the distal shaft. Lichen sclerosus is a common cause of phimosis (Fig. 11-1), but the presence of this disease may not be appreciated before circumcision since the distribution hides the obvious areas of involvement. Involvement of the scrotum and perianal area is notably absent. Meatal stenosis, fragility, and purpura may occur on the penis as on the vulva. Scarring may obliterate the normal demarcation of the corona and shaft, and narrowing of the meatus may occur (Fig. 11-11). This late and severe lichen sclerosus of the penis is called balanitis xerotica obliterans.

Unfortunately, lichen sclerosus may sometimes present with less specific skin findings (Fig. 11-12). Lesions are not always discernably hypopigmented. In patients whose normal skin color is light, or when the area is illuminated by a very bright light, subtle

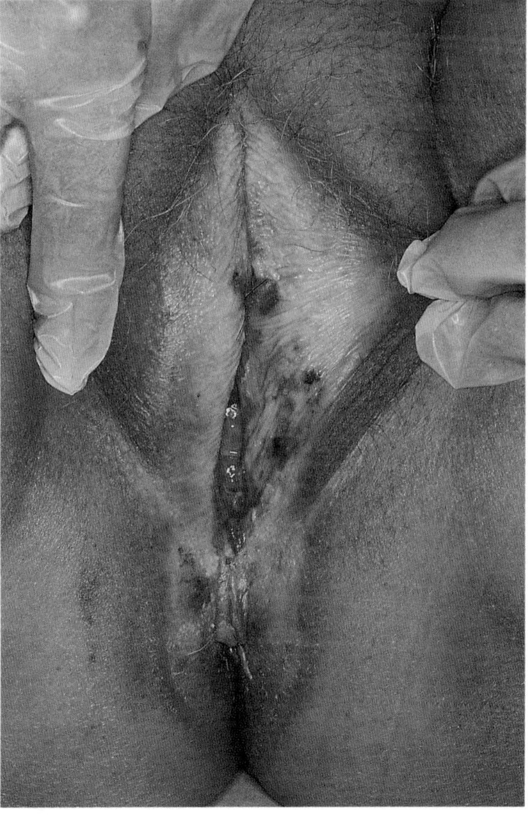

Fig. 11-4. Hypopigmented plaque with marked purpura and erosions showing the typical involvement of the vulva and perianal area in women. Atrophy of the involved skin with wrinkling and shininess is obvious.

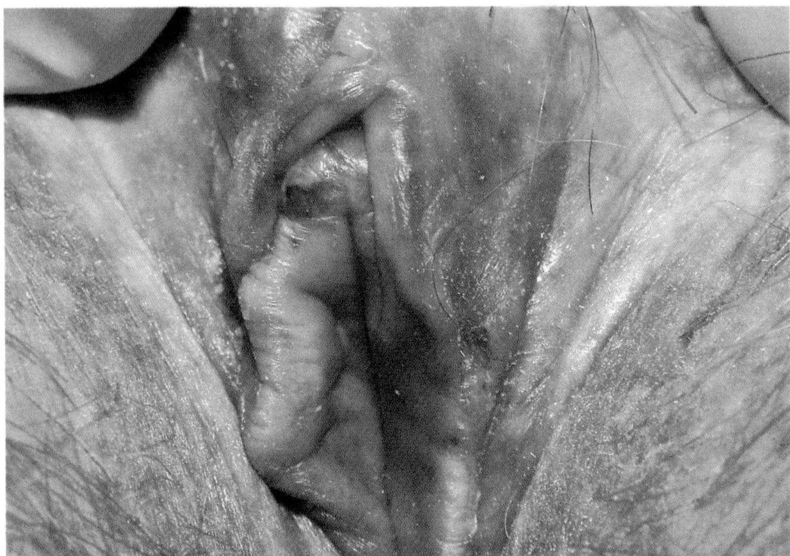

Fig. 11-5. More subtle changes of early lichen sclerosus include the edema seen here, but the mild hypopigmentation, erosions, and purpura are helpful in making the diagnosis.

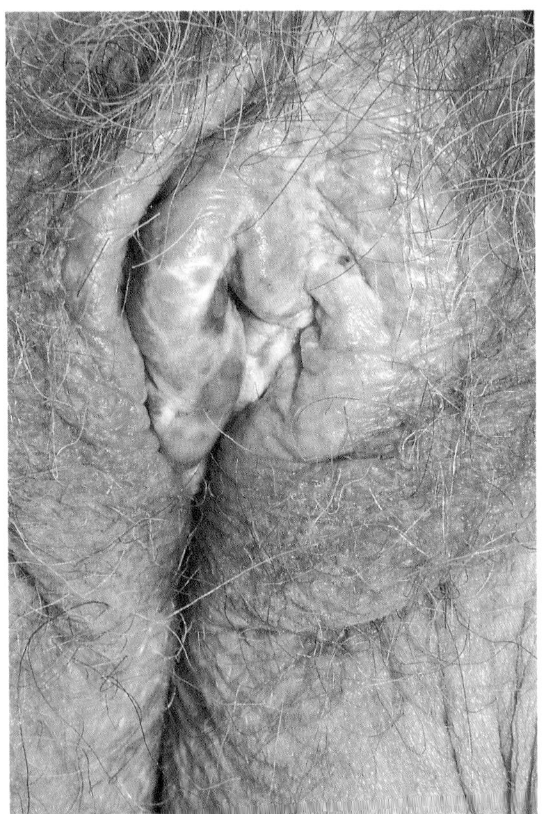

Fig. 11-6. The white hyperkeratosis and erosions associated here with lichen sclerosus can be easily mistaken for lichen planus because of the reticulate pattern, or for neurodermatitis because of the thickening, but a biopsy and lack of other mucous membrane disease indicated the correct diagnosis. Compare with Figures 5-8 and 6-11.

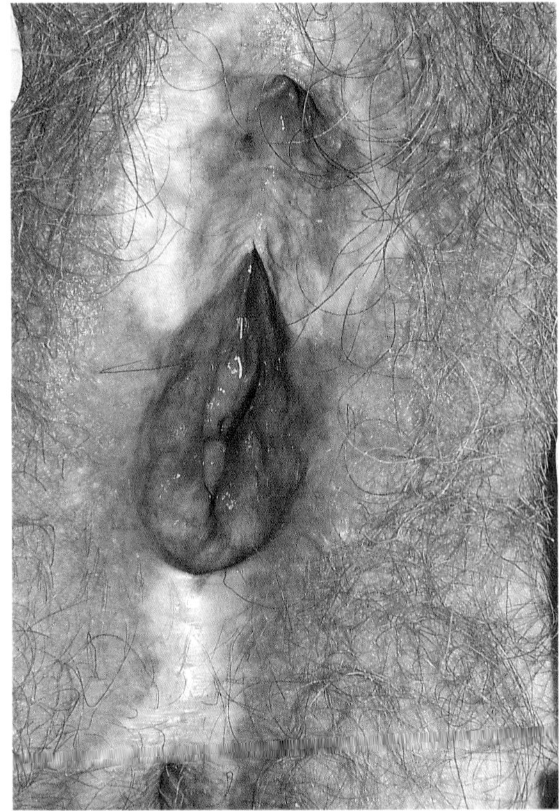

Fig. 11-7. This well-demarcated, white plaque shows not only fine wrinkling and purpura, but also patchy hyperpigmentation in the vestibule bilaterally that occasionally occurs with lichen sclerosus, and the burned-out disease of the midvulva with agglutination of the labia minora.

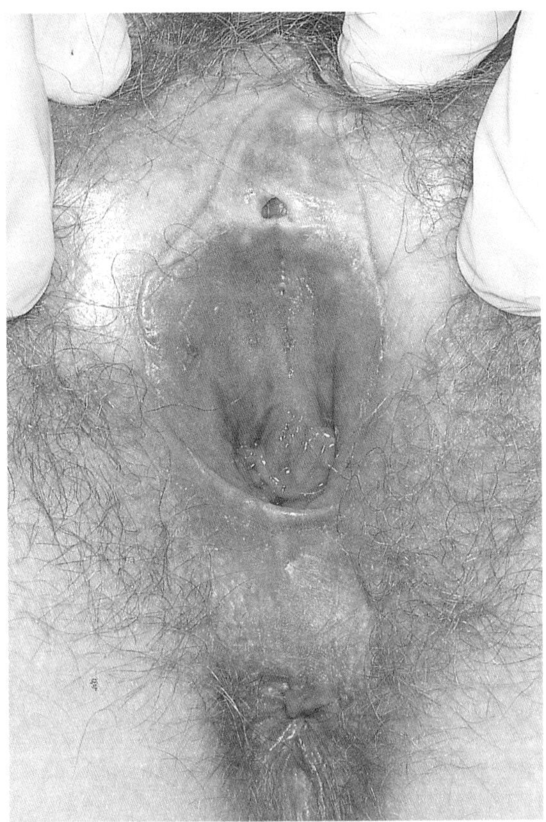

Fig. 11-8. White, shiny, atrophic plaque of lichen sclerosus with loss of labia minora, and agglutination of the clitoral hood to almost completely bury the clitoris.

hypopigmentation may be missed. Both very early lichen sclerosus and late, inactive disease are especially likely to lack the characteristic white color. Before the onset of classic clinical findings, lesions may be edematous and variably erythematous, and purpura, fragility, fine wrinkling, or small areas of typical lichen sclerosus may be discovered only with a very careful examination. Late disease may eventuate into agglutinated skin that has normal color and texture as well as negative histologic findings, and the diagnosis may be impossible if a careful examination does not reveal some areas with characteristic skin findings nearby. Sometimes lichen sclerosus is very localized, and small, distinctive lesions between skin folds are easily missed if the entire area is not inspected meticulously.

Other than the common perianal involvement in women, extragenital disease often is not present. About 20 percent of women exhibit plaques of lichen sclerosus in areas other than the vulva or perianal area. The most common locations are the upper trunk and arms, including the breasts and shoulders. Fewer than 10 percent of patients with penile lichen sclerosus display extragenital disease. Mucous membrane disease, including the vagina, almost never occurs, although there are rare case reports of lichen sclerosus with oral lesions showing suggestive histology.[2a]

Histology

The histology of lichen sclerosus is characterized by hyperkeratosis, thinning of the epidermis, and hydropic degeneration of the basal cells. Subepidermal edema and homogenization of the collagen gives the upper dermis a ground-glass appearance. Subepidermal blisters are common. Blood vessels are often dilated, and extravasated red blood cells are

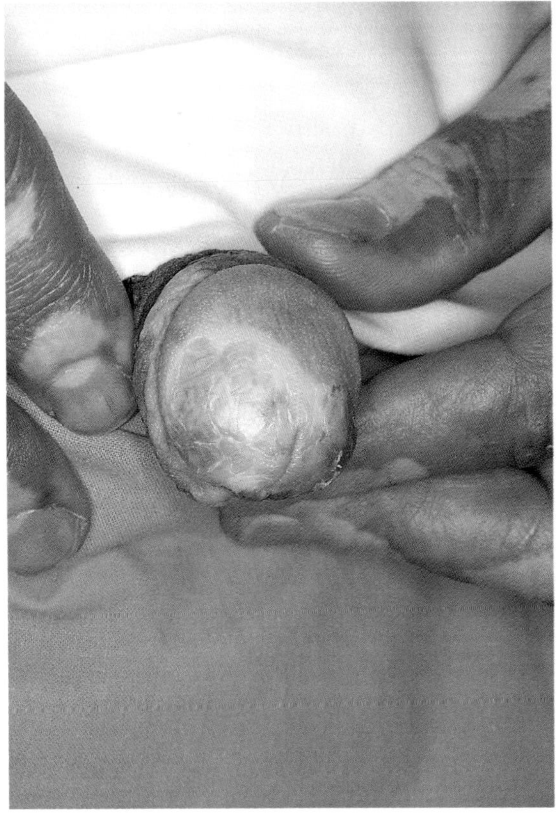

Fig. 11-9. The relatively uncommon occurrence of hyperkeratosis, as manifest by hyperpigmented scale, in genital lichen sclerosus is seen in this man who also has vitiligo.

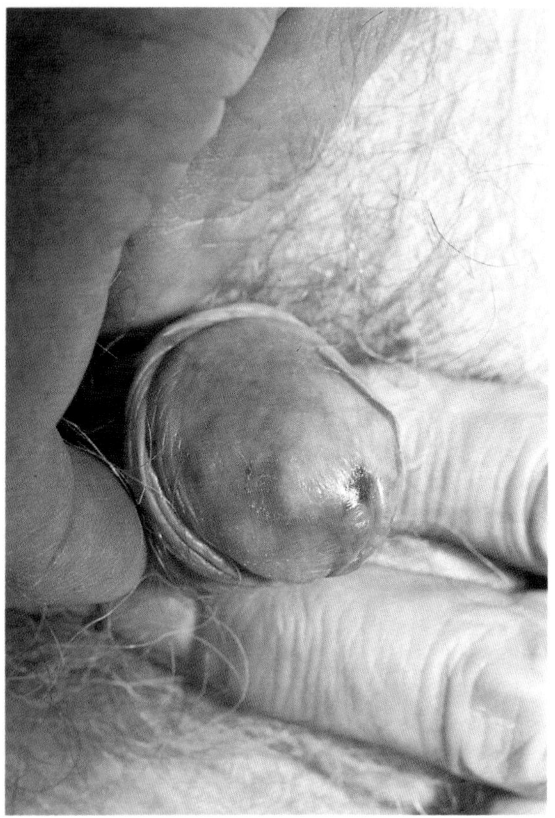

Fig. 11-10. Thin, fragile, shiny skin of lichen sclerosus over the glans penis (balanitis xerotic obliterans).

frequent. A chronic inflammatory infiltrate composed mostly of lymphocytes with some histiocytes is present in the mid-dermis, although younger lesions show a more superficial infiltrate. Some vulvar lesions, especially those present in very pruritic patients, may show thickening of the epidermis, sometimes associated with elongation of the rete ridges. These latter changes may be secondary to rubbing and scratching.

Diagnosis

The differential diagnosis of lichen sclerosus includes other white lesions and scarring diseases. Vitiligo and lichen sclerosus both characteristically exhibit well-demarcated white lesions over the vulva and glans. The presence of fine wrinkling, atrophy, hyperkeratotic papules, purpura, or erosions usually makes the separation easy, but occasionally lichen sclerosus displays only subtle atrophy, making a diagnosis surprisingly difficult. Even more difficult is the differentiation of lichen sclerosus from neurodermatitis with white discoloration due to lichenified, hydrated, hyperkeratotic skin. Because lichen sclerosus is usually pruritic, the resulting scratching and rubbing often produce superimposed neurodermatitis that may obscure the characteristic fine wrinkling and atrophy of lichen sclerosus. Agglutination of the labia minora is not pathognomonic, since this may occur as a result of any ongoing significant inflammation including lichen planus, neurodermatitis, or even as a result of atrophic changes of low estrogen in postmenopausal women. Treatment of the secondary neurodermatitis associated with lichen sclerosus with a topical corticosteroid usually allows visualization of the characteristic features of lichen sclerosus, but a biopsy may be required. End-stage scarring and hypopigmentation from lichen planus can be confusing,

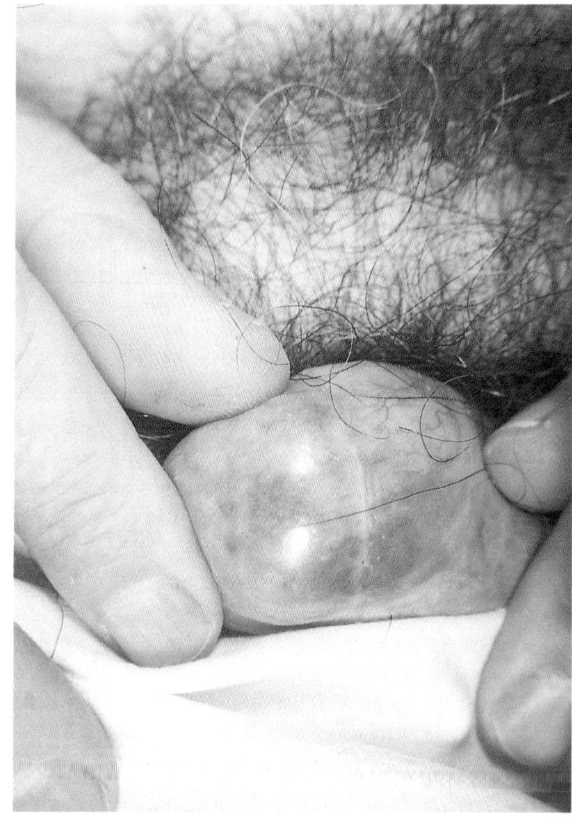

Fig. 11-11. Although less common in men, penile lichen sclerosus can sometimes also result in scarring and atrophy as evidenced by the shiny, thin, and smooth skin (balanitis xerotica obliterans). The coronal sulcus has been obliterated.

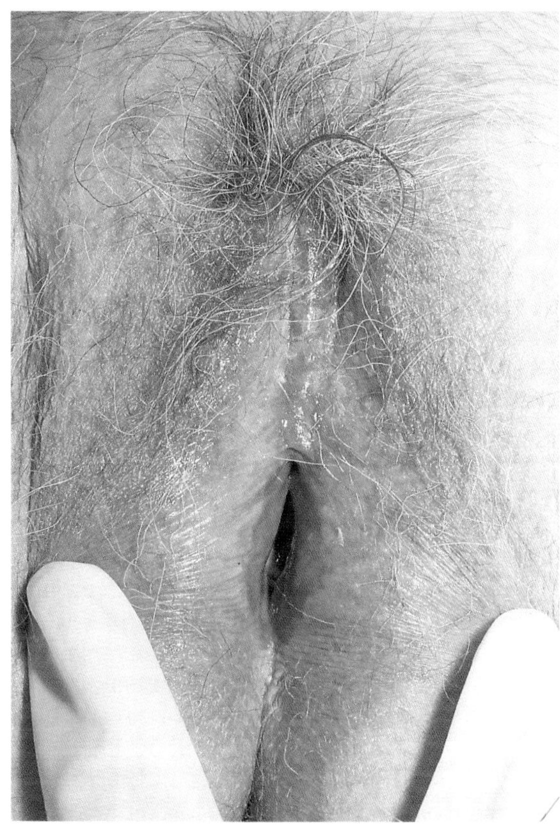

Fig. 11-12. Late, burned-out lichen sclerosus may not exhibit the white, well-marginated plaques with fine wrinkling, but show primarily scarring. Diagnosis may be difficult since biopsies often do not show diagnostic histology, and sometimes several samples must be taken. Compare with Figures 6-14 and 16-9.

and a search for typical vaginal and oral lesions as well as skin biopsy is often necessary. Some diseases producing erosions or end-stage scarring that are occasionally confused with lichen sclerosus are summarized in Table 6-1. Fine crinkling and purpura of the skin are absent in lichen planus as well as in other diseases to be considered, especially cicatricial pemphigoid, epidermolysis bullosa acquisita, and pemphigus vulgaris. Late, scarring lichen sclerosus of the vulva and penis may be nonspecific, and the differential diagnosis is listed in Table 6-1.

Course and Prognosis

Although lichen sclerosus is a chronic condition in all adults, those appropriately treated with proper therapy do very well, with cessation of symptoms and scarring, as well as reversal of the fragility, hypopigmentation, and hyperkeratosis of the skin. On the other hand, there is no reversal of existing scarring, and the disease does not usually remit permanently. Ongoing topical therapy is generally necessary to maintain control of the disease, and occasionally surgery is required to lyse scars that interfere with function.

In the past, prepubital girls with vulvar lichen sclerosus were believed to experience complete resolution at puberty, but this is no longer felt to be true. However, lichen sclerosus in young boys who undergo circumcision often resolves.

Lichen sclerosus affects the skin only, although there is an increased incidence of autoimmune disease. About 20 percent of women have an autoimmune disorder, and almost one half exhibit at least one autoantibody.[3] The most common autoimmune diseases associated with lichen sclerosus in women are alopecia areata, vitiligo, and thyroid disease. It also has been reported to occur in association with morphea (localized scleroderma) and lichen planus. Women with lichen sclerosus have an increased incidence of autoimmune disease present in first-degree relatives.

There is a clear association of vulvar and probably penile lichen sclerosus with squamous cell carcinoma, although the cause-and-effect relationship is debated (Fig. 11-13). Large series of patients with vulvar lichen sclerosus have shown a 4 to 5 percent incidence of malignancy.[4] Although the carcinomas are probably unrelated to human papillomavirus (HPV) infection, these reports predated the availability of sophisticated tests for the presence of this virus, and some reports appeared before the association of HPV and squamous cell carcinoma was known. Many believe that the increased risk of malignancy with lichen sclerosus results from inflammation and chronic rubbing, but this supposition is controversial. The occurrence of squamous cell carcinoma in penile disease is limited to case reports,[5,6] and there seems to be no increased risk of carcinoma development in extragenital disease.

Pathogenesis

The etiology of lichen sclerosus is not known.[7] Some believe it is an autoimmune condition because of its association with other autoimmune diseases. Also, biopsies show the vacuolar degeneration of the

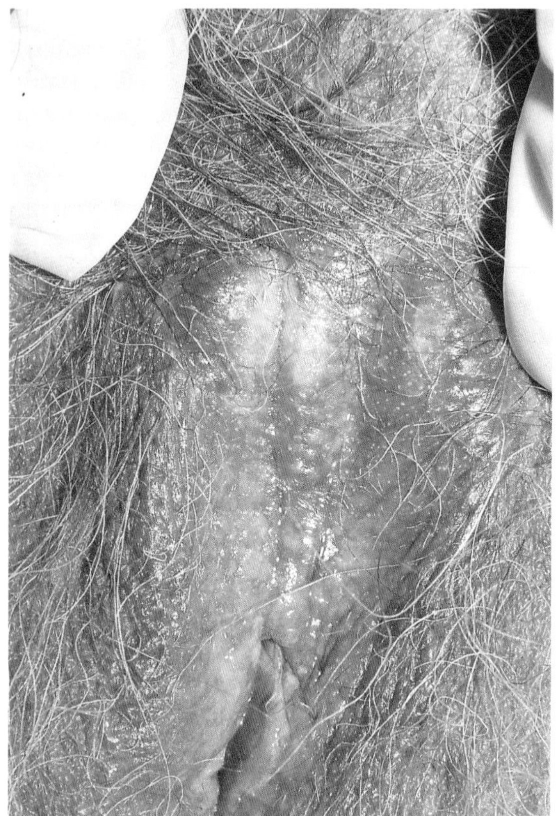

Fig. 11-13. Squamous cell carcinoma occurring in the setting of lichen sclerosus usually presents as persistent hyperkeratosis or thickening as seen here, or as a nonhealing ulcer or erosion.

basal cell layer that is common to other immune-mediated skin diseases such as graft-versus-host disease, lichen planus, lupus erythematosus, and erythema multiforme; the coexistence of lichen sclerosus and lichen planus is well described. Because topical testosterone is a time-honored treatment, an abnormality of testosterone metabolism or receptor responsivity has been suggested, and some published data also suggest this possibility.[8] Other postulated associations and etiologies include an absence of collagenase, increased elastase activity, and an increased collagen-inhibitor enzyme. Abnormal keratins have been reported, and there are variable and conflicting reports of HLA associations, but familial occurrence is well recognized. More recently, an association with *Borrelia burgdorferi* has been suggested, with differing reports on its presence in lichen sclerosus.[9]

Whatever the etiology of this disease, it behaves in an unusual and fascinating fashion that suggests local environment is important. The normal irritation and traumas of the genital area probably is important by precipitating the disease as a result of Köbner's phenomenon. Not only does this disease show a remarkable predilection for the genital area, but skin grafts of normal, distant skin to the affected vulva as an attempt at therapy usually develop lichen sclerosus. This has occurred even when a myocutaneous graft from the thigh with its own neurovascular supply totally replaced all vulvar tissue.[10] However, affected vulvar skin grafted to the thigh has been observed to return to normal.[11]

Treatment

The treatment of lichen sclerosus is gratifying. Although the disease is not curable, it is controllable, and symptoms generally can be completely alleviated. Successful treatment produces reversal of hypopigmentation, thinning, hyperkeratosis, and fragility so that skin texture and color revert toward normal. However, there is no medical therapy that will reverse scarring, agglutination, and narrowing of the introital or meatal openings. Most reports of therapy for lichen sclerosus are based upon trials that examined only vulvar disease.

Corticosteroid therapy is the only treatment that affords prompt improvement in symptoms. Whatever long-term therapy is chosen, symptomatic patients often require initial control of inflammation and pruritus before other sometimes irritating topical medications can be tolerated. Normally, a medium potency topical corticosteroid such as triamcinolone 0.1 percent is all that is required to improve symptoms. An ointment base is usually more soothing, particularly when erosions are present, since the alcohols in creams may produce burning. In patients with extensive erosions or inflammation, the possibility of bacterial and *Candida* superinfection should be addressed. In addition, these patients are at risk during corticosteroid therapy for superinfection, so that reevaluation is important in the event of worsening of symptoms. Although some of these iatrogenic infections can be treated locally, many patients are too inflamed to use topical creams comfortably, and oral antibiotics and anticandidal agents are often a better choice. In patients who initially report inability to sleep because of pruritus and scratching, nighttime sedation is extremely important.

More recently, corticosteroids have been shown not only to improve symptoms initially but also actually to improve the disease process itself.[12] Reversal of skin findings of lichen sclerosus has been demonstrated in women treated with the ultrahigh-potency topical steroid clobetasol propionate 0.05 percent, in spite of the usual rule of avoidance of potent corticosteroids in the genital area. Although there are no reports of its efficacy in men, anecdotal experience suggests beneficial effects in this setting. In patients who are very symptomatic due to erosions and irritation, an ointment base is preferred, but as skin heals, a cream base that is less greasy, macerating, and more cosmetically acceptable often can be substituted. This medication is applied once or twice a day under careful and frequent observation for atrophy and other local adverse reactions. Physicians should be comfortable with their ability to recognize the earliest clinical appearance of atrophy, steroid dermatitis, and striae, and patients should be warned about these possible side effects and necessity for follow-up. Atrophy occurring as a result of the use of an ultrahigh-potency corticosteroid is amazingly uncommon in affected skin, especially considering that lichen sclerosus itself is characterized by atrophy. However, topical medications routinely spread to surrounding, normal skin that is prone to steroid atrophy. Medication should be given in small tubes without refills so that happily asymptomatic patients cannot disappear for prolonged periods. Patients generally require about 12 weeks of treatment with clobetasol propionate, and as signs of the disease abate, the frequency of application may be decreased or a midpotency corticosteroid such as triamcinolone 0.1 percent may be substituted. Those patients who initially do well and then experience a flare should be carefully evaluated for intercurrent infections or for an allergic contact dermatitis to clobetasol propionate.

Although corticosteroid therapy is the treatment of choice for lichen sclerosus outside the United States and is fast becoming first-line therapy within it, the most often used treatment in this country remains topical testosterone. However, recent evidence shows that topical testosterone has little or no place in the treatment of lichen sclerosus today. A compilation of reports that address results of testosterone therapy for lichen sclerosus found improvement in 93 percent of patients.[13] However, some feel that the beneficial effects of testosterone result simply from the lubricating effect of the vehicle. A recently reported trial that compared a 2 percent testosterone propionate cream with the cream vehicle in 58 patients with lichen sclerosus reported that 75 percent of vehicle-treated patients improved symptomatically, compared with 66.6 percent of testosterone-treated patients (Sideri M et al, personal communication, 1989). Objective signs of regression including histologic improvement were generally absent. Another trial that compared testosterone, clobetasol propionate, and placebo showed marked superiority of clobetasol propionate over both other groups.[14] Classically testosterone has been felt to be less effective for genital lichen sclerosus in men and premenopausal women, and it is generally ineffective for all extragenital lichen sclerosus.

There is no commercially available topical preparation of this hormone, so testosterone propionate 2 percent in petrolatum must be compounded by a pharmacist, and it should be replaced every 6 months since the shelf life is not known. This medication is applied to the affected area twice a day for 4 to 6 months, and when definite improvement is present, the frequency of application can be tapered to twice a week. Although most patients improve with this medication, the skin does not return to normal. The most common side effect is local irritation producing a flare of pruritus and soreness, especially when testosterone ointment is begun in a patient with secondary infection or whose inflammation and pruritus has not first been alleviated with a topical corticosteroid. Most patients who are comfortable at the initiation of testosterone therapy do not complain of vulvar irritation. Because significant absorption of this drug occurs, some patients experience systemic side effects. Increased libido is relatively common and can be a problem for postmenopausal women who are embarrassed by this or who have no satisfactory outlet. Clitoral hypertrophy may occur but is generally not a problem, even in those with agglutination of the clitoral hood. Other reported but uncommon adverse reactions include hirsutism and deepening of the voice, both of which may be permanent. This treatment should be avoided in children because of these systemic hormonal effects.

Another time-honored therapy with fewer adverse

reactions but minimal if any beneficial effects is topical progesterone. This medication was used primarily before the beneficial effects of topical corticosteroids were realized. It was prescribed for patients intolerant to or unresponsive to topical testosterone, and for children. It also must be compounded by a pharmacist, by mixing progesterone in oil, 400 mg in 4 oz. of Aquaphor. This is also applied twice a day. Although there are essentially no side effects, this medication is rarely used today because of its lack of efficacy.

Etretinate (Tegison), an oral aromatic retinoid, has been reported to be useful in patients with vulvar lichen sclerosus unresponsive to testosterone therapy.[15] Although this drug is used for disorders of keratinization such as psoriasis and ichythosis, there are reports of beneficial effects on lupus erythematosus and lichen planus, diseases that exhibit some histologic similarities. Several published reports of treatment with etretinate 1 mg/kg/day have shown benefit in most patients. However, in practice this therapy has not impressed clinicians, perhaps because adverse reactions and cost limit its use to those patients with very resistant disease that is most likely to be unresponsive to any therapies. Side effects include but are not limited to cutaneous dryness and fragility, arthralgias, myalgias, headaches, hair loss, and hypertriglyceridemia. It is a potent teratogen that remains stored in body fat for years. Since the first reports of the benefits of etretinate, the superiority of clobetasol propionate in regard to cost, efficacy, and side effects has rendered this retinoid of minimal use in the treatment of lichen sclerosus.

Other therapies discussed in the literature have appeared as case reports or small series and have not been corroborated. These treatments include cryotherapy, oral potassium para-aminobenzoate, and 585-nm flashlamp pulsed dye laser therapy.[16,17,18] The topical retinoid tretinoin (Retin-A) has been found beneficial by some, but its usefulness is limited by its irritant effects. It may be particularly helpful for keratotic lesions.

Excisional and ablative therapies such as vulvectomy and carbon dioxide laser therapy have been used extensively. Lichen sclerosus generally recurs after these aggressive and painful therapies. In the past, some physicians felt that, anecdotally, premenopausal women who were resistant to topical testosterone were likely after surgery to experience recurrent disease that was more responsive to the testosterone. In light of the excellent response of most patients to topical clobetasol propionate, these treatments for lichen sclerosus are outmoded. Interestingly, however, circumcision appears to produce lasting improvement or even resolution in boys with lichen sclerosus, and sometimes improvement in adult men with this disease.

Because medical therapies do not reverse architectural changes, surgery may be indicated in some patients after their disease is controlled. Meatal and introital stenosis and, less often, clitoral entrapment may require and benefit from surgical release. If the disease is not controlled and is receiving ongoing treatment, and if dilators and early lysis of new adhesions is not performed during healing, rapid recurrence of scarring is expected.

Extremely important in the management of women with genital lichen sclerosus is a regular examination for the development of a squamous cell carcinoma that has a very real risk of metastasis. The frequency of visits depends upon the severity and degree of control of the disease. Because malignancy has also been reported in penile lichen sclerosus, men should be aware of this risk and have follow-up. These tumors usually arise in thickened skin or, less often, present as chronic erosions. Any area of thickening suspicious for tumor should be biopsied immediately. If thickening is felt to represent secondary changes from rubbing and scratching, the area can be treated with a high-potency or ultrahigh-potency topical corticosteroid and reevaluated in a month. If still present, a biopsy is indicated. Any patient presenting with a chronic ulcer deserves a biopsy, and if the history suggests recent onset, the patient may be followed up again shortly after intensified therapy and treatment of any superinfections to ensure that healing occurs.

Because lichen sclerosus, is associated with an increased likelihood of other autoimmune disease, a brief examination for alopecia areata and vitiligo and thyroid function tests are warranted, at least in adult women.

VITILIGO

Vitiligo is a disease affecting melanocytes and is characterized by white discoloration of the skin. It often affects the genitalia and may be mistaken for lichen sclerosus (et atrophicus).

Clinical Presentation

Vitiligo occurs in both sexes, in all races, and at any age. The lesions are asymptomatic, and patients may or may not be aware of their existence, depending on the location and the degree of contrast with surrounding skin. Classically, individual lesions are characterized by depigmentation in the absence of erythema, elevation, thinning, purpura, excoriations, scale, or any other surface texture changes. These lesions are completely devoid of color so that the skin is stark white compared with surrounding skin. This lack of color can range from startling contrast in normally darkly pigmented patients, to an almost undetectable color change in very light-skinned individuals. The initial lesions usually develop around orifices, such as the mouth, eyes, and nose, and over bony prominences, such as the knuckles. The genital area is often affected and is sometimes the earliest area of involvement. Genital lesions are most prominent over the hair-bearing skin of the vulva in women (Fig. 11-14), and on the shaft penis of men (Fig. 11-15). Hair in the involved area is sometimes white as well, and this phenomenon is referred to as poliosis. Occasionally, patches of vitiligo are surrounded by a zone of hyperpigmentation (Fig. 11-15), or else areas of intermediate color change between normal and depigmented skin occur, called trichrome vitiligo. Within some white patches, follicular pigmentation may be apparent, heralding local improvement of the disease, while development of the disease may begin with follicular depigmentation that coalesces into patches.

Patients with vitiligo are at risk for involvement of the melanocytes of the ear, leptomeninges, and choroid and retinal epithelium of the eye, although these are almost always asymptomatic. There is a minimally increased risk of iritis that may also be asymptomatic, at least initially. Patients with vitiligo are somewhat more likely to develop other types of autoimmune disease, especially thyroid disease.

Histology

Because the primary abnormality in vitiligo is the destruction of melanocytes, the histologic abnormality in affected skin is seen using special stains that allow visualization of melanocytes. Well-developed lesions show an absence of these cells, whereas early changes include a decrease in the number of melanocytes, and melanin within the basal cell layer.

Diagnosis

Genital vitiligo is often difficult to distinguish from lichen sclerosus, another genital disease characterized by hypopigmentation, and these diseases sometimes occur together (Fig. 11-9). However, lichen sclerosus usually exhibits obvious atrophy and other surface changes discussed below. Postinflammatory hypopigmentation or depigmentation, especially

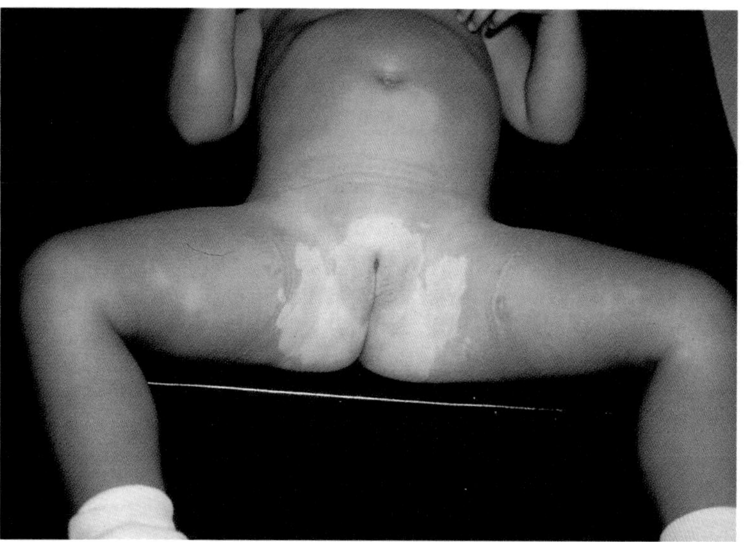

Fig. 11-14. Sharply demarcated, depigmented patches of otherwise normal skin over the vulva are typical of vitiligo.

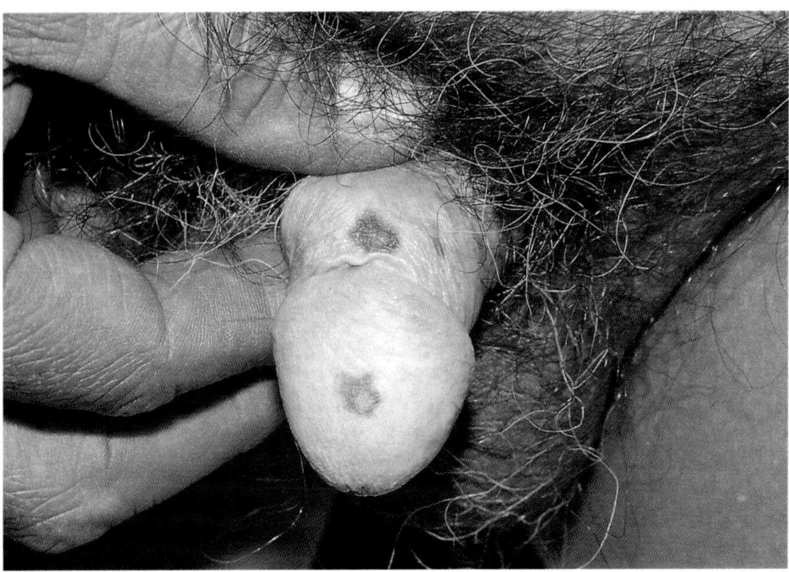

Fig. 11-15. White discoloration without scaling or other surface change surrounding two islands of remaining pigment occur on this penis affected with vitiligo.

that following severe neurodermatitis in black patients, can be extremely difficult to differentiate from vitiligo, although in white patients the lesions exhibit less sharp margination, and both usually report a history of pruritus. Other white genital lesions to be considered, such as lichen planus and other causes of hyperkeratosis, usually can be excluded by the obvious surface changes and associated findings.

The diagnosis of vitiligo is usually made on the basis of the appearance of the lesions and the pattern of involvement over the other body surfaces. In patients who are light complexioned, identification of other involvement may be difficult. These patients can be examined quickly in a dark room with a Wood's light, a long-wave ultraviolet light that enhances the contrast between normal and depigmented skin. This light discloses any depigmented patches as bright white areas on otherwise shadowed skin. A distribution pattern of depigmentation characteristic of vitiligo will make the diagnosis. Occasionally, a patient presents with only genital lesions. A biopsy may help to make the diagnosis, as will following the disease for its pattern of progression.

Course and Prognosis

Vitiligo can be either stable or (usually) slow progressive. It does not generally spontaneously remit, and even successful repigmentation with therapy is normally incomplete.

Pathogenesis

The cause of vitiligo is unknown, but several theories have been advanced. Most feel that this is an autoimmune destruction of melanocytes because of its association with other autoimmune diseases and the presence of autoantibodies both to melanocytes[19] and to other organs.[20] Because of clinical, ultrastructural, and biochemical findings, some feel that neurochemical mediators may induce melanocyte destruction,[21] especially when vitiligo occurs in a segmental distribution. A small subset of patients seems to inherit the predilection for this disease in an autosomal recessive fashion. Finally, toxic metabolites of melanin synthesis are believed by some physicians to cause destruction of the melanocytes.[22]

Treatment

The treatment of vitiligo in any area is difficult, and this is especially true for disease occurring on the genitalia. Some patients respond to chronic topical corticosteroid use, but they should be aware that this medication is associated with the side effects of atrophy, striae, and steroid dermatitis. Patients should be examined frequently and carefully for signs of atrophy both in the involved skin and in surrounding areas where the medication may spread. Hydrocortisone cream 1 percent can be used initially, but a midpotency preparation such as triamcinolone 0.1 percent may be necessary to produce results. In other areas of the skin psoralen and ultraviolet A (PUVA) treatment is beneficial. Oral or topical psoralen, a medication that sensitizes the skin to ultraviolet light, is followed by exposure to ultraviolet A light. Not only is this difficult from a practical standpoint in women, but also cutaneous squamous cell carcinomas of the genitalia have been reported in men treated with PUVA for other diseases without shielding of the genitalia. Small skin grafts of normally pigmented skin into the depigmented areas to allow migration of normal melanocytes to surrounding affected skin is successful in some patients with stable disease. Tattooing and dyeing the skin have also been used.

POSTINFLAMMATORY HYPOPIGMENTATION AND DEPIGMENTATION

Postinflammatory hypopigmentation (lightening) and depigmentation (whitening) of the skin develops as a result of damage to or destruction of melanocytes from inflammation or injury.

The condition occurs most often in dark-complexioned patients who may or may not have symptoms of the original, underlying cause of the inflammation. The degree of lightening of the skin may not correlate with the degree of the cutaneous insult. The distribution depends upon the offending agent. A common cause is a well-scratched vulvar or scrotal neurodermatitis that shows a light or white patch over the area of the dermatitis. For unknown reasons, the white change in this setting is often well demarcated even though the neurodermatitis was not. Black and Hispanic children often experience poorly demarcated hypopigmentation following diaper dermatitis. Cryotherapy for genital warts sometimes produces white macules in the distribution of the treatment.

A biopsy may be helpful by ruling out other diseases. The epithelium is normal. A sparse superficial perivascular lymphocytic inflammatory infiltrate is present with numerous melanophages.

The differential diagnosis includes other white lesions such as vitiligo, lichen sclerosus, and hyperkeratotic conditions that appear white because of hydration of the stratum corneum.

Postinflammatory hypopigmentation usually slowly repigments, but no therapy is available to enhance this process. Depigmented disease may be permanent, and there is likewise no effective therapy.

HYPERKERATOSIS OVERLYING ECZEMATOUS AND MALIGNANT DISEASE

At one time or another you probably have noticed that, following prolonged water immersion, your fingertips turned white. Keratin, the end product of keratinizing epithelial cells, is hydrophilic. When keratin becomes macerated ("waterlogged") it turns white. Not surprisingly, the more keratin and more moisture that is present, the more marked this phenomenon is. Many mucocutaneous diseases are associated with increased keratin formation; histologically this is seen as a thickening of the stratum corneum termed hyperkeratosis. When these diseases are encountered in the moist environment of the anogenital region, both of the factors required for white color are present. Of the many diseases meeting these requirements, two can be viewed as prototypical: squamous cell carcinoma and atopic/neurodermatitis.

Squamous Cell Carcinoma

The pathophysiology of squamous cell carcinoma (SCC) includes uncontrolled proliferation of epithelial cells. When these proliferating cells are well differentiated, an accompaning increase in keratin production occurs. Because of the anatomic configuration of the labia, lesions of both vulvar intraepithelial neoplasia (VIN) and invasive carcinoma are likely to be situated in a persistently moist environment. For this reason, vulvar squamous cell carcinoma frequently presents as a white lesion. Penile squamous cell carcinoma, on the other hand, rarely presents as a white lesion except sometimes in uncircumcised men, when carcinoma occurs on the glans pubis or on the inner aspect of the foreskin.

Atopic/Neurodermatitis

Chronically traumatized skin thickens to protect itself. The best recognized example of this protective response occurs when callus develops on the palms and soles. However, any skin surface that is persistently scratched or rubbed responds in a similar manner. For this reason, acanthosis and hyperkeratosis are an integral part of chronic, pruritic eczematous disease such as atopic/neurodermatitis (also known as lichen simplex chronicus and squamous cell hyperplasia). When this disease occurs in the anogenital region, the lesions frequently are white.

MISCELLANEOUS DISEASES

Other diseases, particularly if they are pruritic enough to result in scratching, may also manifest this white color. Thickened, white lesions are regularly found in lichen sclerosus and are sometimes encountered in psoriasis, lichen planus, Darier's disease, Paget's disease, and Hailey-Hailey disease.

These observations lead to an important conclusion. A thickened, white appearance occurs as a result of moistened hyperkeratosis; this feature is nonspecific and frequently obscures the clinical morphology of the underlying disease. It is therefore risky to make a diagnosis based on only clinical examination when the surface of any lesion is thick and white. These lesions should be biopsied if the diagnosis is not absolutely certain or if there is less than complete response to treatment. Only in this way can both physician and patient be assured that the correct diagnosis has been established and that potentially serious disease has not been overlooked.

REFERENCES

Lichen Sclerosus

1. Chalmers RJG et al: Lichen sclerosus et atrophicus. A common and distinctive cause of phimosis in boys. Arch Dermatol 120:125, 1984
2. Rickwood AMK, Helmaltha V, Batcup G et al: Phimosis in boys. Br J Urol 52:147, 1980

2a. Aravjo VC, Orsini SC, Marcucci G, Arávjo N: Lichen sclerosus et atrophicus. Oral Surg Oral Med Oral Pathol 60:655, 1985

3. Meyrick RH, Ridley CM, McGibbon DH, Black MM: Lichen sclerosus et atrophicus and autoimmunity—a study of 350 women. Br J Dermatol 118:41, 1988
4. Ridley CM: Dermatological conditions. p. 172. In Ridley CM (ed): The Vulva. Churchill Livingstone, New York, 1988
5. Weber P, Rabinovitz H, Garland L: Verrucous carcinoma in penile lichen sclerosus et atrophicus. J Dermatol Surg Oncol 13:529, 1987
6. Pride HB, Miller III OF, Tyler WB: Penile squamous cell carcinoma arising from balnitis xerotica obliterans. J Am Acad Dermatol 29:469, 1993
7. Ridley CM: Lichen sclerosus. Dermatol Clin 10:309, 1992
8. Friedrich Jr EG, Karla PS: Serum levels of sex hormones in vulvar lichen sclerosus and the effect of topical testosterone. N Engl J Med 310:488, 1984
9. Aherer E, Kollegger H, Kristoferitsch W, Stnek G: Neuroborreliosis in morphea and lichen sclerosus et atrophicus. J Am Acad Dermatol 19:820, 1988
10. di Paola GR, Rueda-Leverone NG, Belardi MG: Lichen sclerosus of the vulva recurrent after myocutaneous graft. A case report. J Reprod Med 27:666, 1982
11. Whimster LW: Personal communication. In Jeffcoate TNA: The dermatology of the vulva. J Obstet Gynaecol Commonw 69:888, 1962
12. Dalziel KL, Wojnarowska F: Long-term control of vulval lichen sclerosus after treatment with a potent topical steroid cream. J Reprod Med 38:25, 1993
13. Friedrich EG: Vulvar dystrophy. Clin Obstet Gynecol 28:178, 1985
14. Bracco GL, Carli P, Sonni L et al: Clinical and histologic effects of topical treatments of vulval lichen sclerosus. A critical evaluation. J Reprod Med 38:37, 1993
15. Mork N-J, Jensen P, Hoel PS: Vulval lichen sclerosus et atrophicus treated with etretinate (Tigason). Acta Derm Venereol (Stockh) 66:363, 1986
16. Pennys NS: Treatment of lichen sclerosus with potassium para-aminobenzoate. J Am Acad Dermatol 10:1039, 1984
17. August PJ, Milward TM: Cryosurgery in the treatment of lichen sclerosus et atrophicus of the vulva. Br J Dermatol 103:667, 1980
18. Rabinowitz LG: Lichen scelerosus et atrophicus treatment with the 585-nm flashlamp-pumped pulsed dye laser. Arch Dermatol 129:381, 1993

Vitiligo

19. Naughton GK et al: Detection of antibodies to melanocytes in vitiligo by specific immunoprecipitation. J Invest Dermatol 81:540, 1983
20. Brostoff J: Autoantibodies in patients with vitiligo. Lancet 2:117, 1969
21. Mosher DB, Fitzpatrick TB, Hori Y, Ortonne JP: Disorders of pigmentation. p. 29. In Fitzpatrick TB, Eisen AZ, Wolff K et al (eds): Dermatology in General Medicine. McGraw-Hill, New York, 1993
22. Lerner AB: Neural control of pigment cells. p. 3. In Kawamura T et al (eds): The Biology of Normal and Abnormal Melanocytes. University Press, Tokyo, 1971

SUGGESTED READINGS

Lichen Sclerosus

Ridley CM: Lichen sclerosus. Dermatol Clin 10:309, 1992

This is an excellent review of all aspects of lichen sclerosus, including a brief discussion of possible causes, various presentations and differences in the disease and its management when occurring in children and as well as the classic features of the disease in women. The management of the disease and the association of lichen sclerosus with other disease processes are discussed.

IV Brown, Blue, and Black Lesions

12 Dark-Colored Papules and Nodules

SEBORRHEIC KERATOSES

Seborrheic keratoses are benign lesions frequently encountered in patients over the age of 40 years. Most are easily recognizable as sharply marginated, square-shouldered, pigmented papules 3 to 15 mm in diameter (Fig. 12-1). The color ranges from tan to brown-black. They are usually wider than they are tall and often appear to be so superficial as to suggest "a drop of dirty candle wax fallen on the skin." A rough, keratotic surface is present in many of these lesions and, if present, is a highly characteristic feature. Unfortunately, those that occur in the anogenital region often lack this keratotic surface and feel quite smooth on palpation. Seborrheic keratoses are most numerous on the upper trunk, but lesions on the nonmucosal aspects of the anogenital region are quite common.

Histologically, these lesions show a thickening of the epidermis with a variable degree of overlying hyperkeratosis. Characteristically, pseudohorn cysts are scattered throughout the thickened epidermis.

The differential diagnoses include pigmented nevi, melanomas, warts, and bowenoid papulosis. Scraping the surface of a seborrheic keratosis with a blade (or even the fingernail) reveals the presence of scale; this does not occur when nevi or melanomas are scraped. Sometimes seborrheic keratoses cannot be differentiated clinically from warts and those lesions of bowenoid papulosis that are brown in color. In fact, a recent publication suggests that seborrheic keratoses occuring in a perigenital location may be associated with the presence of human papillomavirus (HPV) infection.[1] It seems likely that the HPV DNA is there coincidentally, since there is no evidence to suggest a viral etiology for these lesions when they occur elsewhere on the body.

The cause of seborrheic keratosis lesions is unknown. Aging appears to be important in their pathogenesis since they first appear in midadult life and thereafter slowly increase in number. Genetic factors also play a role in determining the number of lesions; patients with many lesions tend to have family members with numerous lesions.

Seborrheic keratoses are benign and as such require no treatment. However, shave removal for biopsy is indicated if the diagnosis cannot be established clinically with certainty. Note that some authors believe that under unusual circumstances seborrheic keratoses can undergo malignant degeneration; however, we believe that these lesions were almost certainly HPV induced in situ squamous cell carcinomas from the start.

DERMATOFIBROMA

Dermatofibromas are common, benign lesions that occur in about 20 percent of women and 5 percent of men. Most appear on the lower legs, but they are not infrequently found on the thighs.

They appear clinically as very firm, somewhat indistinctly marginated, smooth papules 5 to 15 mm in diameter (Fig. 12-2). Some of the lesions are elevated

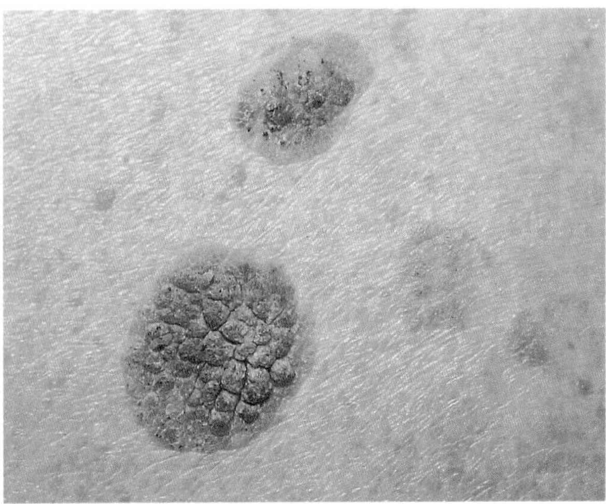

Fig. 12-1. Brown, sharply demarcated, rough, keratotic seborrheic keratoses.

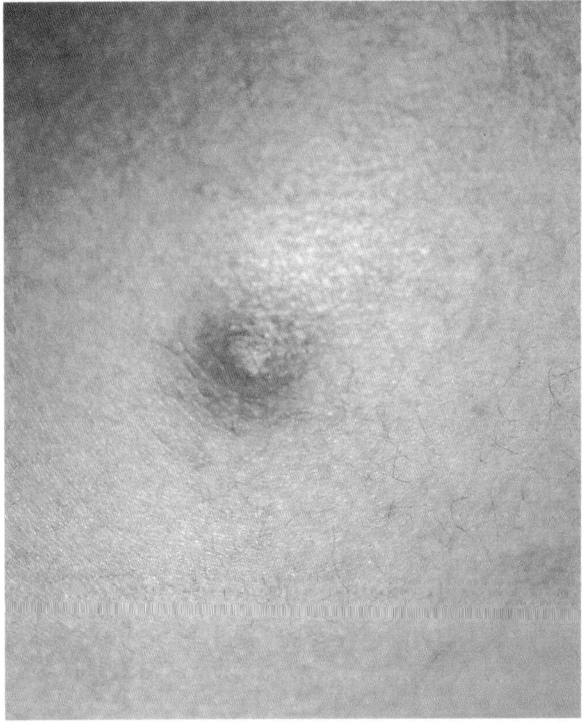

Fig. 12-2. Very firm, brown, deep nodule is distinctive for a dermatofibroma.

above the surface of the skin, in which case the margins are usually slope-shouldered. Others, particularly those that overlie fatty tissue, are level with the surface of the surrounding skin. Color ranges from pink to a fairly dark brown. They develop in early adult life, and usually only a solitary lesion is present.

Microscopically, dermatofibromas consist of a dense collection of fibroblasts with or without accompanying histiocytes. The process is well localized but not encapsulated; it lies in the mid-dermis. Because of this relatively deep location within the dermis, attempts to pick up the lesion between the thumb and forefinger fail and, instead, the lesion appears to invaginate into the skin. This "dimpling" or "puckering" sign is not seen with other skin tumors.

Dermatofibromas are usually easily recognized; occasionally they will be confused with scars because of their firmness. Scars, however, are usually not pigmented, and a history of preceding skin trauma occurring at the involved site can often be obtained. Dermatofibromas are benign lesions and require no treatment. Eliptical excision is required if removal is requested by the patient since lesser procedures result in fairly rapid regrowth. Some clinicians believe that dermatofibromas at least partially regress if they are treated with liquid nitrogen cryotherapy.

EXTRAMAMMARY BREAST TISSUE

Breast tissue can occur in any area along the "milk line," an area of the trunk containing large numbers of apocrine glands. Although common over the lower chest and upper abdomen, genital involvement is rare and is limited to the vulva. Extramammary breast tissue may occur as solitary or multiple lesions. The clinical appearance of extramammary breast tissue depends on whether glandular tissue alone is present, or if the areola with or without smooth muscle is duplicated also. Over the vulva, a single lesion composed only of glandular tissue is the usual presentation. The lesion is a nonspecific skin-colored nodule or more diffuse swelling, without surface change. Ectopic breast tissue is vulnerable to the same hormonal responses and diseases as normal breast tissue. These lesions of the vulva may enlarge with pregnancy and breastfeeding, when extramammary tissue may be noted for the first time. The con-

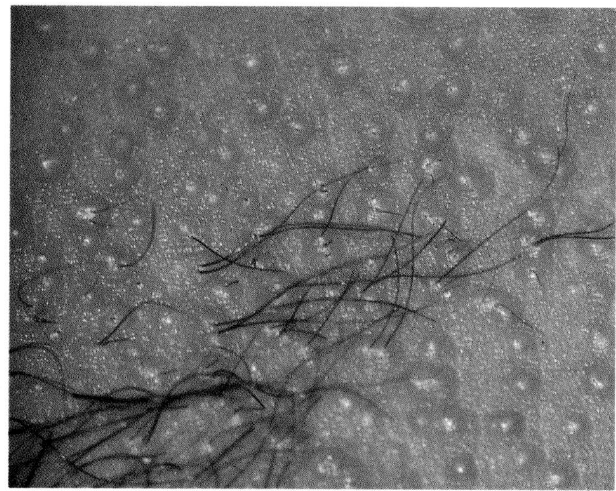

Fig. 12-3. Monomorphous, flesh-colored, dome-shaped follicular papules of Fox-Fordyce disease.

dition is often asymptomatic, but occasionally lactation without a surface outlet or hormonal influences during pregnancy may cause enlargement and discomfort. Surgical removal is often performed for these reasons as well as for diagnosis, since this tumor is not normally diagnosable on clinical grounds alone. Histology shows perifollicular apocrine glands and smooth muscle. Removal also prevents malignant change in tissue that is not likely to be routinely examined.

FOX-FORDYCE DISEASE

Fox-Fordyce disease is an uncommon condition involving apocrine gland-related hair follicles. For this reason, it occurs primarily in the axillae and the anogenital region. It is found primarily in blacks, possibly because of the increased numbers of apocrine glands known to occur in black individuals. It affects women 10-fold more often than men. Onset of the disease usually occurs after puberty, although a few cases in children have been reported.

Clinical Presentation

The individual lesions are smooth-surfaced, skin-colored or slightly pigmented, hemispherical papules 1 to 3 mm in diameter (Fig. 12-3). Each papule closely resembles its neighbors, and, while the papules remain discrete, they are set very closely together. This results in a somewhat cobblestone-like appearance of the clustered papules. The lesions of Fox-Fordyce disease are found only on hair-follicle-bearing aspects of the anogenital region. Thus lesions in women occur primarily on the mons pubis (Fig. 12-4) and labia majora.

Pruritus is usually quite troublesome and as a result, scratching and rubbing may result in the superimposition of lichenification (see Ch. 5).

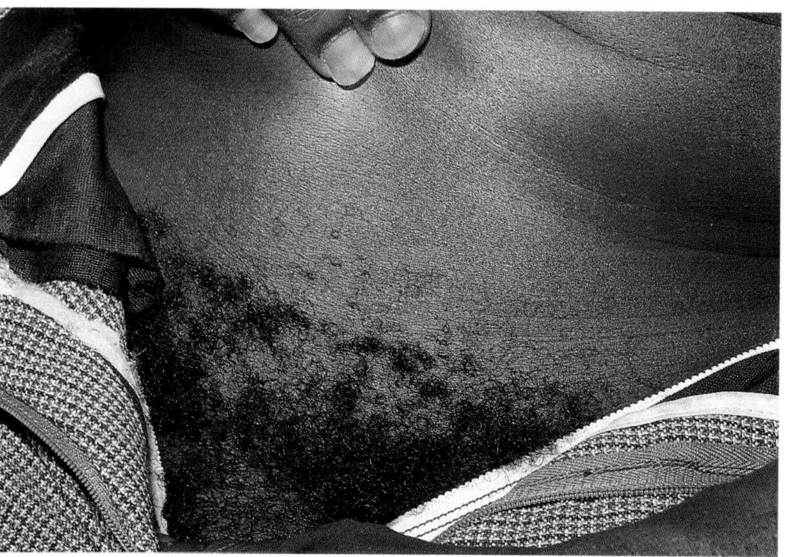

Fig. 12-4. Scattered, dome-shaped, follicular papules of Fox-Fordyce disease occurring in the pubic area.

Histology and Differential Diagnoses

Microscopically there is dilation of the apocrine duct. The ostium of the follicle may contain a keratin plug, and mild perifollicular inflammation may be present. The individual papules look very much like the papules of syringomas, although the latter are always skin-colored, a little larger, and usually not pruritic.

Pathogenesis

The cause of this disease is unknown. The histology suggests that it may be a form of apocrine sweat retention, in which case it would be analogous to eccrine miliaria. Apocrine glands are androgen dependent; this may explain the onset at puberty and involution at menopause. It is not clear why women are affected more often than men but, as for hidradenitis suppurativa, it may relate to the fact that women have more apocrine glands than men.

Course, Prognosis, and Treatment

Fox-Fordyce disease is a chronic problem. It usually lasts for years, and total remission sometimes does not occur until menopause. Treatment is not very helpful. Application of high-potency topical steroids improves the itching and decreases any inflammation that is present. There have been reports of a few cases successfully treated with topical tretinoin (Retin-A) or ultraviolet light, but severe cases may require surgical excision of the involved areas.

NEVI PIGMENTOSUS

A pigmented nevus (mole) is a hamartoma of pigment-producing cells known as nevus cells. These rounded up, nondendritic cells are derived from melanocytes. Nevus cells form in clusters at the dermal-epidermal junction (junctional nevi), in the dermis (dermal nevi), or in both locations (compound nevi). Nevi may be present at birth (congenital nevi) or may appear at any time later in life (acquired nevi). Congenital nevi are discussed in Chapter 22; acquired nevi are discussed below.

Clinical Presentation

Several clinical types of nevi occur. Junctional nevi arise as such, whereas compound and dermal nevi may either evolve from junctional nevi or may develop de novo. Junctional nevi are flat, sharply marginated pigmented lesions 2 to 10 mm in diameter (Fig. 12-5). The color ranges from tan to dark brown, or even black. Compound nevi and dermal nevi are soft, sharply marginated, pigmented papules 4 to 10 mm in diameter (Figs. 12-6 and 12-7). They are usually hemispheric in shape. Compound nevi are similar to junctional nevi in color, but dermal nevi are less intensely pigmented, ranging from skin color to a

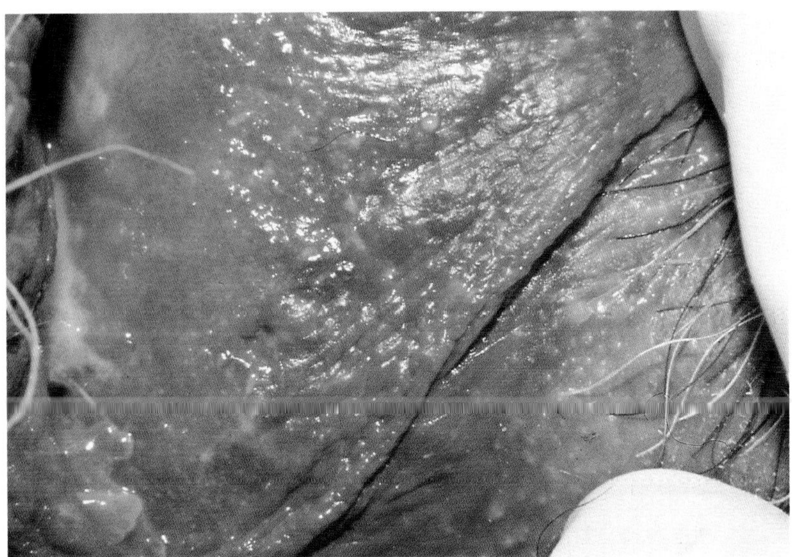

Fig. 12-5. Small, blue macule with the even pigmentation and regular, sharp borders of a benign nevus.

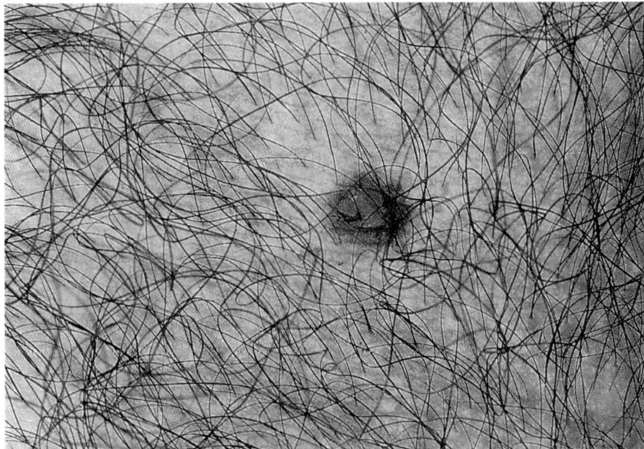

Fig. 12-6. Uniformly brown, small, benign nevus with regular borders.

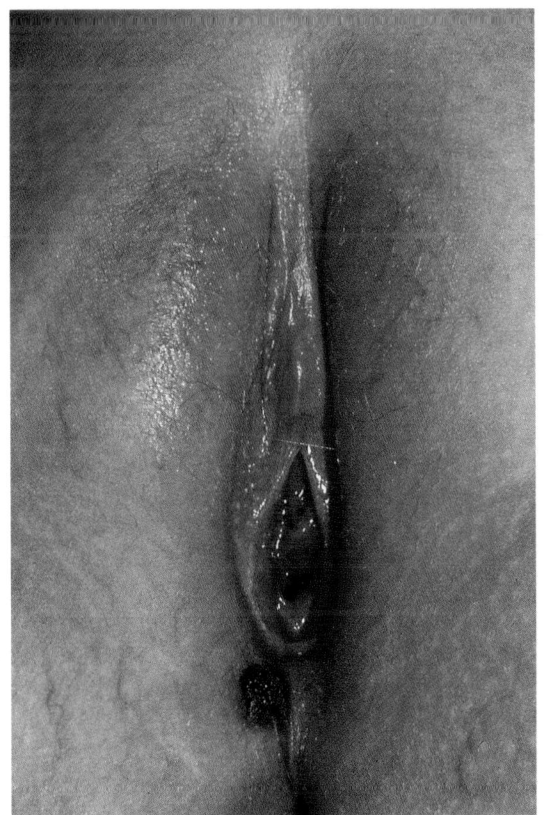

Fig. 12-7. The large size of this dark-brown plaque correctly suggests that it is a congenital rather than acquired nevus.

color slightly darker than the surrounding skin. All three types of nevi are found on the hair-bearing portions of the anogenital region. Nevi occurring on the mucosae are usually junctional in nature.

Differential Diagnoses

The differential diagnoses for elevated nevi include seborrheic keratoses, warts, bowenoid papulosis, dysplastic nevi, and melanoma. The differential diagnoses for flat nevi include lentigenes, postinflammatory melanosis, dysplastic nevi, and melanoma in situ (atypical melanocytic hyperplasia). Dysplastic nevi and melanomas are considered in the following sections.

For some nevi a clinical diagnosis can be established on the basis of homogenous pigmentation, perfect roundness, and a history of long duration and stability in size and shape. However, for many pigmented lesions, biopsy is necessary to ensure that a correct diagnosis has been made.

Pathogenesis

The factors responsible for the development of these lesions are not well understood. Trauma, especially that of ultraviolet light, is recognized as a predisposing factor since nevi arise frequently on sun-exposed skin and infrequently on sun-protected skin. Other forms of trauma may also play a role; for example, nevi seem to arise preferentially at the site of healed blistering skin lesions. Genetics may also be important because the number of nevi in a patient seems to correlate reasonably well with the number of nevi in other members of the family.

Treatment

Removal is not necessary for benign nevi occuring on the genitalia in spite of statements to the contrary found in older textbooks.

DYSPLASTIC NEVI

Dysplastic nevi (Clark nevi, atypical moles) are among the most controversial in all of dermatology; even the name is suspect. A recent National Institutes of Health (NIH)-sponsored Consensus Conference suggested that the preferred term is *atypical mole,* but this point of view has not been widely accepted by the dermatology community. For this reason we have chosen to use the historically preferred term *dysplastic nevus.* In spite of the controversy over nomenclature, a few generalizations of practical importance can be made. Clinically, dysplastic nevi have one or more morphologic features that are clearly atypical. These include speckled pigmentation, asymmetrical (irregular) shape, reddish hues, and indistinct margination. They are usually larger than 7 mm (the diameter of a lead pencil eraser) and are either flat or only slightly elevated.

Clinical Presentation

The microscopic appearance of these lesions does not always correlate with the degree of atypicality that was present clinically. Some clinically dysplastic nevi are totally benign microscopically, whereas others demonstrate features that are generally considered atypical. Such features include elongation of the rete ridges, clusters of nevus cells bridging the tips of adjacent rete ridges, papillary fibrosis, and an inflammatory infiltrate consisting of lymphocytes and melanophages. To many—but not all—dermatopathologists, cellular atypicality is not required as a part of the histologic recognition of dysplastic nevi.

Nevi that are clinically dysplastic occur with appreciable frequency. They may appear as solitary lesions or may be quite numerous. Solitary lesions often occur in individuals lacking a family history of dysplastic nevi, whereas multiple dysplastic nevi are frequently encountered in patients who have a positive family history of the same. Some of these latter individuals also have a family history of melanoma.

Dysplastic nevi in the anogenital region, as in all locations, should usually be biopsied because one cannot absolutely exclude the possibility of a melanoma on a clinical basis. Many clinicians perform these biopsies with a shave technique (see Ch. 2) because of speed and convenience. The shave technique has two drawbacks, however. First, if a melanoma is present, rather than dysplastic nevus, there is concern about removing only the superficial portion of the lesion with consequent inability to measure the depth of the malignancy. Second, dysplastic nevi removed in this manner may recur, having the appearance of "pseudomelanoma" both clinically and histologically.

Treatment

If the atypical features characterizing dysplastic nevus are found microscopically, a decision must be made regarding follow-up. No specific follow-up is necessary if the lesion is a solitary one and if there is a negative family history for dysplastic nevi or melanoma, or both. On the other hand, if the biopsied lesion is one of many with similar clinical morphology or if there is a family history of dysplastic nevi or melanoma, the patient should be followed at 6- to 12-month intervals by a physician skilled in the handling of pigmented lesions. This close observation is required because patients with dysplastic nevi and a family history of dysplastic nevi or melanoma, or both, are at significant risk for the development of melanoma either de novo or through evolution of one or more of their existing dysplastic nevi.

MELANOMAS

Melanomas are malignant tumors of pigment-producing cells. Some appear to arise directly from melanocytes, while others seem to evolve from nevus cells. Melanomas occur most commonly in the skin, but a small percentage develop from adjacent mucous membranes. Thus it is not surprising that melanomas occur not only on the vulva and penis but also in the anus, vagina, and urethra.

Several types of melanoma are recognized: superficial spreading melanoma (Fig. 12-8), nodular melanoma (Fig. 12-9), and lentiginous melanoma (lentigo maligna melanoma and acral lentiginous melanoma). Anogenital melanomas may appear as any of these types, although nodular melanomas occur proportionally more often in this location than they do on sun-exposed skin.

The genitalia account for only about 1 percent of the skin surface area, and yet (at least in women) they are the site for about 3 percent of all melanomas. This finding suggests that the genitalia may be specifically predisposed toward the development of this malignancy. As opposed to melanomas occurring on sun-exposed skin, incidence rates for anogenital melanoma are not rising and may even be falling.[2]

Melanoma of the genitalia is a disease of the elderly. The lesions are often large and clinically atypical at the time of recognition, and 5-year survival

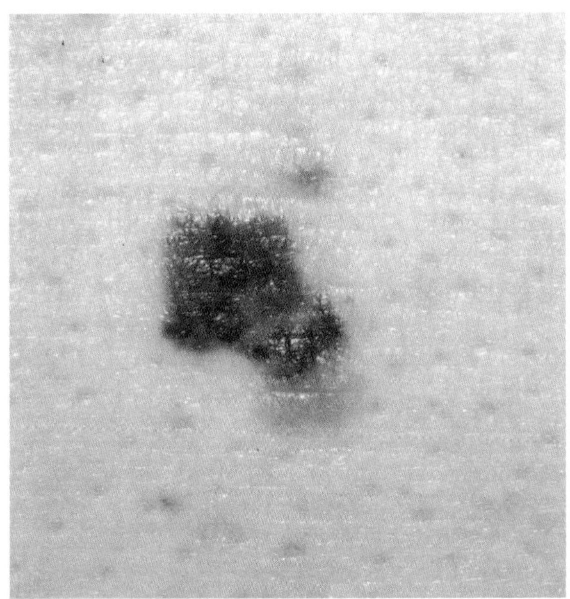

Fig. 12-8. The typical irregular borders, variegate pigmentation, and pink hues of a cutaneous melanoma.

rates are well below those for melanoma occurring on sun-exposed skin.

Clinical Presentation, Course, and Prognosis

Vulvar Melanoma

The most common site of genital melanoma is the vulva. Melanomas here represent about 3 percent of all melanomas and account for 5 to 10 percent of all vulvar malignancies, placing them second in frequency after squamous cell carcinoma.[3] More than 500 cases have been reported. Lesions occur most commonly on the labia majora,[4] but they can be found on the labia minora, vestibule, and clitoris.

Lesions may be nodular or polypoid and tend to be large (often 2 cm or more) at the time of recognition (Fig. 12-9). Most tumors are darkly pigmented, but amelanotic melanoma occurs proportionally more often than is true for melanomas elsewhere. Many are ulcerated and thus present with weeping, crusting, and bleeding.

Histologically about 50 percent are superficial spreading melanomas, 35 percent nodular melanomas, and 15 percent lentiginous melanomas.[3] Data on Clark (or Chung) and Breslow levels are incomplete, but the lesions are deep, averaging 4.75 mm in one series.[3]

Clinical outcomes are not very good; 5-year survival rates averaged about 35 percent in two large series.[2,5] Treatment in the past has primarily involved radical surgery with or without radiation therapy. However, now that it is recognized that prognosis relates directly to tumor depth, thin lesions are more often treated less aggressively, with wide local resection.[4]

Vaginal Melanoma

Melanoma of the vagina is less common than vulvar melanoma. In a large Swedish series only about 10 percent of female genital melanomas occurred in the vagina,[2] and prior to that fewer than 150 cases had been reported in the English literature.[6] The majority of patients are in mid- to late life at the time of diagnosis. The average age at presentation was 66 years in one large series.[2] Presentation is usually that of vaginal discharge with or without bleeding. Presumably because of the hidden site, lesions are large and deep at the time they are found. Correspondingly, in spite of aggressive surgery, there is a very poor 5-year survival rate of 5 to 15 percent.[2,6]

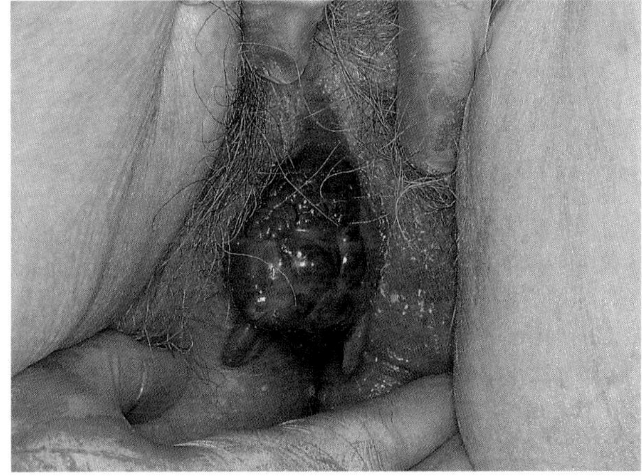

Fig. 12-9. Fungating, black, nodular melanoma of the vulva with amelanotic, pink, polypoid component.

Male Genital Melanoma

Melanoma of the penis is quite uncommon. A review of the literature in 1987 revealed only a total of 66 cases involving the penis and 27 cases involving the male urethra.[7] As does genital melanoma in women, penile melanoma in men occurs later in life; most patients are in their sixth and seventh decades. Nearly all the lesions occurred on the glans penis, with a smaller number occurring on the prepuce. Involvement of the urethra occurs primarily in the fossa navicularis. At the time of Oldbring and Mikulowski's review, only three patients were reported to have had melanoma on the shaft of the penis.[7] In 1992, only five cases of scrotal melanoma had been reported.[8]

Penile melanoma most often presents with a crusted or bleeding nodule. Pigment may or may not be apparent. As for vulvar lesions, the preoperative diagnosis is often squamous cell carcinoma rather than melanoma. The disease is quite advanced at the time of recognition. None of the patients reported by Oldbring and Mikulowski had lesions less than 1.5 mm deep. These authors indicated that about half of the patients had metastatic disease at the time of diagnosis.[7] Accurate data are not available regarding 5-year survival, but it is probably less than 30 percent in spite of aggressive surgery.

Anorectal Melanoma

Anorectal melanoma occurs about as frequently as does vulvar melanoma; several hundred cases have been reported. These lesions make up about 0.5 to 1.0 percent of all anorectal malignancies. Most patients are in mid- to late life at the time of diagnosis.[9] As for other genital melanomas, a large proportion of the lesions are of the nodular and polypoid type. A review of the literature in 1992 indicated that bleeding was the most common presenting sign, that about half of the lesions were 2 cm or more in diameter, and that about half of the patients had metastatic disease at the time of diagnosis.[10] Histologically anorectal melanomas are deep at the time they are removed. Most are more than 5 mm thick,[10] and in an older, large series, only 3 of 26 had lesions less than 2 mm thick.[9] As expected, 5-year survival rates are very poor, averaging less than 10 percent regardless of the type of surgery.[10]

Pathogenesis

The etiology and pathogenesis of melanoma are not understood. As opposed to melanomas occurring elsewhere, sunlight exposure is clearly not playing an etiologic role. Some evidence suggests that, as for melanomas of the plantar aspect of the feet, chronic trauma can be involved, but it is not clear how trauma might be important for anogenital lesions.

Treatment

Treatment for anogenital melanomas has historically been very aggressive, but most reports, as indicated above, do not demonstrate improved cure rates for those treated with radical surgery. Melanomas are at least partially radiosensitive, and thus radiation treatment can be effectively used for palliation. Chemotherapy is of limited usefulness for melanomas in other locations and presumably this would be true for anogenital lesions as well.

Basically the outcome in melanoma depends almost entirely on the histologic depth of the lesion at the time it is removed; if melanomas can be treated when the depth of invasion is less than 1.5 mm, a good outcome can be obtained with wide local resection. Thus the major problem in treatment relates to earlier diagnosis, which in turn requires better education of both patients and physicians.

KAPOSI'S SARCOMA

Kaposi's sarcoma is a proliferative process of spindle cells that are presumably endothelial in origin. It is believed to be a neoplasm, but spontaneous regression in some cases raises the possibility that, in some settings at least, it is a reactive rather than malignant condition. The disease occurs in several settings: a classical form in elderly men (often Jewish) of Mediterranean origin; endemic disease in indigenous Africans; and as a more rapidly disseminated disease in immunosuppressed individuals such as those who are infected with human immunodeficiency virus (HIV) and those who have received solid organ transplants. Men are affected much more often than are women.

Clinical Presentation

Kaposi's sarcoma often involves the genitalia as part of disseminated cutaneous disease. In spite of this, only a handful of cases of genital involvement have been reported.[11] The cutaneous lesions of Kaposi's sarcoma are multiform, consisting of patches, plaques, nodules, and larger tumors (Fig. 12-10). Ulceration may or may not be present. The color of the lesions ranges from deeply violaceous to dusky red. Lesions occurring on the genitalia are similar in appearance to those occurring elsewhere.

While the clinical lesions are quite distinctive, the histologic picture, especially in early lesions, may be quite difficult to recognize. Biopsy reveals a vascular tumor with proliferation of erythrocyte-filled vascular slits and blood vessels with prominent endothelial cells. These vessels are surrounded by a fairly dense concentration of spindle cells. Inflammatory cells, extravasated erythrocytes, and hemosiderin pigment are also generally present. The cell from which these tumors are derived is not known with certainty. Most believe that the tumor arises from endothelial cells, but others favor an origin from perivascular dendritic cells.

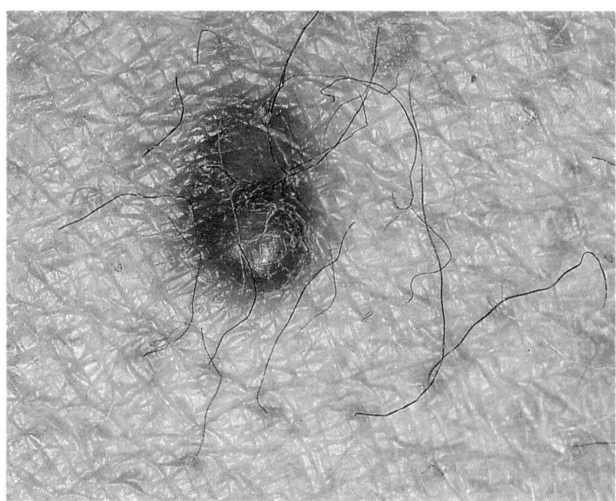

Fig. 12-10. Violaceous nodule of AIDS-associated Kaposi's sarcoma.

Treatment

The initial lesions of Kaposi's sarcoma are usually found on the skin or mucous membranes. Subsequent lesions may appear internally, especially in the lymph nodes and intestine. Treatment depends on the setting and the degree to which dissemination has occurred. When possible, factors leading to the presence of immune suppression should be modified. Systemic chemotherapy will be required if systemic disease is present. Individual small skin lesions can be treated with cryotherapy or intralesional injections of vinblastine.[12] Large lesions and disseminated cutaneous disease are best treated with radiotherapy.

REFERENCES

Seborrheic Keratoses

1. Leonardi CL, Zhu WY, Kinsey WH, Penneys NS: Seborrheic keratoses from the genital region may contain human papillomavirus DNA. Arch Dermatol 127:1203, 1991

Melanoma

2. Ragnarsson-Olding B, Johansson H, Rutqvist LE, Ringborg U: Malignant melanoma of the vulva and vagina. Trends in incidence, age distribution, and long term survival among 245 consecutive cases in Sweden 1960–1984. Cancer 71:1893, 1993
3. Ronan SG, Eng AM, Briele HA et al: Malignant melanoma of the female genitalia. J Am Acad Dermatol 22:428, 1990
4. Look KY, Roth LM, Sutton GP: Vulvar melanoma reconsidered. Cancer 72:143, 1993
5. Bradgate MG, Rollason TP, McConkey CC, Powell J: Malignant melanoma of the vulva: a clinico-pathological study of 50 women. Br J Obstet Gynaecol 97:124, 1990
6. Bonner JA, Perez-Tamayo C, Reid GC et al: The management of vaginal melanoma. Cancer 62:2066, 1988
7. Oldbring J, Mikulowski P: Malignant melanoma of the penis and male urethra. Report of nine cases and review of the literature. Cancer 59:581, 1987
8. Moul JW, McLeod DG: Melanomas that defy clinical recognition. JAMA 267:2605, 1992
9. Wanebo HJ, Woodruff JF, Farr GH, Quan SH: Anorectal melanoma. Cancer 47:1891, 1981
10. Frank W, Kurban RS, Hoover HC Jr, Sober AJ: Anorectal melanoma. A case report and brief review of the literature. J Dermatol Surg Oncol 18:333, 1992

Kaposi's Sarcoma

11. Schmidt ME, Yalisove B, Parenti DM et al: rapidly progressive penile ulcer: an unusual manifestation of Kaposi's sarcoma. J Am Acad Dermatol 27:267, 1992
12. Serfling U, Hood AF: Local therapies for cutaneous Kaposi's sarcoma in patients with acquired immunodeficiency syndrome. Arch Dermatol 127:1479, 1991

SUGGESTED READINGS

Dysplastic Nevi

McBride A, Rivers JK, Kopf AW et al: Clinical features of dysplastic nevi. Dermatol Clin 9:717, 1991

An excellent discussion of the clinical morphology of dysplastic nevi is presented.

Seab JA Jr: Dysplastic nevi and the dysplastic nevus syndrome. Dermatol Clin 10:189, 1992

This article reviews the entire subject of dysplastic nevi but focuses on the histologic aspects.

Tiersten AD, Grin CM, Kopf AW et al: Prospective follow-up for malignant melanoma in patients with atypical-mole (dysplastic-nevus) syndrome. J Dermatol Surg Oncol 17:44, 1991

Five percent of 357 Caucasian patients with dysplastic nevus, who were followed for an average of 4 years, developed melanoma.

Kaposi's Sarcoma

Tappero JW, Conant MA, Wolfe SF, Berger TG: Kaposi's sarcoma. Epidemiology, pathogenesis, histology, clinical spectrum, staging criteria and therapy. J Am Acad Dermatol 28:371, 1993

This review article does not directly discuss genital involvement but does have two color photographs of penile lesions.

13 Pigmented Patches and Generalized Pigmentation

NORMAL AND HORMONE-INDUCED HYPERPIGMENTATION

Different areas of the body naturally exhibit different numbers of melanocytes with different degrees of pigmentation, and patients with different constitutive pigmentation produce different intensities of normal cutaneous pigmentation in these areas. Hormonal stimulation accentuates this hyperpigmentation, and increased pigmentation of the genital area as well as nipples is most marked with pregnancy or at birth when the skin has been exposed to melanocyte-stimulating hormone. The areas of the genitalia most likely to be affected are the scrotum in males and the hair-bearing portion of the labia majora and edges of the labia minora in females. The anal canal is also regularly and normally hyperpigmented. These color changes are asymptomatic and are rarely noticed by the patient.

Hormonal factors are also associated with melasma, or chloasma, an irregular patchy hyperpigmentation occurring most often over the face, but occasionally around the nipples and in the genital area. Also called the "mask of pregnancy" because of its frequent association with pregnancy, it may occur with oral contraceptives, menopause, or occasionally at any time, even in men.

The most difficult condition to differentiate from hormone-induced genital hyperpigmentation is postinflammatory hyperpigmentation. Genital melanosis and pigmented tumors are usually recognizable by pattern and asymmetry.

Treatment is unnecessary and unavailable for normal genital hyperpigmentation and melasma in this area.

POSTINFLAMMATORY HYPERPIGMENTATION

Brown color can occur from several different processes in addition to pigmented tumors. One of the most common is postinflammatory hyperpigmentation. Any injury to the skin that affects melanocytes or disrupts the basal cell layer is likely to cause changes in pigment production or deposition and result in darkening or lightening of the skin, depending on the nature and degree of the insult.

Clinical Presentation

Patients may present with a history of a preexisting inflammatory process or injury, but sometimes they have no memory of such an event. Frequently, they are even unaware of color change in a relatively hidden area until it is pointed out to them, and they may then mistakenly believe that this change is new.

On physical examination, postinflammatory hyperpigmentation consists of color change only, unless frank scarring from the preceding inflammatory insult has occurred. The color change most often is light to dark brown, but may sometimes exhibit tones of gray or blue; in naturally dark skin, the hyperpigmentation may be black. This color change can be even or irregular and is sometimes seen at the periphery of hypopigmentation. The intensity and pattern of the color change depend upon the etiology of the inflammation, which can often be inferred from the color. For example, small, irregular patches of light brown color often result from recurrent herpes simplex infection. Poorly demarcated hyperpigmentation limited to the labia majora or scrotum is often caused by neurodermatitis. More sharply marginated patches of hyperpigmentation over the upper inner thighs may occur following resolution of tinea cruris.

The intensity of hyperpigmentation is related less to the severity of the inflammation than to the nature of the inflammation and the normal constitutive pigment of the patient. Diseases that cause disruption of the basal cell layer of the epidermis or basement membrane such as lichen planus, lupus erythematosus, and fixed drug eruptions routinely cause striking hyperpigmentation as melanin is released into the dermis. Naturally dark-complexioned patients have an increased ability to produce pigment, and they experience exaggerated hyperpigmentation compared with a very light-complexioned patient.

Histology

On biopsy, the number and size of melanocytes are increased, and new dendrites are seen with melanin in transit to epidermal keratinocytes. Melanin is released from injured melanocytes into the dermis, where it is seen within melanophages.

Diagnosis

The differential diagnosis of postinflammatory hyperpigmentation includes ongoing inflammatory processes that appear darker than surrounding skin. Inflammation of black skin often appears clinically as hyperpigmentation rather than redness. Even a conscientious examination by a wary physician may not yield the expected erythema of active inflammation. Important causes of hyperpigmentation of the genitalia to be differentiated from postinflammatory hyperpigmentation are Pityriasis versi-color, pigmented Bowen's disease, or human papillomavirus-associated pigmented squamous cell carcinoma in situ (bowenoid papulosis). Although these conditions are usually slightly elevated or infiltrated on examination, at times they may appear flat. Often, surrounding genital warts are evident on careful examination. Other diagnoses to be considered include accentuation of the normal hormone-induced hyperpigmentation of the genitalia, and the bluish hyperpigmentation of mongolian spots that occur in dark-complexioned patients, especially over the buttocks of children. Early cutaneous melanomas and junctional nevi are usually recognizable as tumors rather than postinflammatory hyperpigmentation because of their localized nature, deeper color, and (sometimes) surface changes. Benign genital melanosis, an idiopathic patch of hyperpigmentation, is sometimes clinically indistinguishable from postinflammatory hyperpigmentation but may more closely resemble a melanoma when striking variegation of colors is present (see below). Other diseases of genital hyperpigmentation are elevated or scaling and obviously represent a neoplastic or inflammatory process.

The diagnosis is usually made by the clinical appearance and, when possible, historical confirmation of preceding inflammation. Patients with black skin should be evaluated carefully for subclinical, active inflammation if the diagnosis is unclear. It is especially important to identify any cause of hyperpigmentation that can be treated, such as active inflammation, or dangerous diseases such as squamous cell carcinoma in situ or melanoma. Any hyperpigmentation not easily diagnosed deserves a skin biopsy.

Clinical Course and Prognosis

Postinflammatory hyperpigmentation usually slowly fades after inflammation has completely resolved. Although the process can be hastened somewhat with medication when most of the pigment is epidermal, dermal pigment is generally not improved by this treatment. Fading of the hyperpigmentation is extremely slow, and patients should be warned not to expect obvious and early improvement. Dermal pigment may require years to fade.

Pathogenesis

Postinflammatory hyperpigmentation is related in part to the reparative process of injured melanocytes, the pigment-producing cells in the basal cell layer of the epidermis.

Treatment

The treatment of postinflammatory hyperpigmentation includes removal of any ongoing inflammatory process. Topical corticosteroids may be useful if there is doubt as to the presence of inflammation. Otherwise, reassurance is usually the only additional intervention needed. In those who are bothered by the color change, hydroquinone 4 percent cream or gel (Eldoquin Forte), or 3 percent solution (Melanex), can be used. This medication acts as a fading agent when applied twice a day if the pigment is primarily epidermal.

BENIGN GENITAL MELANOSIS/ LENTIGINOSIS

Benign genital melanosis or lentiginosis refers to uncommon, idiopathic, asymptomatic macules and patches that are sometimes clinically indistinguishable from cutaneous melanoma.

These lesions may be discovered on routine examinations, or patients may present with concerns about the appearance. The lesions show color change only, usually with irregular borders but without scaling or elevation (Figs. 13-1 and 13-2). This color change ranges from a uniform light or dark brown color to, more often, a remarkable variegation of these colors, sometimes including black or blue hues within the same lesion. Genital melanosis occurs on the glans and shaft of males. This disease in women occurs on all areas of the vulva, as well as in the vagina and on the cervix. Lesions may be single or multiple, and some may be quite large, reaching several centimeters. There has been at least one report of an extensive cutaneous melanoma apparently arising within one of these lesions,[1] balanced by multiple reports of benign courses.

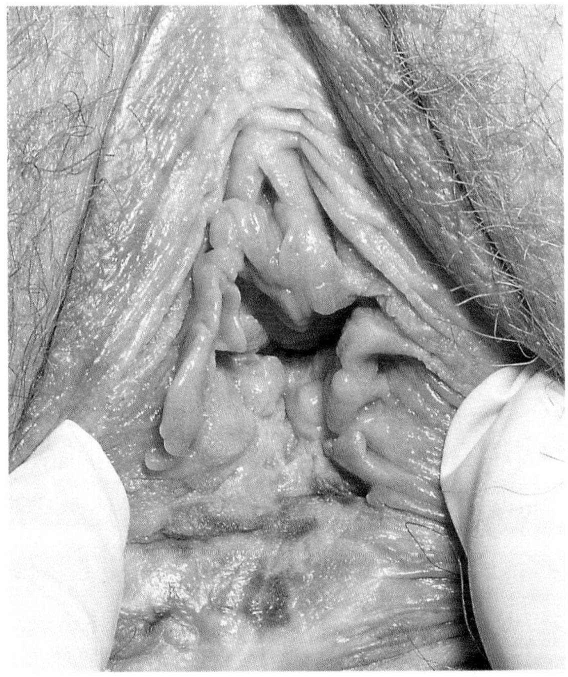

Fig. 13-1. Irregular brown and black macules of benign genital lentiginosis.

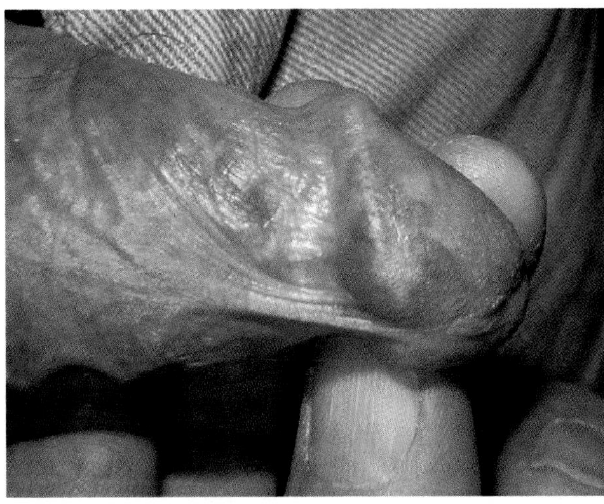

Fig. 13-2. Light brown, irregular patch of benign genital lentiginosis over the glans, corona, and, to a lesser degree, shaft of the penis.

A biopsy, which is usually indicated to rule out cutaneous melanoma, shows no evidence of atypical melanocytes, but rather basilar hyperpigmentation with an increase in the number of solitary melanocytes. Elongation of the rete ridges of the epidermis is common, and melanin is seen within macrophages in the dermis.

The most important conditions that can be confused with genital melanosis are malignant melanoma and pigmented squamous cell carcinoma. Skin biopsies, sometimes from several representative areas in atypical-appearing lesions, should be performed to rule out these more serious diseases. Postinflammatory hyperpigmentation, junctional nevi, and hormonal hyperpigmentation may also mimic genital melanosis.

Excision or destruction of lesions would be required for removal, but treatment for this condition is unnecessary beyond ruling out malignancy. This is almost always a benign condition, and extensive surgery is unwarranted. Most clinicians believe that reassurance alone is appropriate, but the past occurrence of a melanoma indicates that the issue of follow-up is not totally resolved.

ACANTHOSIS NIGRICANS

Acanthosis nigricans is a relatively common skin finding characterized by thickened intertriginous brown plaques that occur primarily in obese people.

Patients with acanthosis nigricans usually are asymptomatic and either are unaware of the presence of this condition or are simply annoyed at the dirty brown color that they cannot wash off. These skin changes are most often found over the lateral aspect of the neck and the axillae, and in the crural creases and proximal, medial thighs (Fig. 13-3). The affected skin shows thickened, brown, velvety plaques that are relatively well demarcated. The papillomatous nature of the plaques often can be appreciated at the center of the plaque, where accentuation of skin folds is most distinct and the disease most prominent. In patients with marked disease, these papillomatous changes can be associated with clinically apparent skin tags, and changes can be seen on other skin surfaces subject to friction such as over the knuckles.

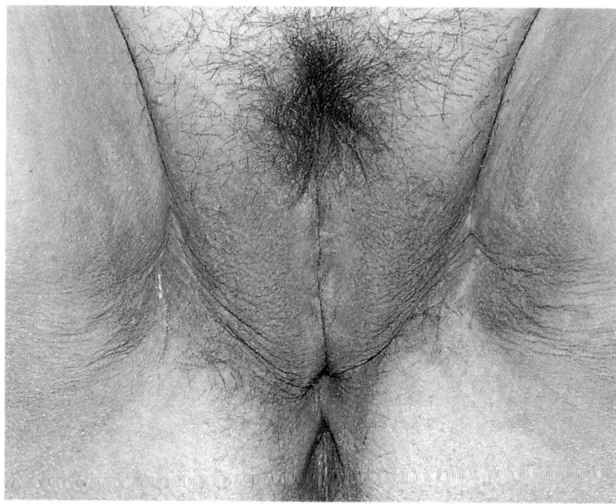

Fig. 13-3. Poorly demarcated, thickened, velvety brown plaques characteristic of acanthosis nigricans.

The majority of patients with acanthosis nigricans exhibit at least chemical evidence of insulin resistance.[2] Much less often than other endocrinopathies, malignancies of the gastrointestinal tract, breast, ovaries, lung, and prostate, and the use of some medications, such as niacin, are associated with this cutaneous finding.

Histologically, the name *acanthosis nigricans* is a misnomer, since neither significant acanthosis nor increased melanin is present. Rather, this condition is characterized by papillomatosis and hyperkeratosis.

There are few other diseases in the differential diagnosis of acanthosis nigricans. In severe disease, skin tags and genital warts may appear to be present.

The treatment for acanthosis nigricans is weight loss and reassurance. In patients who are not obese or who exhibit extensive and remarkable skin disease, a workup for important underlying systemic disease is indicated.

REFERENCES

Benign Genital Melanosis/Lentiginosis

1. Kerley SW, Blute ML, Keeney GL: Multifocal malignant melanoma arising in vesicovaginal melanosis. Arch Pathol Lab Med 115:950, 1991

Acanthosis Nigricans

2. Hud JA, Cohen JB, Wagner JM, Cruz PD: Prevalence and significance of acanthosis nigricans in an adult population. Arch Dermatol 128:941, 1992

SUGGESTED READINGS

Benign Genital Melanosis/Lentiginosis

Barnhill RL, Albert LS, Shama SK et al: Genital lentiginoisis: a clinical and histopathologic study. J Am Acad Dermatol 22:453, 1990

This report is a literature review of the clinical and histologic findings in patients with genital melanosis and adds ten cases to those already reported.

Estrada R, Kaufman R: Benign vulvar melanosis. J Reprod Med 38:5, 1993

The authors describe 11 patients with benign vulvar melanosis; location, size, and treatment are included.

V Pustules, Vesicles, Bullae, and Erosions

14 Pustules and Pseudopustules

FOLLICULITIS

Folliculitis is a common papulopustular eruption resulting from inflammation of the superficial portion of hair follicles.

Clinical Presentation

Patients often present with complaints of pruritus or mild tenderness, although symptoms are sometimes absent. Careful examination of the affected area usually yields a variable number of pustules (Fig. 14-1), sometimes but not necessarily pierced by a visible hair. However, this pustule is short-lived and often not obvious. Scattered, discrete, superficial red papules often predominate (Fig. 14-2). Some of these papules are dome-shaped and nonscaling, while others have a central crust. The lesions of folliculitis range from about 2 to 10 mm. Many patients have associated furunculosis, representing a deeper infection of the follicle. In those individuals with pruritic disease, excoriations or secondary eczema manifested by erythema and scale may be prominent. Folliculitis can occur anywhere on hair-bearing skin, and irritant folliculitis is relatively common in the genital area, especially over the buttocks. Although folliculitis does not occur on the glans penis or in the vulvar vestibule, it can occasionally occur over the modified mucous membrane portions of the labia majora and on the labia minora, where the skin sometimes contains hair follicles microscopically.

Histology

On biopsy, folliculitis shows neutrophils around and within the hair follicle with frequent abscess formation. Special stains may reveal the causative organism in instances where the etiology is due to infection.

Diagnosis

The diagnosis of folliculitis can usually be made clinically, but the identification of the etiologic agent often requires investigation by potassium hydroxide preparation or bacterial culture. The differential diagnosis includes other papular and pustular diseases that occur in the genital area such as *Candida* infection, keratosis pilaris, scabies infestation, insect bites including chiggers and fleas, and a primary herpes simplex virus infection.

Course and Prognosis

Folliculitis is usually eradicated by the appropriate antibiotic or antifungal therapy, except for *Pseudomonas* folliculitis, which is self-resolving. However, folliculitis from any of these causes may recur and require prolonged treatment or retreatment.

Pathogenesis

The follicular inflammation of this disease can result from an infection of the follicular epithelium by bacteria or dermatophytes, or it may be an irritant,

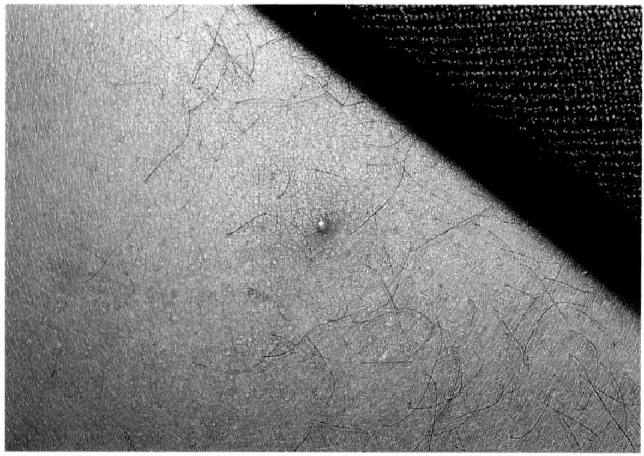

Fig. 14-1. A follicular pustule on a red base typical of folliculitis.

sterile process, often resulting from occlusion or friction. Bacterial folliculitis is almost always due to *Staphylococcus aureus.* However, hot tub folliculitis, found in patients who are exposed to contaminated water, is caused by the bacterium *Pseudomonas aeruginosa.* The lesions are often tender or pruritic and are distributed over areas of occlusion such as the bathing suit area and intertriginous areas. Hot tub folliculitis may be associated with mild constitutional symptoms such as fever, headache, earache, sore throat, and nausea.

Folliculitis of the genital area can be caused by a dermatophyte and is most often seen in men in association with tinea cruris. It may occur within or surrounding well-formed plaques of tinea cruris, or it may remain after a preexisting dermatophyte infection has been treated with a topical agent that did not penetrate into the follicles. Fungal folliculitis of the upper thighs may occur in women who have tinea of the feet and have inoculated the legs and thighs with the organism by shaving.

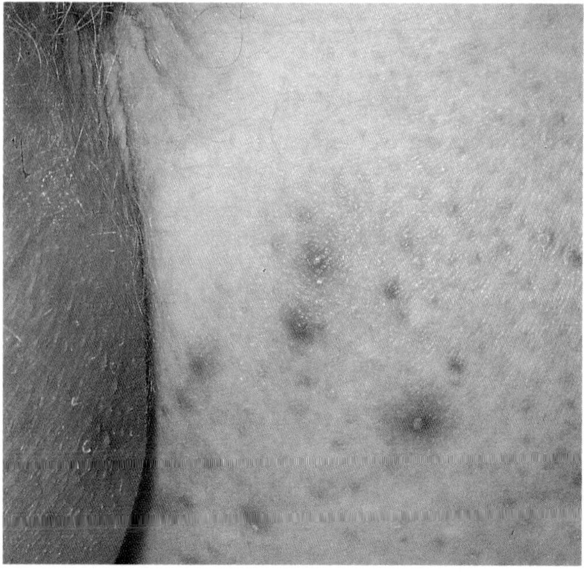

Fig. 14-2. Red papules and pustules of staphylococcal folliculitis on the buttock.

Treatment

The treatment of folliculitis due to infection consists of antibiotics to eradicate the offending organism. Treatment should be oral since topical medications as a rule do not penetrate to the affected levels of the follicle. Oral antibiotics with staphylococcal coverage such as erythromycin, dicloxacillin, or cephalexin for 10 to 14 days are cost-effective treatments. Patients with staphylococcal folliculitis often are carriers of this bacteria, and their eruption may recur with discontinuation of the antibiotic. This risk is minimized by the application of mupirocin ointment into the nose with a cotton-tipped swab four times a day for a week. Patients who experience recurrence often require a longer course of oral antibiotics. Patients with hot tub *(Pseudomonas)* folliculitis require no treatment except avoidance of further hot tub exposure, although recurrences without apparent reexposure occasionally occur. The treatment of fungal folliculitis requires oral griseofulvin or ketoconazole until lesions clear, usually in 2 to 4 weeks. Ongoing topical treatment to control any chronic or recurrent underlying dermatophyte infection is useful in preventing recurrences. For patients with sterile folliculitis, the use of less occlusive clothing, the avoidance of heavy creams and ointments, and attempts to keep the area cool and dry may be beneficial. Sterile folliculitis, like acne, may require chronic treatment with oral antibiotics known for their nonspecific anti-inflammatory properties, including tetracycline and erythromycin at a dose of 500 mg twice a day.

KERATOSIS PILARIS

Keratosis pilaris occurs in approximately 10 percent of the population, with equal frequency in men and women. Onset is usually in late childhood and the disease is uncommonly encountered after 40 years of age.

Clinical Presentation

The presentation is one of a "field" effect. An area of skin, (cheeks, lateral arms, lateral thighs, and buttocks most commonly) is covered by small red papules about 1 mm in diameter (Fig. 14-3). Each papule is of equal size and the papules are equidistant from one another. Most often a hair can be identified at the center of each lesion.

The only break in the "monotony" of the eruption is the occasional presence of a white summit on some of the red papules. In most of these white-capped lesions, the white material is a plug of keratin that blocks the follicular ostia; the firmness of the keratin plugs gives the involved skin a characteristic sandpaper-like feel. These keratin plugs can be "dug out" with a fingernail or a curette, revealing a small white firm concretion. A coiled hair is often present within the removed plug.

A few of the white-topped red papules, however, are usually slightly larger and are capped by a true pustule. These pustules represent a form of sterile folliculitis and as such are identical in appearance to the lesions of bacterial folliculitis. Differentiation of bacterial folliculitis from keratosis pilaris folliculitis can sometimes be difficult. Clues to the presence of keratosis pilaris include the monotonous background of the surrounding red papules, the recurring nature of the process, confinement of the process to the lateral thighs and buttocks, failure to respond to antibiotics, and repeated failure to recover *Staphylococcus aureus* on culture.

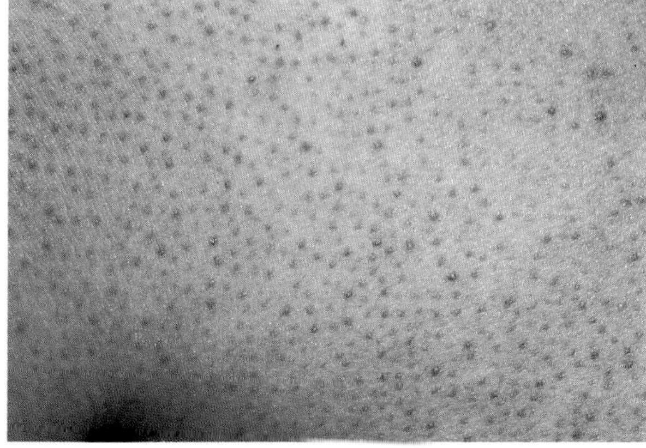

Fig. 14-3. Monomorphous, pink, pinpoint, follicular papules of keratosis pilaris, some with visible white keratin plugs.

Course and Prognosis

Keratosis pilaris is a chronic disease. From the time of its development in late childhood until the time of its spontaneous disappearance in midlife, affected patients are rarely without some evidence of the disease. Individual lesions, of course, come and go, but visible follicular prominence and palpable roughness remain fairly constant. The process is generally more troublesome in the winter when low humidity increases the dryness of the skin. Scarring can occur at the site of the more inflammatory lesions, but this is rarely encountered in the anogenital region.

Pathogenesis

The pathogenesis of the problem involves the development and retention of a keratin plug in the outer portion (ostium) of hair follicles. This whitened plug enlarges the follicle outlet and accounts for the presence of a white-topped, small red papule. A true pustule ensues if the plug distends the follicle to the point of partial rupture, with consequent extrusion of keratin and follicular bacteria into the surrounding tissue. This escape of follicular contents results in a foreign body inflammatory reaction consisting of an influx of neutrophils and the formation of a true pustule.

Hormones may play a role in stimulating the follicles to the point of rupture. This consideration is based on the peripubertal age at onset and the gradual tapering of activity after midlife. There is probably also a genetic component to the process since often there is a family history of similar lesions. Keratosis pilaris is believed by some to be a marker for the presence of the atopic diathesis.

Treatment

In most cases no specific treatment is required. Lubrication with standard hand cream or lotion softens the skin and reduces the degree of sandpaper-like roughness. Antibiotics offer little improvement since the process is not really a bacterial disease. Tretinoin (Retin-A) cream or gel, starting with the 0.025 percent concentration applied once or twice daily, can be tried, but often the irritant reaction caused by this medication is more troublesome than the disease itself. Tub soaks of at least 20 minutes followed by a brisk brushing with a scrub brush will temporarily loosen the keratin plugs, but unfortunately they quickly reform.

SUGGESTED READINGS

Silverman AR, Nieland ML: Hot tub dermatitis: a familial outbreak of *Pseudomonas* folliculitis. J Am Acad Dermatol 8:153, 1983

This article summarizes findings in this disease and has color photographs.

15 Vesicular Disease

HERPES SIMPLEX VIRUS

Herpes simplex virus (HSV) (herpes progenitalis, genital herpes) infection is a sexually transmitted, recurrent neurocutaneous viral infection characterized by vesicles and erosions.

Clinical Presentation

Primary, first-episode genital herpes simplex virus infections most often occur in younger men and women of any race. Patients present with local pain, pruritus, or (rarely) minimal symptoms. Many describe a prodrome of local burning or tingling of the skin before visible skin lesions appear. During this initial event, some patients complain of fever, malaise, headaches, and other constitutional symptoms. Radicular pain extending down a leg may occur, local pain and edema may produce urinary retention, and tender inguinal lymphadenopathy is common. The duration of these initial outbreaks of HSV is usually from 2 to 3 weeks. Early primary HSV infection manifests by scattered and grouped 1- to 2-mm vesicles, usually located over the glans and shaft of the penis or the mucous membrane portion of the vulva, extending to glabrous skin (Fig. 15-1). The cervix is usually affected also, and a purulent vaginal discharge as a result of vaginal or cervical involvement is common. Primary herpes simplex can be limited to the cervix. Because most of the vesicles are short-lived, especially vulvovaginal lesions, the physician sometimes sees few, if any, intact blisters. Instead, scattered small, sharply demarcated, crusted papules on keratinized skin or erythematous erosions on mucous membranes are common. Coalescence of the erosions produced by vesicles results in larger, irregular lesions. The cutaneous findings may be unimpressive compared with the symptoms.

Sometimes the primary HSV infection is subclinical and unrecognized. The patient's first clinical episode is often erroneously believed to be a primary one, and both the unfortunate patient and sexual partner suspect the other of recent exposure. However, first-episode, nonprimary disease more closely resembles a recurrent event clinically.

Recurrent episodes of HSV infection and first-episode, nonprimary disease are usually less painful and generally are not associated with significant systemic symptoms. Reappearances may occur as often as several times a month, or there may be no clinical recurrences. Most often, patients experience a return of the disease several times a year, with disease-free intervals gradually lengthening and symptoms diminishing. Recurrent episodes usually last for 3 to 5 days and are characterized by grouped or even coalescent vesicles that quickly evolve into small, round erosions or larger erosions with scalloped borders (Figs. 15-2 and 15-3). Mucous membrane lesions are sometimes less sharply demarcated, more scattered, and less specific in appearance. Patients become very experienced at recognizing the various manifestations of their own disease and can often correctly identify an outbreak when only banal erosions or linear fissures along skin folds are evident. Immunosuppressed patients generally exhibit clinically atypical ulcers or hypertrophic lesions (see Ch. 24). Occasionally, the herpesvirus may induce a hypersensitivity reaction manifested by erythema multiforme that recurs after each herpes outbreak (see also Ch. 16).

This disease is infectious when active lesions are present, but the risk of transmissibility in the absence

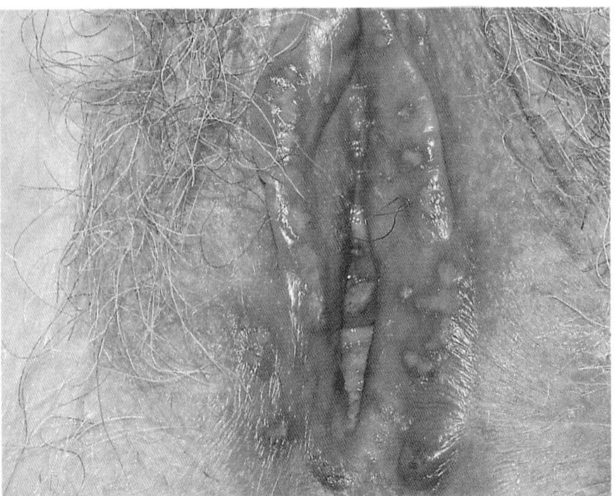

Fig. 15-1. The scattered nature of the round and oval erosions are suggestive of a primary herpes simplex virus infection rather than a recurrent one.

of visible lesions is not clear. Asymptomatic shedding has been documented in women[1] and less often in men. Because viral numbers are low, the risk of infection is probably small but not absent. There is also a risk of transmission from mother to infant during delivery, usually occurring in the setting of an active primary HSV type 2 infection. Neonatal infection can also occur as a result of asymptomatic viral shedding.

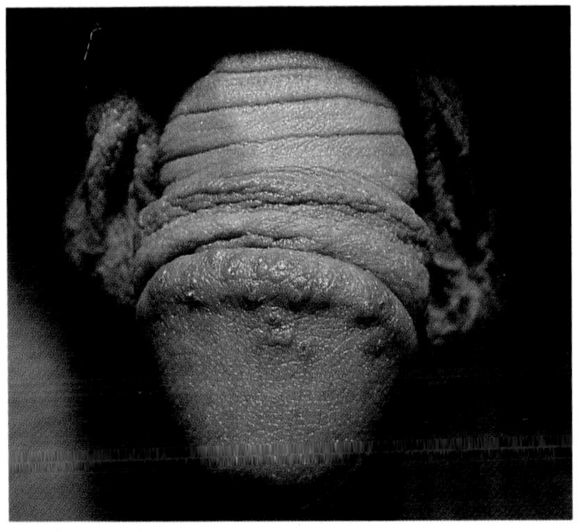

Fig. 15-2. Clustered edematous papules and clear vesicles of recurrent herpes simplex virus infection arising from minimally pink skin.

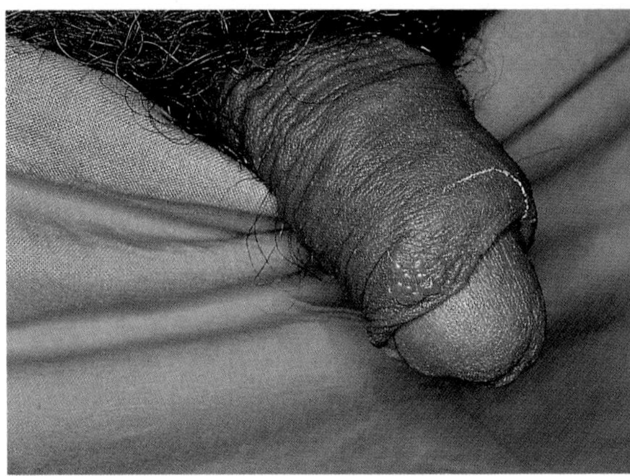

Fig. 15-3. Grouped, confluent vesicles on a pink base classic for recurrent herpes simplex infection.

Although this risk is remote, surviving infected infants generally develop severe neurologic sequelae. Careful attention should then be paid to pregnant women with a history of HSV infection, and even more so to pregnant women with new-onset herpes infection.

Formerly, infection with HSV was believed to be a causative factor in the development of cervical carcinoma. More recently, this role has been attributed to the human papillomavirus, although some evidence exists that the herpesvirus may influence carcinogenesis to some degree. Genital herpes simplex infections are not associated with other diseases except for the logical increased risk of additional sexually transmitted diseases.

Histology

A biopsy of herpes simplex infection shows an intraepithelial blister formed from the detachment and rupture of edematous keratinocytes. As some cells rupture, others transform into distinctive giant cells, and characteristic intracellular eosinophilic inclusion bodies occur in some keratinocytes. An upper dermal inflammatory infiltrate of mononuclear cells and neutrophils is present, and a leukocytoclastic vasculitis is sometimes identified beneath the blister.

Diagnosis

The diagnosis of herpes simplex infection can usually be made on the basis of the appearance of the clinical lesions and the history. Folliculitis, which can occasionally occur on some modified mucous membrane portions of the vulva, can resemble herpes simplex, but the course is generally more chronic and symptoms less severe. The erosions and pustules of candidiasis should be considered in some patients; a potassium hydroxide preparation will show yeast forms. Coalescent erosions may ulcerate, especially in immunosuppressed patients or in those who become superinfected, and these ulcerative lesions should be differentiated from large aphthous ulcerations, chancres, chancroid, and granuloma inguinale. When the diagnosis is in question, a culture for herpes simplex, a skin biopsy, or the polymerase chain reaction test for HSV DNA (after taking a swab sample) should be performed. Herpes simplex cultures yield a high number of false-negative results in many laboratories. A skin biopsy is highly sensitive in early lesions but does not differentiate between herpes simplex and herpes zoster infections, although these diseases are usually clinically distinguishable. The polymerase chain reaction technique is sensitive and specific but of limited availability. The diagnosis is more difficult in patients with healing lesions. Although some physicians request determinations for the presence of serum antibodies against HSV, the high rate of background positivity in adults usually makes this test unhelpful. On the other hand, a persistently negative test is helpful in eliminating this disease. Some physicians and patients request HSV typing. Because either of the two types may be found in the genital area as well as on the lip, this is not useful in most patients. However, HSV type 1 (HSV-1) usually pursues a milder course and is less likely to produce peripartum infant infection, so typing is sometimes of interest to the patient. However, it does not change management or advice.

Course and Prognosis

HSV remains in the host permanently, but predominantly in a latent state. Patients should be advised that, whereas acyclovir suppresses clinical outbreaks, viral shedding may continue and, although less likely, transmission of the disease may occur. The proper use of a condom at all times and avoidance of intercourse and oral sex when lesions are present are the most reliable methods of avoiding transmission. In most patients herpes simplex virus infection is an annoyance and an embarrassment but not a significant medical illness. Some patients, however, have frequent and severe recurrences that are major disruptions to their comfort, life-style, and sense of well-being.

Pathogenesis

HSV infection is caused by *Herpesvirus hominis,* a double-stranded DNA virus. Genital herpes is usually related to HSV type 2 (HSV-2), but HSV-1, the usual etiologic agent for labial herpes (herpes of the lip) is responsible for a distinct minority of infections. When HSV-1 produces genital herpes, the resulting disease is usually milder, and recurrences are less common. The virus is introduced by direct inoculation from skin-to-skin contact into the epidermis by friction or through an abrasion, and it subsequently replicates within keratinocytes. With viral replication, intracellular edema and eventual rupture of the cell and release of the virus occurs. The virus spreads along axons to ganglia and then back to the skin by sensory nerve pathways, producing disease in areas innervated by them. Although the cutaneous lesions heal, the virus becomes latent, harbored in nerve ganglia to await a precipitating event to trigger another outbreak. The most common initiating factors are emotional stress, local trauma or inflammation, illness, and hormonal fluctuations.

Treatment

The management of genital HSV infections consists of patient education, early treatment of more severe disease with oral acyclovir, and chronic, suppressive oral acyclovir treatment in patients with frequent recurrences. For patients with severe disease or a superinfection, local and supportive care are beneficial.

This condition carries a social stigma and produces an emotional impact disproportionate to the severity of the disease, making patient education extremely important. The necessary explanations and reassurances are time-consuming but essential for the patient's sense of self-worth and ability to cope with this disease. Patients often volunteer that they feel ashamed and dirty, more so than patients with other sexually transmitted diseases. Patients should be warned to avoid intercourse and skin-to-skin contact during active outbreaks. They should be aware that oral-genital contact during either genital herpes or labial herpes recurrences can spread disease. The process of informing new partners and the role of condoms during asymptomatic disease should be discussed. Women with HSV infection should be counseled about the risk of neonatal transmission, so that future pregnancies can be monitored carefully.

Primary HSV infection is shortened and ameliorated by treatment with oral acyclovir 200 mg five times a day for about 10 days if medication is started in the first few days of illness. Topical acyclovir is of very limited benefit in the treatment of any herpes infection. In recurrent disease that is mild and short-lived, local care of the skin is the only treatment needed. For those patients with severe recurrences, immediate treatment with acyclovir at the first symptom of a prodrome sometimes shortens the duration and lessens symptoms. When the disease is very severe, frequently recurrent, or associated with erythema multiforme, ongoing suppressive acyclovir at 200 mg three to five times a day[2] or 400 mg twice a day[3] generally prevents outbreaks and can be used safely for years. However, this medication does not exert any influence on the future course of the disease. Rare, usually immunosuppressed, patients harbor a virus resistant to acyclovir. Intravenous foscarnet, which is not approved by the U.S. Food and Drug Administration for this purpose, is nevertheless effective and may play a role in treatment of such patients.[4]

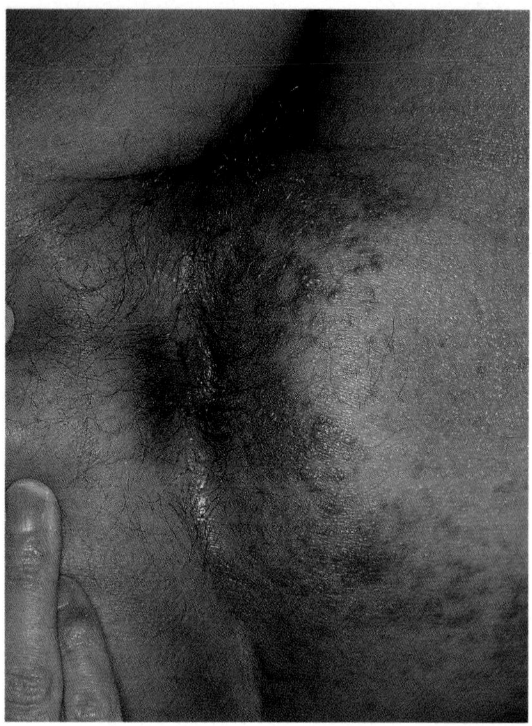

Fig. 15-4. Unilateral erythematous, edematous papules, and plaques of herpes zoster. Vesiculation is often absent early, and can sometimes even be subtle in later disease, as seen here.

HERPES ZOSTER

Herpes zoster (shingles) is an acute blistering eruption that occurs along a cutaneous dermatome. Although most often affecting the trunk and the face, the buttocks and genital areas can be involved, especially in the elderly.

Clinical Presentation

Herpes zoster infection is most common in elderly and immunosuppressed patients. The initial symptom is usually intense pain in the affected area for 1 to several days before skin lesions appear. A rare patient does not complain of pain, even after the appearance of striking skin lesions. Although some patients exhibit low-grade fever, malaise, and headache, usually constitutional symptoms are not marked. Urticarial papules and plaques develop along the involved dermatome (Fig. 15-4). Vesicles and small bullae then appear over the erythematous plaques, coalescing and often becoming hemorrhagic. As these areas heal, crusting occurs over the plaques on keratinized skin, and postinflammatory hyperpigmentation is common, especially in people with dark skin. The total time to healing is about 3 weeks, but lingering pain is a major complication in some people. Postherpetic neuralgia is most common in patients over 60 years of age, and the pain can be incapacitating and very long-lasting. An unusual complication of this disease is dissemination, occurring in some immunosuppressed patients. In addition to typical dermatomal blisters, the generalized appearance of small, nongrouped vesicles indistinguishable from varicella develops. Viral pneumonia or meningoencephalitis rarely occurs.

Histology

A biopsy is identical to that of HSV infection, showing an intraepithelial blister formed from the rupture of edematous cells. Giant cells formed from infected keratinocytes are also characteristic. An underlying leukocytoclastic vasculitis may be present.

Diagnosis

Herpes zoster in the genital area must be differentiated from herpes simplex. The blisters of herpes zoster are unilateral, larger than those of herpes simplex, and often hemorrhagic, and herpes zoster is more likely to occur in older patients. Although herpes zoster classically occurs in a dermatomal distribution, some zosteriform vesicular eruptions are due to herpes simplex. A viral culture or assay by the polymerase chain reaction technique will discriminate between these two diseases when clinical differentiation is difficult.

Course and Prognosis

The lesions of herpes zoster heal spontaneously in all immunocompetent hosts. However, chronic pain that remains after healing may occur, especially in older patients, so that pain control becomes a major consideration. Unlike herpes simplex, zoster is not normally recurrent, although immunosuppressed individuals may experience more than one episode.

Pathogenesis

The etiologic agent for herpes zoster is the varicella-zoster virus, the same virus that causes varicella, or chicken pox. After infection with this virus, usually as a child, the virus becomes sequestered in a latent state in the ganglia of nerves. A precipitating event such as severe illness, local injury, or immunosuppression allows reactivation of the virus with subsequent reappearance of herpes zoster.

Treatment

The most important aspect of herpes zoster management is pain control. Combinations of acetaminophen or aspirin with codeine, hydrocodone bitartrate, or oxycodone are usually sufficient to manage pain, but these frequently must be given regularly rather than on an as-needed basis. Immunocompetent patients seen after the first 2 days of rash need no further specific treatment. However, oral acyclovir at 800 mg five times a day, when given in the first 2 days, slightly shortens the duration and lessens the severity of the disease. When given early, treatment with acyclovir may provide a marginal decrease in the incidence of postherpetic neuralgia. This is primarily a consideration in elderly patients, who are at higher risk for this unfortunate complication. Although treatment with oral corticosteroids has been reported to decrease long-lasting pain following zoster infection, other studies have shown no significant advantage.[5] In the event that chronic pain does occur, oral amitriptyline or desipramine and topical capsaicin are beneficial in long-term control. Unfortunately, capsaicin is irritating and generally not tolerated on genital skin.

The care of the genitalia affected with herpes zoster is limited to gentle debridement with sitz baths or tepid water flushes to minimize superinfection and maceration. Lubrication with an antibiotic ointment or petrolatum may be soothing in some.

LYMPHANGIOMA CIRCUMSCRIPTUM

Lymphangioma circumscriptum, a tumor of lymph channel and often blood vessel origin, appears during childhood and clinically resembles an inflammatory blistering disease. Patients present with asymptomatic, small, clear yellow vesicles, some of which may be hemorrhagic. Vesicles may coalesce, but scattered, discrete lesions are common over the nearby skin surface. The affected area may be either limited or relatively extensive, but, especially when lesions are scattered, deep involvement is usual so that removal of the visible lesions usually results in recurrence. Lymphangioma circumscriptum may occur in any area, but the perineum, axillae, neck, proximal extremities, and mouth are preferential sites. Histologic examination reveals dilated lymphatic vessels in the upper dermis, sometimes enclosed by epidermis. The overlying epidermis may be thinned, thickened, papillomatous, or hyperkeratotic. The lymphatic vessels may extend into fat and empty into enlarged deep lymph channels.

This condition is generally not associated with other abnormalities, although local skeletal abnormalities have been reported. Treatment is necessary only for cosmetic reasons, but this should be discouraged because of the extensive surgery required for removal and the high recurrence rate. Dermabrasion may produce good short-term results with less scarring than surgical excision, but recurrences are usual. Laser therapy may also be considered.

REFERENCES

Herpes Simplex Virus

1. Koutsky LA, Stevens CE, Holmes KK et al: Underdiagnosis of genital herpes by current clinical and viral-isolation procedures. N Engl J Med 326:1533, 1992
2. Straus SE, Takiff HE, Seidlik M et al: Suppression of frequently recurring genital herpes. N Engl J Med 310:1545, 1984
3. Kaplowitz LG, Baker D, Gelb L et al (Acyclovir Study Group): Prolonged and continuous acyclovir treatment of normal adults with frequently recurring genital herpes infections. JAMA 265:747, 1991
4. Safrin S, Crumpacker C, Chatis P et al: A controlled trial comparing foscarnet with vidarabine for acyclovir-resistant mucocutaneous herpes simplex in the acquired immunodeficiency syndrome. N Engl J Med 325:551, 1991
5. Portenoy RK, Duma C, Foley FM: Acute herpetic and postherpetic neuralgia: clinical review and current management. Ann Neurol 20:651, 1986

SUGGESTED READINGS

Herpes Simplex Virus

Maccato ML, Kaufman RH: Herpes genitalis. Dermatol Clin 10:415, 1992

This review discusses the prevalence, clinical features, treatment, and special issues associated with genital herpes simplex virus infection.

Sweet RL, Gibbs RS: Herpes simplex virus infection. p. 144. In: Infectious Diseases of the Female Genital Tract. 2nd Ed. Williams & Wilkins, Baltimore, 1990

The authors review updated information on the epidemiology and diagnosis of herpes simplex virus infections, and discuss the special issue of pregnancy and herpes simplex infection.

16 Bullous Disease

BULLOUS IMPETIGO

The warmth and moisture of the anogenital region favor the growth of infectious organisms such as *Staphylococcus aureus.* Usually, infection with this bacterium results in folliculitis or furunculosis. Certain strains of *S. aureus,* however, contain toxins that cause intraepidermal lysis and the formation of fragile blisters.

Clinical Presentation

The blisters of bullous impetigo are fragile. For this reason patients often present with a mixture of bullae and erosions or even solely with erosions (Fig. 16-1). Intact blisters are filled with clear fluid and are not purulent, as one might expect. They arise primarily from normal skin, although occasionally there is a thin ring of erythema surrounding the blister. One to three or four lesions may be present. Most of the blisters are 1 to 2 cm in diameter.

Erosions, as noted, are also usually present. They are circular, with remnants of the blister roof ("collarette") encircling the periphery of the erosion. The base of the erosion may be red and moist, or it may be covered with loosely adherent yellow crust.

The blisters and erosions of bullous impetigo develop on hair-bearing skin, and thus they are usually found on the upper inner thighs, pubic triangle, or nonmucosal aspects of the genitalia. Bullous impetigo is usually asymptomatic, although sometimes mild itching is present.

Histology

The blister cavity in bullous impetigo is located within the epidermis, at or just below the level of the granular layer. A few neutrophils are found in the cavity, but they are less numerous than might be expected. Occasionally a small number of acantholytic epidermal cells are noted; these presumably form because of the action of enzymes released by the neutrophils. A mild inflammatory infiltrate consisting of neutrophils and lymphocytes is present in the upper dermis.

Diagnosis

Clinical diagnosis can be difficult because the blisters are similar in appearance to those of the immunobullous diseases discussed below. The fragility of impetigo blisters helps to rule out the subepidermal blistering diseases of the pemphigoid family, and the restriction to a localized area helps to exclude pemphigus. Gram stain from the blister fluid is often negative due to the sparsity of organisms, but culture from the fluid is usually positive for *S. aureus.* Biopsy, as indicated above, demonstrates a quite characteristic picture.

Course and Prognosis

Individual blisters and erosions heal spontaneously in a week or two, but all the while, new lesions are forming. Thus the overall course is rather chronic. No scarring occurs at the lesion sites. Eventually,

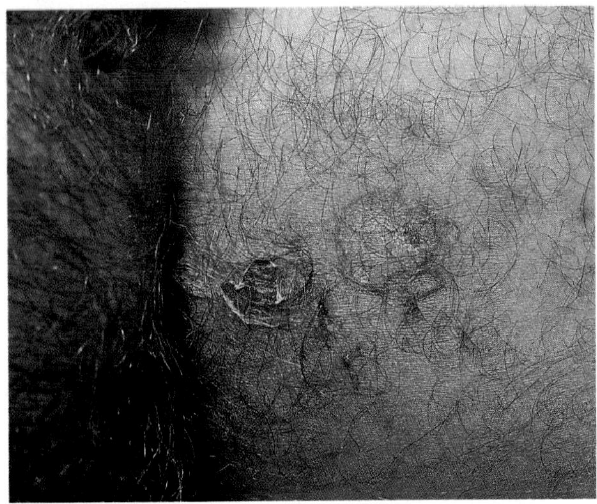

Fig. 16-1. Fragile, collapsed bullae of bullous impetigo. The roof of the blister on the left is torn and partially missing.

even without treatment, the disease resolves spontaneously.

Pathogenesis

Bullous impetigo is caused by *S. aureus* infection; rarely a few streptococcal organisms, as part of a mixed infection, will also be recovered. Generally the staphylococcal organisms are of phage group II. An epidermolytic toxin has been recovered from the blister fluid in a few cases, suggesting that the organisms responsible (and the disease itself) is closely linked to staphylococcal scalded skin syndrome.

Treatment

Good hygiene is, of course, important. On the other hand, washing should not be so vigorous as to cause damage, and thus increased susceptibility for infection, to the surrounding skin. Topical antibiotic treatment with mupirocin (Bactroban) is recommended by some,[1] but most authorities prefer orally administered antibiotics. Penicillin derivatives such as dicloxacillin given in a dose of 250 mg four times a day work well except in the very rare instance of methicillin-resistant infection. Erythromycin can be used,[2] but the proportion of staphylococcal organisms resistant to this antibiotic is fairly large. Hydrogen peroxide and other similar home remedies are not helpful and may even slow down the rate of healing.

FIXED DRUG ERUPTION

A fixed drug eruption is an annoying but benign cutaneous reaction to a systematically administered medication, resulting in one to several round, erythematous plaques, blisters, or erosions.

Clinical Presentation

Occurring without age, race, or gender predilection and located on both skin and mucous membranes, this eruption boasts several peculiar clinical features. Patients usually report that previously affected skin lesions recurrently "puff up" or blister, sometimes in association with genital or oral sores. On physical examination, nonmucous membrane lesions are strikingly round, although mucous membrane involvement may be irregular in shape. Finally, hyperpigmentation of affected skin is usually remarkable and increases with each new episode. Genital lesions are common and occur most often on the glans penis. Although there are few published reports of vulvar fixed drug eruptions, these are seen relatively often and occur primarily on the clinically non-hair-bearing genital skin. Genital lesions generally present as erosions rather than blisters because of the fragile nature of skin in this area (Figs. 16-2 and 16-3). The erosions are well demarcated and usually 2 to 3 cm in size. Although genital lesions are often single, oral and cutaneous lesions are frequently present as well (Fig. 16-4). A brief cutaneous examination is useful because the hyperpigmented and round nature of the affected areas is much better appreciated on hair-bearing skin.

Histology

A biopsy of an acute lesion shows a superficial and deep perivascular inflammatory infiltrate with lymphocytes, neutrophils, and eosinophils. Superficial dermal edema is generally present and, when a blister is present, it is located subepidermally. The epidermis shows necrotic keratinocytes and sometimes extensive necrosis. Vacuolar degeneration of the basal cell layer is usual. Older lesions show evidence of past basement membrane disruption including dermal pigment incontinence.

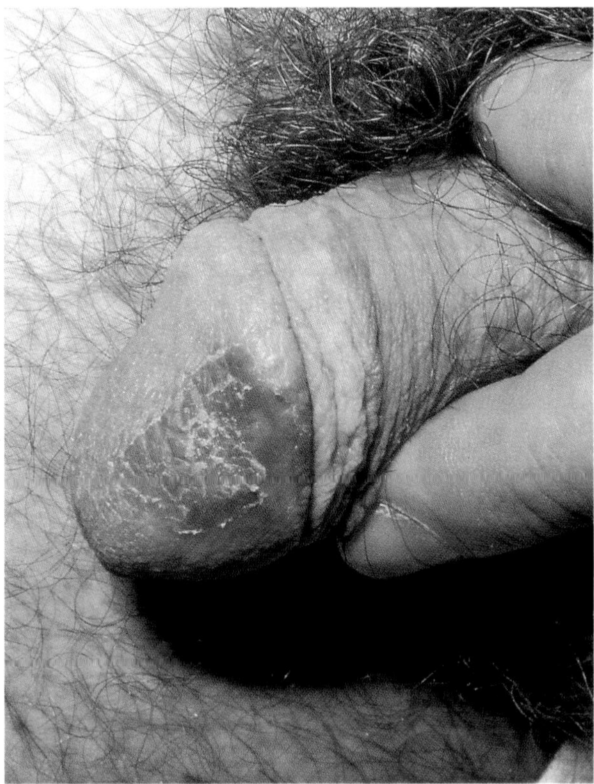

Fig. 16-2. Well-demarcated, healing erosion of a fixed drug eruption in its typical location on the glans. (Courtesy of Ronald C. Hansen, M.D.)

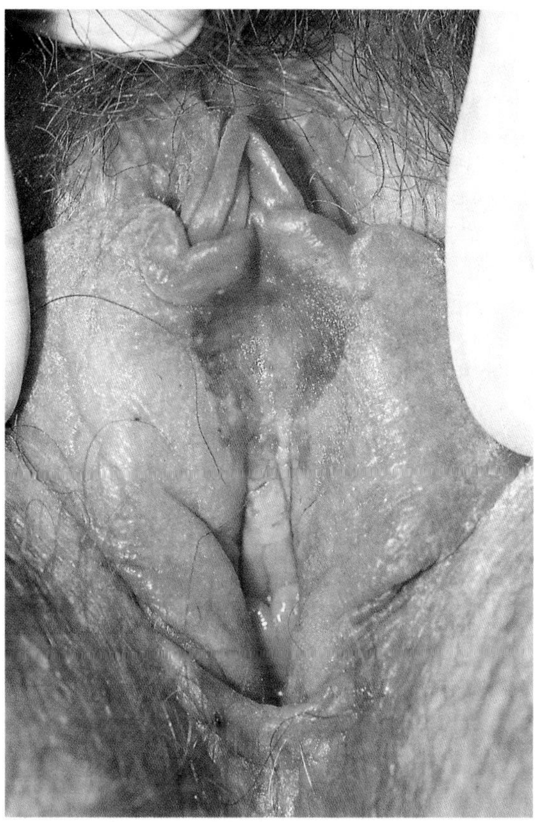

Fig. 16-3. This round erosion over the anterior vestibule associated with oral lesions represents a fixed drug eruption.

Diagnosis

This diagnosis is made on the basis of the clinical appearance, often confirmed by a history of intermittent use of a medication known to cause a fixed drug eruption. The most common diseases confused with this condition include herpes simplex virus infection because of the history of recurrence at the same site, although herpes produces small, grouped vesicles and erosions. Erythema multiforme can mimic a fixed drug reaction since both are characterized by morphologically similar round, edematous, or blistering lesions associated with mucous membrane involvement. However, erythema multiforme exhibits more numerous and smaller skin lesions that do not recur exactly superimposed over previously affected skin.

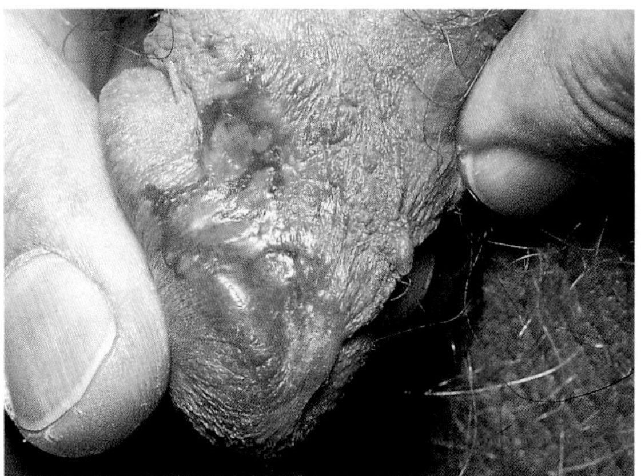

Fig. 16-4. Only the presence of classic, round, hyperpigmented patches and blisters on distant skin enabled the clinician to make the diagnosis of a fixed drug eruption from this nonspecific erosion.

Course and Prognosis

The postinflammatory hyperpigmentation from each recurrent lesion darkens with each reexposure to the offending medication and reactivation of the lesion. With removal of the responsible agent, the hyperpigmentation gradually resolves.

Pathogenesis

The medications that cause fixed drug eruptions are many (Table 16-1). Most common are phenolphthalein, tetracycline, sulfonamides, and barbiturates.

Treatment

The treatment of a fixed drug eruption is removal and subsequent avoidance of the offending agent. Lesions heal spontaneously, and local care to minimize pain and secondary infection is the only necessary intervention.

BULLOUS ERYTHEMA MULTIFORME

Erythema multiforme (erythema multiforme major, Stevens-Johnson syndrome, toxic epidermal necrolysis) is a hypersensitivity reaction usually occurring in response to a medication or infection. Classic disease is characterized by red, nonscaling, round papules or small plaques that often acquire varying degrees and shades of erythema in a concentric pattern producing a bull's-eye appearance. However, this disease exists on a spectrum of clinical severity, with more serious forms resulting in blistering of mucous membranes that include the genitalia, often with widespread skin involvement and a significant risk of mortality and morbidity. Bullous erythema multiforme (erythema multiforme major, Stevens-Johnson syndrome) represents erythema multiforme of sufficient severity to cause epithelial necrosis and blistering in association with mucous membrane lesions. Toxic epidermal necrolysis (TEN, Lyell's disease) features confluent skin involvement with large denuded areas and, most often, mucous membrane lesions, causing death in up to 50 percent of those affected. Because these conditions represent varying degrees of intensity, many patients do not fit neatly into one niche.

Table 16-1. Common Causes of Fixed Drug Eruption

Acetaminophen
Acetylsalicylic acid
Barbiturates
Metronidazole
Nonsteroidal anti-inflammatory medications (many)
Oral contraceptives
Penicillins
Phenolphthalein
Phenothiazines
Salicylates
Sulfonamides
Tetracycline

Clinical Presentation

This disease occurs in all ages and races, and in both genders. The onset is usually abrupt, and patients often exhibit constitutional symptoms including fever, malaise, myalgias, and sore throat. The history is important, often revealing recent treatment with a medication, or symptoms of a preceding viral or bacterial infection. Although the genitalia are usually affected with bullous erythema multiforme and TEN, this involvement typically is overshadowed by disease in other areas. Nonspecific mucous membrane erosions are often the first lesions recognized. In men, erosions occur at the meatus (Fig. 16-5) and then extend to involve the glans and prepuce particularly (Fig. 16-6); sometimes the entire genitalia and even the whole skin surface are affected. Exudation and crusting is marked. Late scarring occasionally produces phimosis. Women first experience erosions over the labia minora, inner labia majora, and vestibule (Fig. 16-7). The vagina may also be affected, sometimes producing vaginal adhesions. Here again, nonmucous membrane skin lesions often develop and show intensely erythematous plaques with central dusky necrosis that forms a blister. The red color is often difficult to appreciate in black skin, in which the lesions appear hyperpigmented. In patients with severe disease, lesions may become confluent so that sheets of epithelium are denuded. Sometimes mucous membrane erosions, especially of the mouth but also of the genital area, occur without generalized skin involvement. A fairly typical pattern includes mucous membrane erosions with palmar and plantar lesions only.

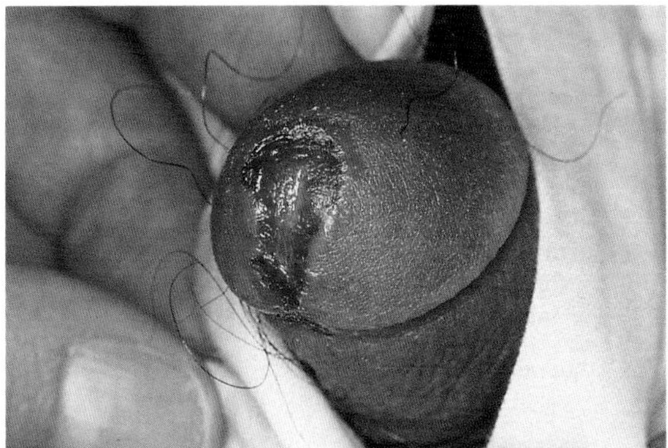

Fig. 16-5. The correlation of this meatal erosion with other mucous membrane lesions of sudden onset indicates the diagnosis of Stevens-Johnson syndrome.

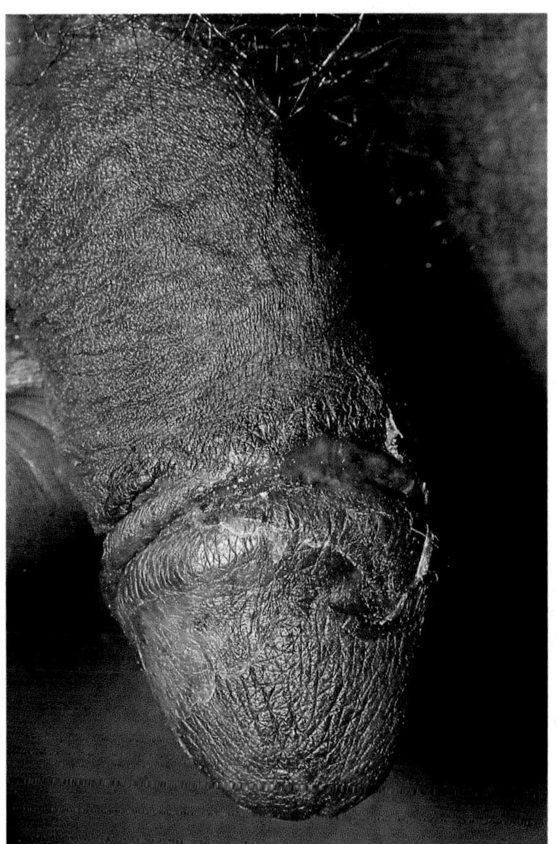

Fig. 16-6. This nonspecific erosion of bullous erythema multiforme (Stevens-Johnson syndrome) on the glans penis and corona is accompanied by oral erosions and target lesions with central blisters on the palms and soles.

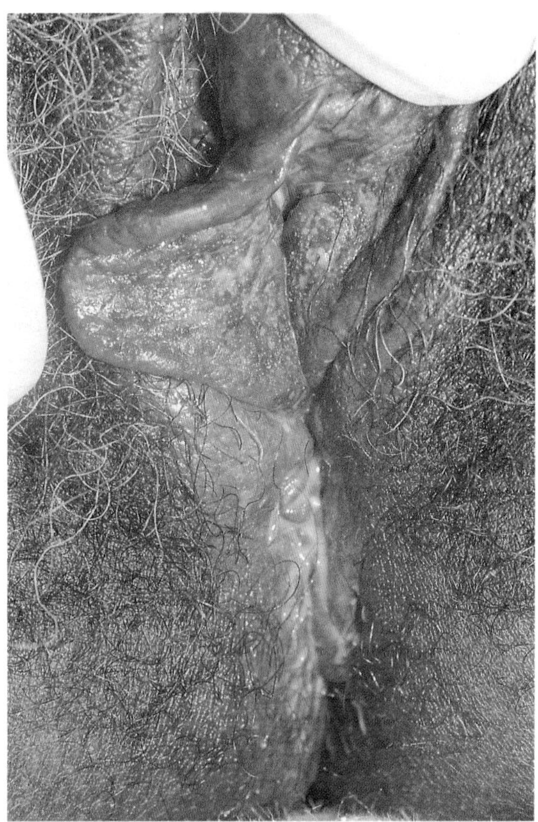

Fig. 16-7. Nonspecific erosions of erythema multiforme, with a purulent vaginal discharge characteristic of vaginal involvement.

The oral mucosa is a principal target, with erosions extending anteriorly to include the lips. The nasal mucosa and conjunctiva are often involved as well, and, in severe disease, the pharynx, esophagus, and upper airways may be affected.

Histology

The skin biopsy of erythema multiforme shows a perivascular and upper dermal lymphocytic infiltrate. The epidermis contains necrotic keratinocytes and shows hydropic degeneration of the basal cell layer. If a blister is sampled, a resulting subepidermal blister is seen. In some, full-thickness necrosis of the epidermis with detachment from the dermis is present.

Diagnosis

The diagnosis of bullous erythema multiforme and TEN can usually be made on historical and clinical grounds. The abrupt onset and intense erythema of the affected skin usually differentiate bullous erythema multiforme from the other cutaneous blistering diseases that are summarized in Table 6-1. However, TEN can sometimes mimic widespread immunobullous disease, primarily pemphigus vulgaris. Staphylococcal scalded skin syndrome can also present with extensive denuding of skin associated with constitutional signs, but sloughing is more superficial, mucous membrane lesions are absent, and children are the most often affected. A skin biopsy of affected but non-eroded skin generally confirms the diagnosis of erythema multiforme or a variant in unclear cases.

Table 16-2. Common Causes of Erythema Multiforme

- Medications
  - Allopurinol
  - Barbiturates
  - Carbamazepine
  - Cephalosporins
  - Furosemide
  - Nonsteriodal anti-inflammatory medications
  - Penicillins
  - Phenytoin
  - Phenothiazines
  - Sulfonamides
  - Salicylates
  - Thiazide diuretics
- Infections
  - Viral
    - Herpes simplex virus
    - Epstein-Barr virus
  - Bacterial
    - Streptococcal
  - Mycobacterial
    - Tuberculosis
  - Mycoplasmal
  - Fungal
    - Histoplasmosis
    - Coccidioidomycosis
- Connective tissue diseases
- Lymphoreticular malignancies
- Immunizations
- Envenomations

Course and Prognosis

The usual course of bullous erythema multiforme is one of abrupt onset with blistering and loss of epithelium, cessation of new lesion formation, and gradual healing. Future retreatment with an offending medication or a chemically similar drug may result in a recurrence, as also occurs when erythema multiforme results from herpes simplex virus infection that is usually recurrent. Severe disease may result in death or permanent scarring that can produce, in addition to the genital sequelae discussed above, blindness.

Pathogenesis

The underlying pathogenesis of erythema multiforme and its variants is not known, but the disease appears to result from an immune response to antigenic sensitization. The underlying antigenic stimuli are many (Table 16-2). In severe disease, the most common precipitating agents are medications. Whereas an enormous number of drugs have been reported to induce erythema multiforme, Stevens-Johnson syndrome, and toxic epidermal necrolysis, a more limited number produce these diseases with regularity. The medications most often implicated include sulfonamide and penicillin antibiotics, the anticonvulsants phenytoin and carbamazepine, as well as barbiturates and allopurinol. Infections can also result in erythema multiforme and its variants. Herpes simplex virus infection is responsible for nearly all episodes of recurrent disease in those not taking offending medications. Much less often, other conditions characterized by misdirected immune responses produce this spectrum of diseases. These include lymphoreticular malignancies, particularly those affecting B cells, and autoimmune diseases such as lupus erythematosus and rheumatoid arthritis.

Treatment

The management of erythema multiforme includes the identification and removal of the inciting factor, general supportive care, and scrupulous local management of mucous membrane disease. The use of systemic corticosteroids is debated, and there are no prospective controlled trials that address this issue.[3] Patients with minor blistering often respond well to oral prednisone at a dose of 40 to 60 mg a day with abrupt discontinuation when disease progression has ceased. Corticosteroid use is more controversial in those patients with widespread disease. When patients with toxic epidermal necrolysis treated with systemic corticosteroids have been compared retrospectively with those untreated, treated patients have experienced a worse outcome. However, many of these patients were treated late, when beneficial effects would be expected to be less, and they experienced anticipated adverse reactions and an increased risk of infection. It is the experience of many clinicians that systemic corticosteroids can significantly minimize the intensity of the disease when given early in the course of severe erythema multiforme variants. However, the risk of infection probably outweighs the benefit of steroids after large areas have been denuded.

Nonspecific supportive care is crucial, and patients with widespread denuded skin can best be treated in a burn center. Attention to fluid loss, the early recognition and treatment of superinfection, and good nutrition is imperative. Regular debridement of necrotic skin removes an important source of infection.

Local care of the genitalia in patients with severe disease is necessary to prevent possible late complications. Unfortunately, these patients are sometimes in an intensive care setting, and attention is diverted by necessary ongoing and aggressive supportive measures. However, in the week or two during the acute phase of the disease, severe scarring can occur. The most common late complications in men, meatal stenosis and phimosis, can be avoided by daily careful retraction of the foreskin and flushing of the glans with tepid water for debridement, as well as lubrication with an antibiotic ointment and treatment of any superinfections. If significant meatal involvement in either sex causes dysuria and urinary retention, urinating while in a sitz bath or tub bath may obviate the need for a urinary catheter, which can be extremely painful to insert. However, any signs of urinary outlet obstruction should be treated with a catheter that both empties the bladder and provides patency of the urethra and meatus during healing. Sitz baths or flushing of the vulva periodically with tepid tap water for cleaning debrides the area and provides the opportunity to inspect the vulva regularly for superinfection. The vagina should be examined for involvement and, if affected significantly, a vaginal mold can be inserted during the acute phase to maintain patency.[4] The physician should remember that younger women may experience menses, so that local hygiene should be managed. The development of vulvovaginal endometriosis and vaginal adenosis may be related to the contact of menstrual fluid with eroded skin, so that suppression of menses with parenteral progesterone has been suggested.[4] Early scarring, strictures, or adhesions of the genitalia should be gently separated manually, and the area well lubricated regularly with an antibiotic ointment. Patients with a local bacterial or yeast infection should be treated systemically rather than locally to avoid local irritation caused by alcohol-containing medications on denuded skin.

BULLOUS PEMPHIGOID

Bullous pemphigoid is an uncommon autoimmune blistering disease that occurs equally in men and women, predominantly during the sixth to eighth decades of life. However, this disease can affect patients at any age, including childhood.

Clinical Presentation

Patients present with blisters, erosions, and often intense pruritus. The hair-bearing skin of the inner thighs, inguinal crease, perineum, scrotum, and labia majora are the most affected areas of the genitalia. Tense, straw-colored blisters are most common, but in these areas of friction, many blister roofs will have been denuded, leaving erosions and collarettes (Fig. 16-8). Older blisters may become cloudy, and some blisters may be hemorrhagic. Mucous membrane involvement of the anogenital area may occur but is uncommon and presents as erosions more often than intact blisters because of the fragile nature of non-hair-bearing genital skin. Mucosal genital lesions are often asymptomatic and therefore undiscovered. Although bullous pemphigoid is usually regarded as a nonscarring disease, chronic, uncontrolled disease of the vulva can produce adhesions when modified mucous membranes and mucous membranes are affected.

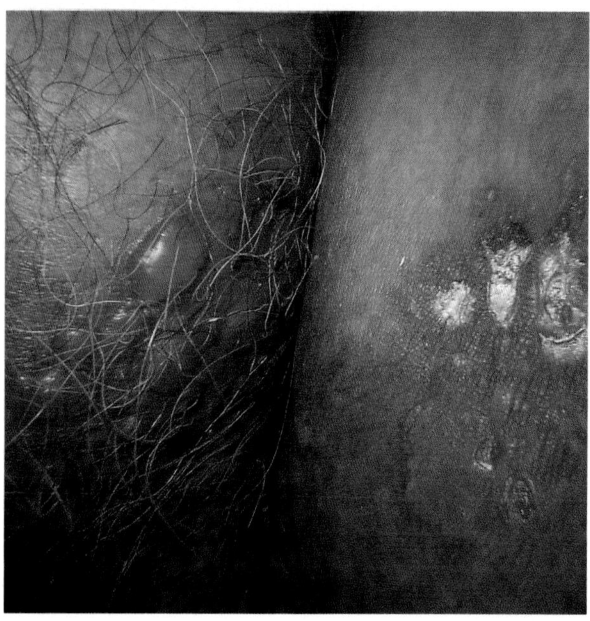

Fig. 16-8. Intact bulla with clear, yellow fluid and erosions are characteristic of bullous pemphigoid.

Skin involvement is more common than mucosal disease. Most often, tense bullae that generally range from about 1 to 5 cm begin over the distal extremities and gradually extend to include other skin surface areas. Blisters arise from both erythematous and normal uninflamed skin. Intertriginous areas such as the axillae and groin are especially affected. Sometimes, blisters and erosions remain localized, and bullous pemphigoid can affect the vulva alone.

Oral involvement develops in about one third of patients, primarily over the palate, buccal mucosa, and tongue, although desquamative gingivitis also occurs. Other mucous membrane involvement generally is absent. Early bullous pemphigoid may exhibit no blistering. Some patients initially develop fixed, circinate, urticarial plaques without blistering, and several weeks later acquire clinical bullae. Still other patients exhibit a nonspecific eczematous eruption that represents early chronic pemphigoid. Although, like other autoimmune diseases, bullous pemphigoid may confer an increased risk of concurrent autoimmune diseases, this increase is minimal. An association of bullous pemphigoid with an internal malignancy has been debated and, if present, is weak.[5]

Histology

The diagnosis of bullous pemphigoid should be confirmed by a biopsy that includes the edge of a blister. The characteristic findings for bullous pemphigoid include a subepidermal blister with a variable degree of dermal inflammation. In some patients, only slight inflammation is present, consisting of upper dermal eosinophils that may also occur in the bullae. A perivascular infiltrate of mononuclear cells and eosinophils is present. In inflammatory lesions, many eosinophils as well as mononuclear cells and polymorphonuclear leukocytes are found in these locations. A biopsy for direct immunofluorescence is confirmatory (see Pathogenesis).

Diagnosis

The differential diagnosis of genital bullous pemphigoid includes any blistering and erosive diseases that affect the genitalia, some of which are listed in Table 6-1. Other immunobullous diseases such as epidermolysis bullosa acquisita, cicatricial pemphigoid, and pemphigus vulgaris should be considered, especially when intact blisters are present, but the latter two diseases almost always exhibit marked mucous membrane involvement. Bullous impetigo may be confused with bullous pemphigoid, but blisters appear more superficial and are usually more localized. Herpes simplex virus infection also presents with blistering, but is more vesicular and localized, and lesions are clustered and short-lived. Bullous erythema multiforme can sometimes be confusing, but blisters usually arise from much more inflammatory skin, and mucous membrane lesions are more prominent. A biopsy for routine histology and direct immunofluorescence should be performed for confirmation. Because the direct immunofluorescent findings do not differentiate bullous pemphigoid from epidermolysis bullosa acquisita or cicatricial pemphigoid, some feel that immunoelectron microscopy or immunofluorescence on split skin is indicated for absolute differentiation and optimal treatment. Circulating IgG antibodies directed towards the pemphigoid antigen in the lamina lucida of the dermal-epidermal junction are usually detectable by indirect immunofluorescence in patients with bullous pemphigoid.

Course and Prognosis

Bullous pemphigoid is a chronic disease that only rarely remains in remission following termination of successful treatment. Much of the morbidity of the disease relates to the fragile health of the older patients most at risk of this disease and to the side effects of corticosteroids.

Pathogenesis

Bullous pemphigoid is a autoimmune disease. As can be seen on a biopsy for direct immunofluorescence, IgG or C3, or both, are deposited in a linear pattern at the basement membrane. As a result of immunoglobulin deposition, complement activation occurs with the generation of mediators of inflammation and the influx of inflammatory cells. This process results in tissue injury and blister formation.

Treatment

The management of genital bullous pemphigoid includes both treatment for the underlying disease and local supportive care. Corticosteroids are the mainstay of treatment for this disease. Although occasional patients with local disease can be controlled with topical preparations, oral prednisone at 40 to 80 mg a day is nearly always necessary, with slow tapering after cessation of new blister formation. In those patients refractory to treatment or who cannot be tapered to lower doses, a corticosteroid-sparing agent such as azathioprine or cyclophosphamide can be added. It should be noted that the action of these medications is delayed by about 1 month. Oral methotrexate is useful in some, and pulse doses of intravenous methylprednisolone or cyclophosphamide in various dosing schedules are sometimes used in resistant cases.

Patients with mild or localized disease sometimes can be treated successfully with more conservative regimens. The anti-inflammatory effect of oral tetracycline at 500 mg qid is useful for some patients, as is oral niacinamide at 500 mg tid alone or in combination with tetracycline.[6] Those patients whose biopsies show marked neutrophilic inflammation may respond to oral dapsone at 100 mg a day.[7] The benefit of all treatments except for corticosteroids is not seen for weeks.

Most patients with significant genital bullous pemphigoid have widespread disease and require systemic corticosteroids. Therefore, care of the genital area consists primarily of supportive treatment rather than control of the primary disease process. Local care of the genitalia is especially important for the occasional woman or uncircumcised man with mucous membrane lesions, both of whom are at risk for scarring. Erosions and maceration increase the risk of infection, which in turn increases scarring. Careful cleansing of the area with clear water flushes and treatment of any secondary infection help to minimize long-term problems. Regular retraction of the foreskin is also useful to reduce scarring and the need for late circumcision or other surgical correction. Because the genital area is not usually the first or worst area affected by bullous pemphigoid, the possibility of genital involvement and the need for local care often does not occur to the physician. However, the sometimes marked disease of the genital area should be emphasized to ensure that proper attention is paid to local care.

CICATRICIAL PEMPHIGOID

Cicatricial pemphigoid (benign mucous membrane pemphigoid) is an autoimmune blistering disease that targets the mucous membranes of the mouth, the eyes, and often the genitalia. Nonmucous membrane skin involvement may occur. This disease results in scarring that can produce major morbidity in some patients.

Clinical Presentation

Cicatricial pemphigoid develops most often in patients between the ages of 50 and 70 years, of any race. Women are affected about twice as often as men. Although approximately 20 percent of patients exhibit nonmucous membrane involvement, most symptoms and morbidity result from mucous membrane disease that often begins insidiously but then may produce rapid scarring. About one half of patients exhibit genital lesions, and these are occasionally the presenting feature. Women with genital cicatricial pemphigoid frequently describe a chronic purulent vaginal discharge, vulvar pain, pruritus, or dyspareunia. Men may report painful penile erosions and, if uncircumcised, difficulty retracting the foreskin. Patients also may complain of dryness, burning, or grittiness of the eyes or painful mouth lesions. However, these extragenital symptoms are often not volunteered because patients frequently do not realize the association.

Early genital disease shows nonspecific erosions and (rarely) blisters of the clinically non-hair-bearing portion of the vulva, and of the glans penis and inner aspect of the prepuce. The vagina may be affected and show erosions. Scarring occurs, sometimes producing hypopigmentation and loss of the normal skin texture. The skin may become smooth, but inflammation around erosions can induce mild perilesional thickening of the skin and hyperkeratosis. Agglutination of the labia minora to the labia majora, or to each other, may occur, as well as scarring of the prepuce to the clitoris and stenosis of the introitus (Fig. 16-9). However, the fine crinkling and purpura typical of lichen sclerosus is missing. Cicatricial pemphigoid also produces fragility so that fissures at the introitus may occur with introduction of the speculum. Scarring of the vaginal walls can produce obliteration of the vaginal space. In uncircumcised males, erosions of the glans and inner prepuce can result in phimosis and adhesion of these two epithelia. Meatal stenosis may occur in both sexes.

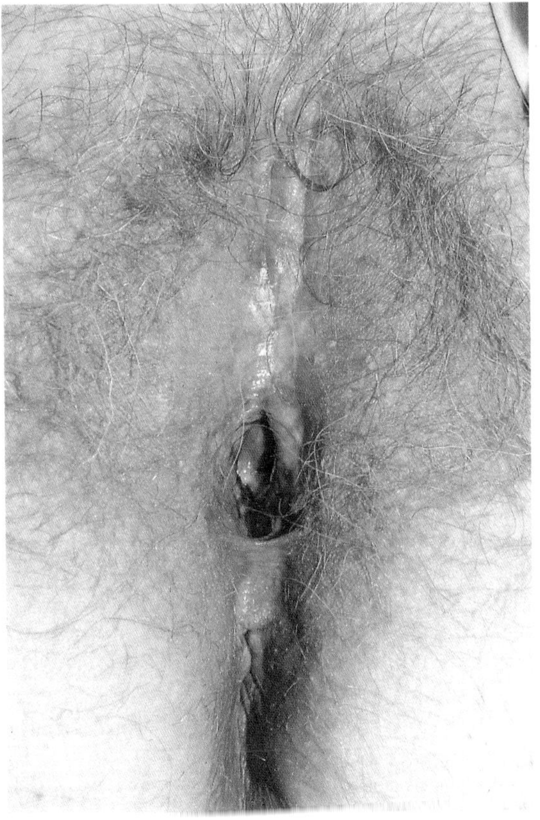

Fig. 16-9. This patient with cicatricial pemphigoid shows nonspecific scarring manifested by smoothness of skin texture, loss of the labia minora, and covering of the clitoris by a scarred clitoral hood. Fragility is demonstrated by the fissure at the posterior vestibule. Note similarities with Figures 6-14 and 11-12. (From Edwards,[8a] with permission.)

The most common areas affected by cicatricial pemphigoid are the mouth and eye. Although a blister is the primary lesion, erosions are much more often seen. The gingiva are often the first site of involvement, producing the erythema, fragility, and erosions that constitute desquamative gingivitis. Scarring is usual, and retraction of the gingivae frequently results in dental disease. The palate, tongue, and lips are also often affected, while involvement of the esophagus and larynx with scarring may occur but is less common. Early but quite symptomatic eye disease may be undetected by the unsuspicious, untrained, or naked eye, but a careful examination by an ophthalmologist usually shows early decreased lacrimation and symblepharon formation, or adhesions of the bulbar and palpebral conjunctiva. More advanced disease may exhibit neovascularization, complete scarring of conjunctival surfaces, adhesions of the upper to the lower lid, and scarring of the cornea that produces blindness. Entropion formation may direct eyelashes inward to rub against the cornea, causing further scarring. Those patients who have nonmucous membrane disease show straw-colored vesicles and bullae that may or may not scar. There are no significant associations with malignancy or other autoimmune disease.

Histology

A skin biopsy is characteristic. The biopsy should include the edge of a new blister when possible. If no blisters are present, then the edge of an erosion is most likely to show the characteristic pathologic features. The biopsy of cicatricial pemphigoid can be identical to that of bullous pemphigoid; it shows a subepidermal blister with a mild to moderate mixed perivascular infiltrate of predominantly mononuclear cells with scattered neutrophils and often eosinophils. In areas of chronic disease, scarring in the dermis often can be appreciated. Direct immunofluorescent biopsies of perilesional skin are positive in most patients, showing a linear deposition of immunoglobulins and complement along the basement membrane. Most common are IgG and C3, although IgM and IgA may be present occasionally, and some show C3 alone. Circulating antibodies are not usually seen, especially in early disease and when present exist in low titers.

Diagnosis

The diagnosis is made by ruling out other scarring mucous membrane diseases. If frankly bullous lesions are present, the diseases most likely to be confused with cicatricial pemphigoid are pemphigus vulgaris, bullous erythema multiforme, epidermolysis bullosa acquisita, and, less often because of the usually minor mucous membrane involvement, bullous pemphigoid. Some of these diseases are summarized in Table 6-1. The clinical characteristics or a skin biopsy can differentiate these diseases except for epidermolysis bullosa acquisita; this differentiation requires immunoelectron microscopy or immunofluorescence on split skin. Usually causing less confusion is a herpes simplex virus infection. For patients with erosions in the absence of blisters, erosive lichen planus and erosive lichen sclerosus should be excluded.

Course and Prognosis

Cicatricial pemphigoid is a chronic disease that generally does not remit. Although some patients respond well to conservative treatment, some experience ongoing active disease and progressive scarring and morbidity in spite of aggressive management.

Pathogenesis

Cicatricial pemphigoid is an autoimmune disease that develops as a result of circulating autoantibodies that bind to the target antigen in the lamina lucida of the basement membrane at the dermal-epidermal junction. This initiates complement activation, resulting in the production of inflammatory mediators with recruitment of inflammatory cells that effect separation of the basement membrane. With loss of the attachment of the epidermis and dermis, a blister forms.

Treatment

The management of cicatricial pemphigoid usually requires systemic treatment, predominantly corticosteroids, to control the underlying disease, in addition to multidisciplinary aggressive local care of the genital area, gingivae, and eyes to minimize scarring and loss of function. Prompt control of this condition is important, especially in those with rapidly progressive disease and aggressive scarring. Oral prednisone at 60 to 80 mg a day arrests the process in many patients, and when the disease is quiescent, the dose can be tapered. Oral azathioprine and cyclophosphamide are useful in some patients as steroid-sparing agents. These should be added to corticosteroid therapy in patients who are refractory to treatment, require high doses of prednisone, or do not tolerate a taper of prednisone. Beneficial effects of these steroid-sparing medications are not appreciated for the first month of treatment. Adjunctive treatment with topical corticosteroids applied to the affected mucous membranes can be useful in some. Oral dapsone at 100 mg a day is also sometimes effective.[8] In case reports and small series, oral cyclosporine has been reported helpful in some patients but useless in others. Because of its toxicity, cost, and variable effectiveness, this medication should be tried only as a last resort.

While control of the underlying process is being achieved, local care of affected mucous membranes is imperative to minimize serious and permanent morbidity. When the skin is eroded and exudative, topical medications may not stay in contact with the affected area, and the addition of an ointment or cream only increases pain and maceration. Sitz baths or gentle flushing of the area with tap water are often useful for cleaning and gently debriding the area. Frequent retraction of the foreskin and use of a vaginal dilator or regular sexual intercourse may help to prevent permanent scarring of these structures. With chronic erosive disease, bacterial superinfection is common. A purulent vaginal discharge generally is a sign of superinfection and clears, at least temporarily and with an improvement in symptoms, with an antibiotic. However, these patients are at high risk for vaginal candidiasis, especially if they have also received a corticosteroid (see Desquamative Vaginitis in Ch. 7). Chronic, nonhealing erosions may respond to intralesional triamcinolone acetonide at a concentration of 5 mg/ml. In patients with intact skin, the addition of a high-potency topical corticosteroid ointment in the genital area may be useful. If a topical corticosteroid is indicated, frequent follow-up to assess the area for the development of resulting atrophy or other adverse reactions is needed.

If significant genital scarring occurs and interferes with function, reparative surgery may be helpful. However, the disease must first be controlled since otherwise scarring immediately recurs and surgical injury can precipitate worsening of the disease locally.

Patients must be followed by an ophthalmologist for eye involvement, even if asymptomatic. Lubrication of the eyes should be provided, as scarring prevents natural lacrimation, and early treatment of eye infections helps to minimize scarring. Oral disease, like genital disease, can occasionally be helped by the addition of topical corticosteroids. Careful dental hygiene and frequent follow-up by a dentist may lessen the loss of teeth from gingival disease and retraction.

EPIDERMOLYSIS BULLOSA ACQUISITA

Epidermolysis bullosa acquisita is an uncommon autoimmune blistering and scarring disease that often exhibits marked mucous membrane involvement and can be clinically indistinguishable from cicatricial pemphigoid.

Clinical Presentation

Occurring most often in middle-aged or elderly patients, this disease usually presents with cutaneous blisters, but about 50 percent of patients have mucous membrane lesions. Initial blisters in the genital area quickly evolve into nonspecific erosions, especially on non-hair-bearing skin. With chronic or more severe disease, scarring becomes a predominant feature. Narrowing of the introitus and obliteration of the normal vulvar structures may occur, including resorption of the labia minora and clitoral hood with disappearance of the clitoris under scar. The normal skin texture often disappears, and the skin becomes smooth. Fragility of the skin may become marked, and uncircumcised men may develop phimosis. The late clinical appearance of epidermolysis bullosa acquisita can be indistinguishable from that of cicatricial pemphigoid and other erosive or blistering, scarring diseases.

Similarly, many other clinical findings are common to cicatricial or bullous pemphigoid. Scarring of the conjunctiva with late blindness can develop, and other mucous membrane involvement including esophageal and laryngeal disease with scarring may occur. Bullae of glabrous skin occur in virtually all patients. The blisters are tense, with straw-colored or hemorrhagic fluid. They may arise from either red or normal skin, often in response to friction or injury. As scarring develops over the hands, the fingers become tapered, reminiscent of scleroderma. Affected skin acquires a cigarette-paper texture with hypo- and hyperpigmentation and milia. Some patients exhibit much less scarring and more closely resemble those with bullous pemphigoid.

Histology

The biopsy of epidermolysis bullosa acquisita should include the border of a fresh blister, but if a blister is not present, the edge of an erosion should be sampled. Histologically, this disease shows a subepidermal blister with or without significant inflammation. Biopsies of inflammatory lesions demonstrate neutrophils and, less often, lymphocytes, macrophages, or eosinophils in the superficial dermis and within the blister. Direct immunofluorescence is usually positive, showing IgG and C3 along the basement membrane in a linear pattern. Less often, IgM or IgA are present. Indirect immunofluorescent assays reveal circulating antibodies in about 40 percent of patients, but levels do not correlate with the disease course. Immunofluorescence of split skin and immunoelectron microscopy reveal differences in the binding sites of antibodies within the basement membrane compared with other similar autoimmune blistering diseases.

Diagnosis

Diseases that can cause similar nonspecific erosions and late scarring of the genitalia include pemphigus vulgaris, cicatricial pemphigoid, bullous erythema multiforme, lichen planus, and lichen sclerosus. The extragenital, cutaneous blistering can be confused with the other autoimmune blistering diseases discussed in this chapter, and cicatricial and bullous pemphigoid in particular may present a diagnostic challenge. Biopsies, including immunoelectron microscopy or immunofluorescence of split skin, are needed to differentiate this disease from cicatricial and bullous pemphigoid.

Course and Prognosis

Epidermolysis bullosa acquisita can be an annoying, chronic condition that is limited to small areas of the body, or it can be widespread and painful with progressive scarring, disfigurement, and dysfunction. Specific treatment is poor, so supportive care is essential in this ongoing disease.

Pathogenesis

Epidermolysis bullosa acquisita results from autoantibodies to type VII collagen beneath the basement membrane zone. Complement activation produces inflammatory mediators that attract neutrophils, and resulting tissue damage produces blistering.

Treatment

The treatment of epidermolysis bullosa acquisita is very difficult. Unlike most autoimmune blistering diseases, this condition is not predictably responsive to corticosteroids or, indeed, any other modalities. However, a course of oral prednisone as well as the other treatments used to treat similar conditions can be tried to assess the individual patient's response.

Local care of the genitalia is important to minimize pain and scarring in this chronic disease. Topical corticosteroids may be useful in some patients. Regular retraction of the foreskin in men and the use of a vaginal dilator or regular coitus for women may prevent scarring that can interfere with function (see Desquamative Vaginitis in Ch. 7). Sitz baths or tepid water flushes to eroded and macerated areas may enhance healing and minimize the increased risk of superinfection. A high index of suspicion for superinfection and prompt treatment can minimize discomfort and scarring.

Patients with epidermolysis bullosa acquisita deserve an ongoing high index of suspicion for other mucous membrane disease. Careful local management of any involved areas by experienced specialists may minimize morbidity such as blindness and esophageal strictures.

CHRONIC BULLOUS DISEASE OF CHILDHOOD

Chronic bullous disease of childhood (childhood linear IgA dermatosis) is an autoimmune blistering disease that shows a predilection for the genitalia.

Clinical Presentation

This disease usually begins abruptly during the preschool years and always begins before puberty. There are no racial or gender proclivities. Children often describe pruritus, and there is sometimes a history of a preceding infection. The lesions consist of bullae that usually occur first over the genitalia, upper medial thighs, and lower abdomen, but the disease may spread and occasionally becomes generalized. Involvement of genital mucous membranes and modified mucous membranes generally does not occur, although about half of patients exhibit oral disease, and eye lesions have been reported.[9]

Individual lesions are tense bullae filled with straw-colored fluid arising from either red or noninflamed skin. There is a tendency for lesions to cluster and form rosettes of annular or arcuate blisters around old erosions or healing plaques. Postinflammatory color changes are common.

Histology

A biopsy shows a subepidermal blister with a neutrophilic or, less often, eosinophilic inflammatory infiltrate. The biopsy can be indistinguishable from bullous and cicatricial pemphigoid, and from dermatitis herpetiformis. Direct immunofluorescence of perilesional skin shows a homogeneous linear deposition of IgA and, less often, IgG, IgM, and/or C3 along the dermal-epidermal junction.

Diagnosis

Chronic bullous disease of childhood occurring in the genital area is most easily confused with bullous impetigo, although the more fragile nature of impetigo produces fewer tense blisters, and a culture reveals *S. aureus.* Other autoimmune diseases, bullous erythema multiforme (Stevens-Johnson syndrome), insect bites, and occasionally herpes simplex virus infection can also be confused with this disease. A biopsy is indicated to confirm the diagnosis.

Course and Prognosis

This disease usually remits spontaneously in 2 to 3 years, and nearly always by puberty, although there are case reports of ongoing disease.[10] The active disease is generally well controlled with oral dapsone or sulfapyridine.

Pathogenesis

The mechanism of blister formation is not known, although an etiologic role for IgA is presumed because it is located at the area of blister formation.

Treatment

Chronic bullous disease of childhood generally responds within several days to oral dapsone or sulfapyridine, and some patients may derive partial benefit from oral corticosteroids. Local supportive care including soaks and treatment of superinfection is useful. Fortunately, the disease remits spontaneously in almost all children.

PEMPHIGUS VULGARIS

Pemphigus vulgaris and its variant pemphigus vegetans are serious autoimmune blistering diseases that affect both mucous membranes and skin.

Clinical Presentation

Pemphigus vulgaris affects men and women equally and is most common in middle age. This disease has a higher incidence in Jewish patients but is seen in all races. The earliest symptoms are often mouth pain and sore throat from oral erosions; although pain or itching from genital involvement may also occur, these are frequently overshadowed by oral symptoms. In more advanced cutaneous pemphigus vulgaris, flaccid bullae and large erosions produce pain and, when extensive, constitutional symptoms associated with fluid and protein loss as well as intercurrent infections.

Initial genital lesions consist of nonspecific erosions, usually of the glans and prepuce of men, and the vestibule, labia minora, and inner labia majora of women (Fig. 16-10). The vagina and cervix may be affected as well. These erosions are very superficial and often unimpressive until superinfection and maceration worsen them secondarily. As the disease progresses, flaccid blisters and erosions may occur on the hair-bearing portions of the genitalia and distant skin. Although pemphigus vulgaris generally does not produce scarring, the thin, non-hair-bearing skin of the genitalia is an exception. Chronic disease and significant genital disease in the absence of careful local management occasionally result in the loss of genital landmarks with an end-stage picture indistinguishable from other scarring processes. Scarring of the labia minora to the labia majora or to each other, resorption of the clitoral hood with disappearance of the clitoris, narrowing of the introitus, and fusion of the vaginal walls that narrow or eradicate the vaginal

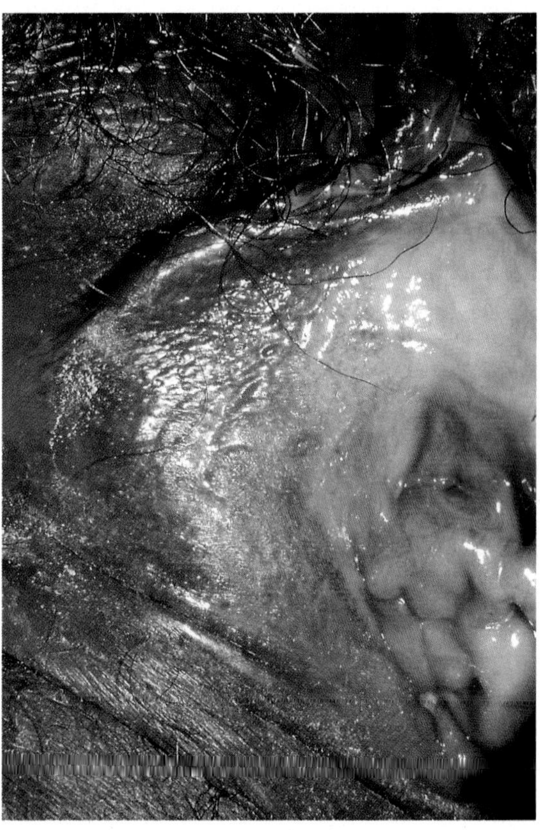

Fig. 16-10. Superficial erosions of the vestibule and inner labium minus in a patient with pemphigus vulgaris of the mouth and vulva only.

space all may occur. Scarring of the inner prepuce to the glans of uncircumcised men may occur. The skin may lose its normal texture and become smooth.

Oral lesions are prominent and occur early. The first involvement occurs in the posterior pharynx, with round, often coalescing erosions. Intact blisters are not seen because of their superficial nature and the fragility of mucous membrane epithelium. The palate, buccal mucosa, gingivae, and tongue may all be involved. Other mucous membranes may become involved, including the conjunctiva, nasal mucosa, and esophagus. Cutaneous lesions show large, flaccid blisters or areas of denuded skin left by evanescent bullae. The skin is fragile and friction strips off the upper epidermis or creates blisters.

The initial lesions of pemphigus vegetans are indistinguishable from those of pemphigus vulgaris. In more advanced pemphigus vegetans, pustules develop at the periphery of erosions, and finally hyperkeratotic plaques cover affected areas and obscure the underlying blistering character (Fig. 16-11).

Histology

The skin biopsy of pemphigus vulgaris shows suprabasal acantholysis. Basal cells remain anchored to the basement membrane but are no longer attached to each other or to overlying cells and present a "row of tombstones" appearance forming the floor of the blister. Except in very early lesions that may show intraepidermal eosinophils, inflammation is nearly absent. Late lesions of pemphigus vegetans show a nonspecific picture of hyperkeratosis, papillomatosis, and pseudoepitheliomatous hyperplasia. However, intraepithelial eosinophilic abscesses are often present and give an important clue to the diagnosis. Direct immunofluorescence of skin shows the intercellular deposition of IgG and C3 on keratinocyte membranes. Indirect immunofluorescence usually detects circulating IgG antibodies that correlate with the activity of the disease and can be followed to assess the patient's response to treatment.

Diagnosis

The diagnosis of pemphigus vulgaris is made on the clinical appearance with histologic confirmation on a sample that includes the border of a blister if possible, and otherwise the edge of an erosion. Early oral and genital erosive disease may mimic cicatricial pemphigoid, lichen planus, and erythema multiforme, whereas later, intact bullae of hair-bearing skin may also suggest bullous pemphigoid. The distribution and appearance of lesions, appearance of surrounding skin, and clinical setting usually yield the correct diagnosis, but a skin biopsy is indicated because of the possibility of error in this serious disease that requires chronic, high-risk treatment.

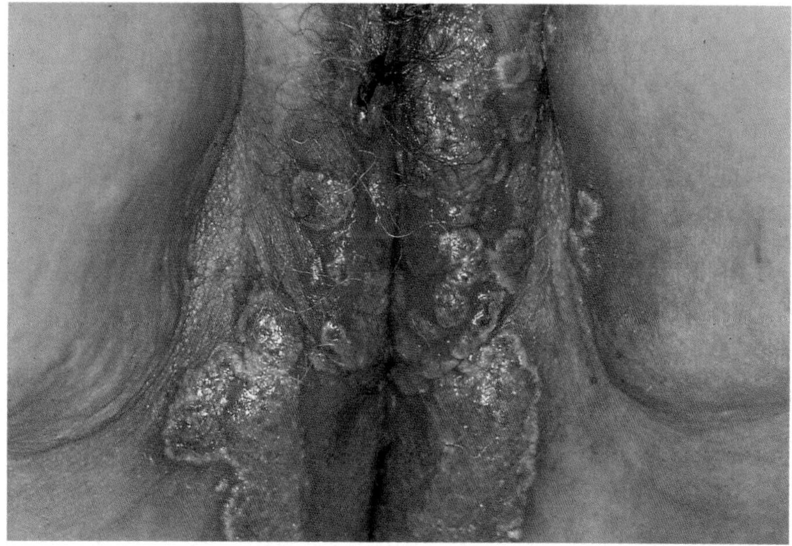

Fig. 16-11. Round and arcuate superficial erosions surrounded by pustules are representative of well-developed early pemphigus vegetans. (From Edwards,[12] with permission.)

Course and Prognosis

Although pemphigus vulgaris is a life-threatening disease, most patients can be controlled with proper management. Also, most patients eventually maintain a remission as medication is tapered to safe levels and sometimes entirely discontinued.

Pathogenesis

Pemphigus vulgaris is an autoimmune disease caused by circulating autoantibodies to normal adherence points of the epidermal cell membranes. These antibodies produce acantholysis and a suprabasalar blister in skin explants exposed to the IgG antibody, both with and without the addition of complement. Because this process is facilitated by complement as well as other evidence, many feel that complement plays an important role in pathogenesis.

Treatment

Untreated pemphigus vulgaris has a mortality rate of about 80 percent, resulting from fluid loss, infection, and an inability to eat, with subsequent wasting. The primary treatment for pemphigus vulgaris and vegetans is systemic corticosteroids in higher doses than are usually required for other skin diseases. In patients who are otherwise healthy, oral prednisone at 80 mg a day can be started, with increases of 20 mg a day every 4 or 5 days if new lesions continue to appear. In patients with severe and widespread disease, initial pulsed doses of intravenous methylprednisolone may be more efficient. Once new lesions do not appear and old erosions are healing, the corticosteroid can be tapered. This should be done carefully, since too rapid tapering, with a reappearance of skin lesions, often requires a return to the original controlling corticosteroid dose. Because some patients require 200 mg of prednisone or more each day to suppress their disease, and some patients cannot tolerate tapering of medication, azathioprine or cyclophosphamide may be added as steroid-sparing agents.[11] However, the benefits of these medications are not usually appreciated for about 1 month. Patients not controlled with these regimens may benefit from the addition of plasmapheresis accompanied by pulsed intravenous methylprednisolone. Monthly pulse intravenous cyclophosphamide is also effective in some refractory patients when added to daily oral cyclophosphamide and prednisone.

Because the mortality and morbidity of pemphigus vulgaris is now related primarily to adverse reactions to corticosteroids, an initial attempt to treat indolent pemphigus vulgaris with other, less aggressive but less effective treatments is reasonable. Alternate day oral corticosteroids, systemic gold, systemic methotrexate, and oral anti-inflammatory antibiotics such as tetracycline and erythromycin are useful in some patients.

Local care of the genitalia is important in this as in all blistering and erosive diseases. Patients with severe or poorly controlled disease are the most likely to experience the occasional local scarring and morbidity. Unfortunately, these are the patients whose other complications and systemic effects from the disease are most likely to divert the physician's attention away from the genitalia. The genital area should be followed carefully and treated for any secondary infections. The foreskin of uncircumcised men should be retracted daily and the glans inspected, flushed with water, and lubricated with a topical antibiotic ointment. If significant vaginal involvement is present in an ill, hospitalized patient, a vaginal mold may be inserted to prevent stenosis, but it must be removed and cleaned periodically to prevent infection. Alternatively, the daily insertion of a vaginal dilator helps to prevent vaginal synechiae (see also Ch. 7). Lubrication of vulvar lesions enhances healing and minimizes adhesions of skin folds. In patients with active genital disease who are otherwise largely controlled so that further systemic intervention is not planned, the addition of a high-potency topical corticosteroid ointment to genital lesions may be beneficial. Close follow-up to identify local adverse reactions is needed. Patients who develop scarring and adhesions may benefit from surgical repair after the underlying disease is inactive.

NON-BULLOUS EROSIVE DISEASES

Lichen Sclerosus

Although lichen sclerosus normally presents with thinned, hypopigmented, finely crinkled plaques, fragility is often prominent. Consequently, mild trauma from scratching, intercourse, or intercurrent infections may produce primary erosions or blisters that quickly become eroded. When lichen sclerosus exhibits prominent erosions, especially when the affected skin is not especially hypopigmented, the differentiation of this disease from other erosive diseases may be difficult. A careful search for an area of typical lichen sclerosus either on the genital area or on extragenital skin may be useful. An examination of the vagina or other mucous membranes that reveals the presence of lesions rules out lichen sclerosus as a diagnosis. Finally, a biopsy from the edge of an erosion may yield a definitive diagnosis (see Ch. 11).

Lichen Planus

Lichen planus regularly presents as scarring, erosive disease over the vulvar vestibule, often over other nonkeratinized skin of the vulva, and on the glans penis. Thus differentiation from other erosive diseases can be difficult. Careful scrutiny of surrounding skin or, even more important, the oral mucosa usually reveals classic white, lacy papules that clinch the diagnosis. Sometimes violaceous or dusky flat-topped papules of lichen planus may be visible on nearby genital skin. Like immunobullous diseases, but unlike lichen sclerosus, vaginal, oral, and gingival involvement is common, and a biopsy may be essential for diagnosis (see Ch. 6).

Chronic Excoriation from Neurodermatitis

Patients with atopic or neurodermatitis who are extremely pruritic often produce excoriations from vigorous scratching. In the damp, occluded environment of the genitalia, especially if superinfected, chronic erosions can develop. Scarring usually does not occur, as it does in lichen sclerosus, lichen planus, and immunobullous diseases. The erosions are often more sharply circumscribed, angular, and deeper than those of other erosive conditions. The skin is usually thickened in response to rubbing and scratching, but epithelium bordering any chronic inflammation or trauma (including blistering or erosive diseases) can thicken and appear similar. The vagina and other mucous membranes are not affected with atopic dermatitis. Again, a biopsy is often useful (see Ch. 5).

Erosive Candidiasis

Although *Candida* infection is usually manifested by a vaginal discharge or by very superficial pustules, this infection can sometimes be erosive. Patients at risk of maceration because of incontinence, obesity, sweating, or other local skin infections are more likely to develop erosive candidiasis. Also at increased risk are patients immunosuppressed by virtue of disease, systemic medications, or even topical corticosteroids. Small pustules become confluent and produce shallow erosions. Usually these erosions show circinate borders and exhibit satellite, round, 1- to 2-mm erosions that can be confused with herpes simplex infection, especially on the uncircumcised glans penis. Unlike some erosive diseases, erosive candidiasis is nonscarring. Normally, only the vagina, the uncircumcised glans, and sometimes the vulva are affected, with other mucous membranes spared. A potassium hydroxide preparation is positive. In women with erosive vulvar candidiasis, the vagina should be evaluated. Erosive vulvar *Candida* infection alone sometimes occurs after the vagina is treated without attention to the vulva or after a topical corticosteroid is added for lingering symptoms or irritation (see Ch. 5).

REFERENCES

Bullous Impetigo

1. Mertz PM, Marshall DA, Eaglestein WH et al: Topical mupirocin treatment of impetigo is equal to oral erythromycin therapy. Arch Dermatol 125:1069, 1989
2. Barton LL, Friedman AD, Portilla MG: Impetigo contagiosa: a comparison of erythromycin and dicloxacillin therapy. Pediatr Dermatol 5:88, 1988

Bullous Erythema Multiforme

3. Fritsch PO, Elias PM: Erythema multiforme and toxic epidermal necrolysis. p. 585. In Fitzpatrick TB, Eisen AZ, Wolff K et al (eds): Dermatology in General Medicine. McGraw-Hill, New York, 1993
4. Wilson EE, Malinak LR: Vulvovaginal sequelae of Stevens-Johnson syndrome and their management. Obstet Gynecol 71:478, 1988

Bullous Pemphigoid

5. Lindelof B, Islam N, Eklund G, Arfors L: Pemphigoid and cancer. Arch Dermatol 126:66, 1990
6. Berk MA, Lorincz AL: The treatment of bullous pemphigoid with tetracycline and niacinamide. A preliminary report. Arch Dermatol 122:670, 1986
7. Venning VA et al: Dapsone as first line therapy for bullous pemphigoid. Br J Dermatol 120:83, 1989

Cicatricial Pemphigoid

8. Foster CS: Cicitricial pemphigoid. Trans Am Ophthalmol Soc 84:527, 1986

8a. Edwards L: Vulvar cicatricial pemphigoid as a lichen sclerosus imitator. J Reprod Med 37:562, 1992

Chronic Bullous Diseases of Childhood

9. Wojnarowska F: Chronic bullous disease of childhood. Semin Dermatol 7:58, 1988
10. Burge S et al: Chronic bullous disease of childhood persisting into adulthood. Pediatr Dermatol 5:246, 1988

Pemphigus Vulgaris

11. Lever WF, Schaumberg Lever G: Immunosuppressants and prednisone in pemphigus vulgaris: therapeutic results obtained in 63 patients between 1961 and 1975. Arch Dermatol 113:1236, 1977
12. Edwards L: Desquamative vulvitis. Dermatol Clin 10:334, 1992

SUGGESTED READINGS

Bullous Impetigo

Williams REA, MacKie RM: The staphylococci. Importance of their control in the management of skin disease. Dermatol Clin 11:201, 1993

This is a good review article covering impetigo and other aspects of staphylococcal disease.

Fixed Drug Eruption

Sehgal VN, Gangwani OP: Fixed drug eruptions. Current concepts. Int J Dermatol 26:67, 1987

This article reviews the clinical features, the pathogenesis, and the many medications responsible for the fixed drug eruption.

Sehgal VH, Gangwant OP: Genital fixed drug eruptions. Genitourin Med 62:56, 1986

Twenty-seven men and two women with fixed drug eruptions of the genitalia are described, including their presentations, other areas of involvement, work-ups, and offending medications.

Bullous Erythema Multiforme

Rohrer TE, Ahmed AR: Toxic epidermal necrolysis. Int J Dermatol 30:457, 1991

The authors review the definition and history, etiologies, clinical manifestations, and management of this disease.

Bullous Pemphigoid

Mutasim DF: Bullous pemphigoid: review and update. J Ger Derm 1:62, 1993

This extensively referenced article on bullous pemphigoid is a concise and readable review of the clinical presentation, associations, course, pathogenesis, and treatment of this disease.

Cicatricial Pemphigoid

Ahmed AR, Kurgis BS, Rogers RS III: Cicatricial pemphigoid. J Am Acad Dermatol 24:987, 1991

This is a comprehensive review of the clinical and laboratory findings of cicatricial pemphigoid, with especially detailed plans for both systemic treatment and local management of this disease. A concise table compares cicatricial pemphigoid with epidermolysis bullosa acquisita.

Epidermolysis Bullosa Acquisita

Woodley DT, Briggaman RA, Gammon WR: Acquired epidermolysis bullosa. A bullous disease associated with autoimmunity to type VII (anchoring fibril) collagen. Dermatol Clin 8:701, 1990

The authors discuss the clinical spectrum, etiology, and management of this disease.

Chronic Bullous Diseases of Childhood

Wojnarowska R: Chronic bullous disease of childhood. Semin Dermatol 7:58, 1988

The author reviews the clinical findings and cause of this disease.

Autoimmune Bullous Diseases

Crosby DL, Diaz LA: Bullous diseases. Dermatol Clin 11:373, 1993

The entire issue consisting of 18 manuscripts includes updated reviews of all major blistering diseases, including chapters on bullous pemphigoid, cicatricial pemphigoid, pemphigus vulgaris and vegetans, epidermolysis bullosa acquisita, and linear IgA dermatosis.

Marren P, Wojnarowska F, Venning V et al: Vulvar involvement in autoimmune bullous diseases. J Reprod Med 38:101, 1993

This is a useful survey of the frequency and characteristics of vulvar disease in a large group of women with blistering disease who were specifically examined for genital involvement.

VI Ulcers

17 Infectious Primary Ulcers

PRIMARY SYPHILIS

The annual incidence of newly reported syphilis in the United States reached a nadir 40 years ago, but it increased appreciably 10 years ago in homosexual men. The rate in this group is now falling, but this is more than balanced by a rise in crack smokers and intravenous drug users. In these latter individuals, the increase relates to the practice of trading sex for drugs.[1] The disease today is somewhat more common in men than women,[2] although the actual occurrence in women may be underestimated because their primary lesions are so often missed.

Clinical Presentation

Syphilis is a remarkably contagious disease; approximately 30 percent of those exposed become infected. Approximately 1 month (range, 10 to 90 days) after exposure, the first clinical signs of infection occur. The initial lesion develops at the site of inoculation as a small papule, which immediately breaks down to form a slowly enlarging ulcer. Classically only a single ulcer is present, but in at least 35 percent of patients, two or even three ulcers may be present.[3] The ulcer usually has a noncrusted ("clean") base and lacks undermining of the ulcer edges. On palpation it has a firm base and is relatively nontender. Palpable lymphadenopathy, often unilateral, is usually present in men with penile lesions and in women with anterior vulvar lesions.

In men, the ulcer most commonly occurs on the distal penis, in women, the labia majora are the most frequently observed site. Cervical lesions probably occur even more often, but in this relatively hidden site they resolve spontaneously before they are discovered. Anal ulcers are also encountered relatively often; not surprisingly, these lesions are particularly likely to be found in gay men as a result of anal intercourse.[3] Anal ulcers should be sought in patients who indicate discomfort on defecation and in those who have bloody or mucus-stained stools.

The main lesions in the list of differential diagnoses include herpetic erosions (less deep; quite painful), aphthous ulcers (more painful; base soft), and chancroid (more painful; base soft and crusted). The other ulcers listed in this chapter and in Chapter 18 would not likely be confused with primary syphilis.

Diagnosis of a clinically suspicious lesion is achieved through dark-field examination, serologic testing, or biopsy. Dark-field examination provides a rapid answer and is the diagnostic test of choice if suitable facilities and well-trained personnel are available. This microscopic examination is both sensitive and specific; nearly all untreated chancres are positive, although care must be taken to differentiate *Treponema pallidum* from the nonpathogenic spirochetes that can be found on all moist mucous membranes. The techniques for performing dark-field examinations and the less commonly used direct fluorescent microscopy can be found in standard textbooks on sexually transmitted diseases.

Serologic testing is the most widely used diagnostic technique. The rapid plasma reagin (RPR) test has almost replaced the Venereal Disease Research Laboratory (VDRL) test because of the ease with which it can be automated. This test is used primarily for screening purposes; a positive result is usually confirmed with a test that uses a specific *T. pallidum* antigen such as the fluorescent treponemal-antibody absorption (FTA-Abs) test or the microhemagglutination assay for *T. pallidum* (MHA-TP). The RPR test usually becomes positive a week or so after the appearance of the chancre. For this reason, the RPR is positive only about 70 to 80 percent of the time when a clinical diagnosis of a chancre is made.[4] A false negative RPR test is particularly likely to occur in patients with human immunodeficiency virus (HIV) infection. The FTA-Abs test and the MHA-TP become positive before the RPR does, and therefore it may be appropriate to obtain either one or the other of these tests when a patient with a clinically suspicious ulcer is RPR negative. Alternatively, and with a reliable patient, the RPR can be repeated several days later.

Biopsy of a genital ulcer should be carried out if a patient with a clinically suspicious ulcer is seronegative and a dark-field examination is negative or not available. The histopathology is rather distinctive because of the large number of perivascular plasma cells. In this setting, an alert pathologist can then identify the etiologic spirochetes using the Warthin-Starry silver stain.

Course and Prognosis

Treatment of primary syphilis results in rapid disappearance, usually without scarring, of the chancre. Secondary lesions of syphilis only develop in those whose primary disease is either untreated or is inadequately treated. Secondary lesions can occur as early as 6 weeks after infection but more typically develop after an interval of several months.

It is very important to note that *untreated* chancres resolve spontaneously within a month or two. For this reason, clearance of a chancre is not of itself sufficient to demonstrate the adequacy of treatment; the titer of the RPR serology should also be followed. Titers begin falling within 2 months and usually decline by 2 dilutions in 3 months and 3 dilutions in 6 months.[5] A similar rate of decline occurs in patients with secondary syphilis and, in both forms of syphilis, a return to seronegativity in 2 years is noted in at least 75 percent of patients. Suspicion of inadequately treated syphilis is suggested by a recurrence of lesions, a rising serology, or a failure to revert to seronegativity within 3 years.

Primary syphilis in patients with concomitant HIV infection is particularly problematic. Serologic tests are less often positive in the early weeks of infection, and adequacy of response to therapy is more difficult to determine. Many outright failures to respond to conventional therapy have been documented in HIV patients.[6] In such circumstances early advancement to neurosyphilis is all too likely to occur. For this reason it is prudent to follow the serologic titers as often as monthly in HIV-positive patients.

Pathogenesis

Syphilis is caused by the spirochete *T. pallidum*. Related treponemal species are responsible for the tropical diseases yaws and pinta. Spirochetes of *Borrelia* spp. cause Lyme disease and occasionally false-positive RPR tests; other nonpathogenic *Borrelia* spp. are regularly found on moist human mucosae. Accurate morphologic identification of these various spirochetes is possible but is unreliable in most clinical laboratories.

T. pallidum spirochetes are present in the moist lesions of primary and secondary syphilis. They are transferred from an infected person to an unaffected person by direct skin-to-skin contact. Early studies indicated that as few as 10 spirochetes were sufficient to result in infection about 25 percent of the time. Infection is possible through intact mucous membranes, but it is facilitated by the type of microbreaks and erosions that occur during the frictional trauma of sexual activity.

Once inoculated, organisms move quickly to the regional lymph nodes. Thus systemic infection has already occurred by the time the first clinical lesions develop. Clinical evidence of wide spread systemic infection, however, is not noted until the secondary stage of the disease, at which point most patients begin to develop fever, malaise, pharyngitis, and musculoskeletal symptoms. Infection of the central nervous system (CNS) was once thought to occur only late in the course of the disease, but recent experience with HIV-infected patients suggests that early

CNS involvement is possible and may even be common. Lumbar puncture for analysis of cerebral spinal fluid may be warranted early on for patients with concomitant HIV infection.

Treatment

Penicillin is the treatment of choice for syphilis. Treponemicidal levels of the drug must be present, uninterrupted, for at least a week because of the long intervals between mitotic divisions of the spirochete. For this reason the depot form of penicillin, benzathine penicillin G (Bicillin L-A), is the preferred product. Care must be taken in ordering Bicillin by brand name lest Bicillin C-R be administered instead. This latter product is a mixture of benzathine penicillin and procaine penicillin; it is not recommended for use in the treatment of syphilis. The dose for both primary and secondary syphilis is 2.4 million U IM. However, because of concern over possible treatment failure, especially in HIV-positive patients, most physicians administer a second dose of 2.4 million U a week after the first. For patients allergic to penicillin, oral administration of doxycycline (100 mg twice daily) or tetracycline (500 mg four times daily) for 28 days is the preferred alternative treatment.

As indicated above, the results of treatment are monitored by the disappearance of clinical symptoms and signs as well as by a falling titer of the RPR test. In the event of treatment failure, as judged by these criteria, retreatment is necessary. In HIV-positive patients who fail treatment, many prefer to switch from benzathine penicillin to daily intramuscular or even intravenous penicillin.[7] Treatment of latent syphilis and neurosyphilis lies outside the scope of this book.

CHANCROID

Chancroid is a sexually transmitted disease with an incubation period of 5 to 14 days in men and 5 to 30 days in women. The incidence of chancroid in America 25 years ago was less than 1,000 reported cases a year. Since then there has been a gradual increase, until 5,000 cases were reported in 1987.[8] Most of the documented increase has occurred as a result of mini-iepidemics in localized geographic areas such as Dallas, New York City, and South Florida.[9] Most of the cases of chancroid in America occur in males of low socioeconomic status who frequent prostitutes. Male to female ratios in reported series range from a low of 3:1 to as high as 50:1.

Clinical Presentation

The initial lesion in chancroid is a small red macule or vesicopapule that rapidly breaks down to form a painful ulcer 1 to 2 cm in diameter. The ulcer may be solitary, but in a majority of cases, two or three clustered ulcers develop (Fig. 17-1). Individual ulcers usually have undermined edges with a crusted gray or purulent base that bleeds easily. The shape of the ulcer is often somewhat irregular. Ulcers in men are usually found on the penis; those in women are often located in the vagina and on the cervix. The "hidden" nature of the lesions in women may partially explain the wide discrepancy in prevalence noted between men and women.

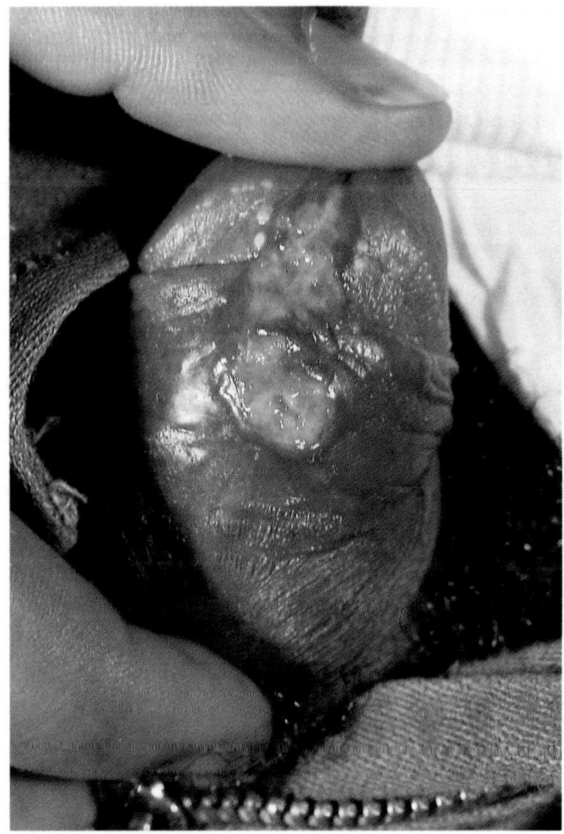

Fig. 17-1. Large, irregular, well-demarcated, clustered ulcers of chancroid.

Lymphadenopathy, usually unilateral and often of massive size, is found in 50 percent of patients. One or more of these enlarged nodes often develop areas of fluctuance forming the so-called bubo. A fluctuant area may then break down and drain purulent material, usually through a single site (Fig. 17-2).

Clinically suspicious lesions are best confirmed with culture; smears from the ulcers are helpful only if the classical "linked chains" or "school of fish" arrangement of gram-negative rods is visualized. Controversy exists regarding the most appropriate form of culture media to be used, but most authorities agree that the use of defibrinated blood (chocolate agar) or Mueller-Hinton media work best.[10] Direct plating of the culture swab, rather than placement in transport media, results in appreciable higher rates of positive cultures.

Many uncommon variants of chancroid have been reported over the years, including (1) small, shallow herpetiform ulcers; (2) confluence of small ulcers to form giant ulcers with serpiginous borders; (3) draining, furuncle-like nodules; (4) lymph node involvement without recognizable mucocutaneous lesions; and (5) urethritis in the male.

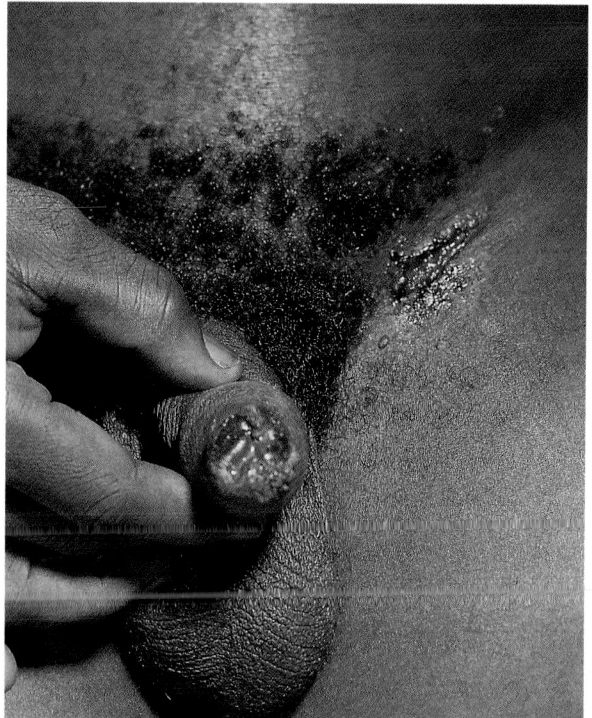

Fig. 17-2. Irregular, slightly undermined ulcer of the glans with a crusted appearance is characteristic of chancroid, and is seen here with an enlarged, ulcerated lymph node.

Histology

Biopsy provides helpful, though usually not diagnostic information. Three zones are situated microscopically at the ulcer base. The first is a narrow zone of necrotic tissue with plentiful neutrophils. The second is a vascular zone in which the blood vessels show marked proliferation of their endothelial cells. The third is an inflammatory band with numerous plasma cells. Unfortunately, stains for *Hemophilus ducreyi* (the causative organism) in biopsy tissue are usually negative.

Differential Diagnoses

Diseases to be considered clinically in the list of differential diagnoses include primary syphilis, aphthous ulcers, Crohn's disease and, in the immunosupressed, genital herpes. The chancre of syphilis is less tender, has a firmer base, will be dark-field positive, and usually will occur in a patient with a positive serologic test for syphilis. Aphthous ulcers have a "cleaner" base, are less likely to be associated with lymphadenopathy, are periodically recurrent, and are separable histologically. Ulcers of Crohn's disease are less "punched out" in appearance and usually occur in the setting of bowel disease. Viral cultures will identify herpetic ulcers.

Course and Prognosis

Untreated, the ulcers persist for 2 or more months before healing spontaneously, usually with scar formation. With appropriate treatment, ulcers heal in about 10 days with little or no scar formation. No immunity develops; for this reason, reinfection occurs easily.

Pathogenesis

Chancroid is a bacterial infection caused by *H. ducreyi*. This organism is a gram-negative rod that is rather difficult to culture dependably. Because the organism is so difficult to recover, the earlier literature often reported series of cases in which the diagnosis was made on a clinical basis. Many of these reports in reality probably described herpes genitalis before this virus was recognized as a common cause of sexually transmitted disease.[11] Moreover, it is unclear whether or not *H. ducreyi* can be found as a colonizing, nonpathogenic organism. If *H. ducreyi* can exist as a commensal organism, the frequent finding of so-called mixed infections, usually with primary syphilis or genital herpes, would be more easily explained.

Treatment

The currently recommended treatment consists of orally administered erythromycin (2 g/day for 7 days) or ceftriaxone, 250 mg administered as a single intramuscular injection.[8] Historically, long-acting sulfa drugs such as Bactrim DS twice daily for 7 days have been used effectively as well. If fluctuance of enlarged nodes is present, needle aspiration is preferred to incision and drainage because chronic sinus formation may sometimes develop following the latter procedure.

GRANULOMA INGUINALE

Granuloma inguinale (donovanosis) is a very rare disease in Europe and North America. Fewer than 100 cases are reported annually in the United States. It does, however, remain as a disease of some importance in Third World countries.[12] It is presumably a sexually transmitted disease, but infectivity between marital partners is actually quite low. The incubation period is highly variable but averages 2 to 4 weeks. Men appear to be infected more frequently than women by a ratio of at least 2 or 3:1.[13]

Clinical Presentation

The initial lesion is a papule that quickly erodes to form a painless, slowly expanding, irregularly shaped ulcer. The base of the ulcer is filled with granulation tissue that bleeds easily with even minor trauma. Linear ulcers, appearing as slits can occur in intertriginous folds. Usually only a single ulcer is present, but multiple lesions can occur. Verrucous, necrotizing, and sclerosing variants of these primary lesions have been reported.[13] The genitalia are most often the site of involvement, but 10 percent of the lesions occur in a perianal location. Lesions in other than an anogenital distribution occur in about 5 percent of infected individuals. Lymphadenopathy is not usually present; this absence of enlarged nodes (except in the setting of secondary infection) is a helpful diagnostic sign.

Histology

Diagnosis is established by tissue smears or biopsy, or both. A smear is obtained by taking a small piece of tissue from the ulcer and crushing it between two glass slides. The material on the slides is then spread out and is first fixed and then stained with Wright's or Giemsa stain. The presence of Donovan bodies (cytoplasmic coccobacilli) in mononuclear cells confirms the diagnosis. Unfortunately, although smears are quite specific, they lack sensitivity, especially early in the course of the disease. Biopsy reveals a granulomatous reaction with neutrophils and plentiful plasma cells. Donovan bodies may be identified but often only with some difficulty. Overlying epithelial hyperplasia may raise a question of associated squamous cell carcinoma.

Differential Diagnoses

Ulcerated carcinoma and the ulcers and fistulae of Crohn's disease can be clinically mistaken for granuloma inguinale. Histologically, other granulomatous diseases such as Crohn's disease and hidradenitis suppurativa should be considered.

Course and Prognosis

Untreated, the ulcers persist and enlarge for years; secondary exudative infection of the ulcers with a variety of bacteria sometimes occurs. In the late stages of the disease, sclerosis of tissue and stenosis of the urethra, vagina, and anus may develop. Lymphatic damage may lead to chronic edema and elephantiasis.[14] Squamous cell carcinoma occurring in chronic lesions has been reported with some frequency. Moreover, untreated patients are at risk for the development of systemic infection, usually in the form of osseous lesions. Early treatment prevents all of these complications.

Pathogenesis

The causative agent is a gram-negative bacterial organism, *Calymmatobacterium granulomatis,* that may be either coccal or bacillary in morphology. The organism is antigenically related to *Klebsiella* spp. Recovery of the bacteria in culture is extremely difficult.

Treatment

Granuloma inguinale responds well to a variety of antibiotics.[15] Tetracycline (2 g/day), doxycycline (100 mg twice daily), and sulfa-trimethoprim (Bactrim DS) twice daily for 14 days are the agents most often used. Since the ulcers may not be completely healed after 2 weeks, some authorities recommend extension of treatment until healing occurs.

LYMPHOGRANULOMA VENEREUM

Lymphogranuloma venereum (LGV) is a very uncommon sexually transmitted disease; fewer than 500 cases are reported annually in the United States. The disease occurs 5 to 10 times more frequently in men than in women, but this ratio most likely reflects inadequate recognition of the disease in women. The incubation period is variable, but it is generally stated to be 3 to 30 days. It is uncertain whether an asymptomatic carrier state exists.

Clinical Presentation

LGV reportedly begins with a papule or shallow ulcer. Because these lesions are painless and transient, only 25 percent of patients are aware of having had these primary lesions. Most male patients do not seek medical attention until lymph node enlargement (bubo formation) becomes apparent.

Lymphadenopathy is the cardinal feature of the disease and is unilateral 70 percent of the time. Inguinal nodes are regularly involved; femoral nodes are involved less frequently. When both inguinal and femoral nodes are enlarged, they are separated by Poupart's ligament (Fig. 17-3). The separation is visible as a groove between the two sets of nodes. This groove sign is believed to be pathognomonic of LGV. Inflammation within the involved nodes frequently leads to the development of fluctuant areas, which may subsequently break down and drain purulent material through multiple sites. The presence of multiple fistulae helps to distinguish the bubos of LGV from those of chancroid, in which only a single site of drainage develops.

Women with vulvovaginal infection may present with lymphadenopathy as described above. However, because of differences in lymphatic drainage, perirectal nodes may be involved instead. Lymphadenopathy in the perirectal area is relatively inapparent unless perirectal abscesses develop.

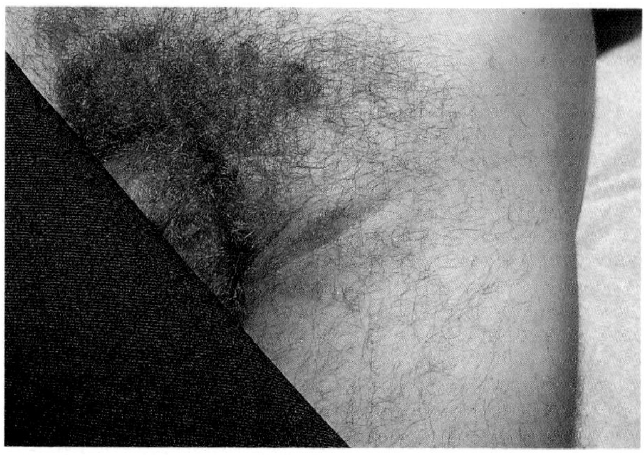

Fig. 17-3. The groove sign of Greenblatt, classic for lymphogranuloma venereum, produced by lymphadenopathy bisected by Poupart's ligament.

When primary infection in women and gay men occurs in the anus via anal intercourse, the presenting signs and symptoms are likely to be those of ulceration and granulation tissue formation simulating the changes of ulcerative colitis. Primary infection in extragenital sites may lead to regional lymphadenopathy similar to that described in the inguinal and femoral nodes.

Most patients with LGV will experience systemic symptoms and signs such as fever, malaise, headache, and arthralgia. A small percentage of patients develop erythema nodosum or erythema multiforme. White blood cell counts are elevated; anemia and increased levels of gamma globulins are sometimes present.

The best test for diagnosis is culture of the causative organism from pus aspirated from the enlarged nodes. Complement fixing and microfluorescent antibody serologic tests are available, but they lack specificity and thus can only be used when the clinical features are classical for the disease. The Frei skin test is no longer used.

Differential Diagnoses

LGV is the major sexually transmitted disease in heterosexual men that presents solely with lymph node enlargement. Male patients with chancroid may have bubos, but generally one or more genital ulcers are also present. Moreover, the bubos in chancroid (as noted above) drain through only a single site. The list of differential diagnoses for those patients who present with proctitis is much longer and includes ulcerative colitis, Crohn's disease of the rectum, and a multiplicity of common and uncommon infections.

Course and Prognosis

LGV, if left untreated, persists for years. Architectural distortion of the external genitalia with fistulae, scarring, and chronic edema (elephantiasis) is regularly present; these changes, when they occur in women, are known as esthiomene. Anal stenosis and rectal strictures are also found. Treatment prevents these sequellae.

Pathogenesis

Lymphogranuloma venereum is caused by *Chlamydia trachomatis.* This organism is similar to, but distinct from , the agents that cause ocular trachoma and genitourinary (urethritis and cervicitis) disease. The serovars responsible for LGV have been identified as L1, L2, and L3. However, there is considerable overlap in antibody formation between the LGV serovars and those of chlamydial organisms responsible for others forms of urogenital disease. For this reason some of the information published in the past regarding antibody levels in LGV is likely to be erroneous.

Treatment

A variety of antibiotics have been successfully used in the treatment of lymphogranuloma venereum. The preferred treatment at the present is doxycycline 100 mg orally two times a day for 3 weeks. Alternatively, tetracycline or erythromycin, both in a dose of 2 g a day for 3 weeks, can be used. Fluctuant nodes should be aspirated with a syringe and needle as often as is necessary. Incision and drainage of fluctuant nodes is to be avoided lest nonhealing fistulae develop.

HERPES SIMPLEX IN THE IMMUNOSUPPRESSED

For a full discussion of herpes simplex in the immunosuppressed, see Chapter 24.

REFERENCES

Primary Syphilis

1. Hutchinson CM, Rompalo AM, Reichert CA, Hook EW III: Characteristics of patients with syphilis attending Baltimore STD clinics. Arch Intern Med 151:511, 1991
2. Mindel A, Tovey SJ, Williams P: Primary and secondary syphilis, 20 years' experience. 1. Epidemiology. Genitourin Med 63:361, 1987
3. Mindel A, Tovey SJ, Timmins DJ, Williams P: Primary and secondary syphilis, 20 years' experience. 2. Clinical features. Genitourin Med 65:1, 1989
4. Anderson J, Mindel A, Tovey SJ, Williams P: Primary and secondary syphilis, 20 years' experience. 3. Diagnosis, treatment, and follow up. Genitourin Med 65:239, 1989
5. Romanowski B, Sutherland R, Fick GH et al: Serologic response to treatment of infectious syphilis. Ann Intern Med 114:1005, 1991
6. Musher DM, Hamill RJ, Baughn RE: Effect of human immunodeficiency virus (HIV) infection on the course of syphilis and on the response to treatment. Ann Intern Med 113:872, 1990
7. Hook EW III: Management of syphilis in human immunodeficiency virus-infected patients. Am J Med 93:477, 1992

Chancroid

8. Felman YM: Recent developments in sexually transmitted diseases: chancroid—epidemiology, diagnosis, and treatment. Cutis 44:113, 1989
9. Schmid GP, Sanders LL, Blount JH, Alexander ER: Chancroid in the United States. Reestablishment of an old disease. JAMA 258:3265, 1987
10. Jones CC, Rosen T: Cultural diagnosis of chancroid. Arch Dermatol 127:1823, 1991
11. Salzman RS, Kraus SJ, Miller RG et al: Chancroidal ulcers that are not chancroid. Arch Dermatol 120:636, 1984

Granuloma Inguinale

12. Niemel PLA, Engelkens HJH, van der Meijden WI, Stolz E: Donovanosis (granuloma inguinale) still exists. Int J Dermatol 31: 244, 1992
13. Sehgal VN, Prasad ALS: Donovanosis. Current concepts. Int J Dermatol 25:8, 1986
14. Sehgal VN, Jain MK, Sharma VK: Pseudoelephantiasis induced by donovanosis. Genitourin Med 63:54, 1987
15. Richens J: The diagnosis and treatment of donovanosis (granuloma inguinale). Genitourin Med 67:441, 1991

SUGGESTED READINGS

Primary Syphilis

Hook EW III, Marra CM: Acquired syphilis in adults. N Engl J Med 326:1060, 1992

This review article covers the epidemiology, laboratory diagnosis, therapy, and interaction with HIV infection very well. It has relatively little material on the clinical features of primary and secondary disease.

Chancroid

Buntin DM, Rosen T, Lesher JL Jr et al: Sexually transmitted diseases: bacterial infections. J Am Acad Dermatol 25:287, 1991

This article contains a short but up-to-date review of chancroid.

McCarley ME, Cruz PD, Sontheimer RD: Chancroid: clinical variants and other findings from an epidemic in Dallas County, 1986–1987. J Am Acad Dermatol 19:330, 1988

This article describes the epidemic of cases that occurred in the mid 1980s in Dallas. It also contains an excellent review of the literature to that point.

Granuloma Inguinale

Buntin DM, Rosen T, Lesher JL Jr: Sexually transmitted diseases: bacterial infections. J Am Acad Dermatol 25:287, 1991

This is a good, short review of the subject.

Wysoki RE, Majmudar B, Willis D: Granuloma inguinale (donovanosis) in women. J Reprod Med. 33:709, 1988

The authors review 13 cases seen in a 10-year period at Grady Memorial Hospital in Atlanta, Georgia.

Lymphogranuloma Venereum

Buntin DM, Rosen T, Lesher JL Jr et al: Sexually transmitted diseases: bacterial infections. J Am Acad Dermatol 25:287, 1991

This article contains a short up-to-date review of lymphogranuloma venereum.

Schacter J, Osoba AO: Lymphogranuloma venereum. Br Med Bull 39:151, 1983

This article provides a very good summary of the information available on lymphogranuloma venereum up to 1982.

18 Noninfectious Primary Ulcers

APHTHOUS ULCERS

Aphthous ulcers (aphthae) of the mouth are extremely common; about 50 percent of the population will develop one or more such lesions. Rarely, similar lesions develop on the genitalia. Exact epidemiologic data regarding the occurrence of these genital ulcers are not available, but our experience suggests that the disease is confined almost entirely to women and that the peak age of onset is from late childhood to early adulthood. Usually patients with genital aphthae have a history of oral lesions as well, but lesions in these two sites do not necessarily occur concomitantly. The occurrence of oral and genital aphthae in the same patient is sometimes termed *complex aphthosis.*[1]

Clinical Presentation

Aphthae begin as small painful red macules that evolve into ulcers within hours. Small ulcers on moist parts of genitalia have a white center similar to those found in the mouth. Larger ulcers and those in drier locations have a clean (noncrusted) base of normal granulation tissue. Ulcer size ranges from 3 mm to 2 cm in diameter. The perimeter of the ulcer may have a thin ring of erythema, but often the ulcer appears to have arisen from totally normal skin without visible evidence of inflammation. The ulcers are very sharply marginated and are surprisingly deep. Little or no undermining occurs (Fig. 18-1). Small ulcers are round; larger ones may be irregular in shape (Fig. 18-2). Aphthae are at least moderately painful; sometimes the pain is described as excruciating.

In women, aphthous ulcers are located most frequently within the vulvar vestibule, but aphthae can occur within the vagina, on the external aspect of the labia minora, and anywhere on the labia majora. In men, the penis and scrotum are most often involved. Perianal ulcers occasionally occur in both sexes. One or several lesions may be present. Palpable lymphadenopathy is usually absent.

Most patients have no associated systemic symptoms and signs. In fact, if more than fatigue and mild malaise are present, one should consider the possibility that aphthae are occurring in the setting of Behçet's or Crohn's disease.[1]

Diagnosis

To some degree the diagnosis is one of exclusion; there are no pathognomonic laboratory tests. Biopsy reveals mostly nonspecific dermal inflammation. Diseases to be considered in the list of differential diagnoses are described below. The chancre of primary syphilis is similar in appearance but has a firm base on palpation and is much less painful; dark-field examination, if available, and serologic tests for syphilis are generally positive. The erosions of genital herpes are more numerous, shallow, and clustered; viral cultures will usually be positive. The ulcers of chancroid are similar to aphthous ulcers, but patients with chancroid have prominent lymphadenopathy, and cultures for *Hemophilus ducreyii* are positive.

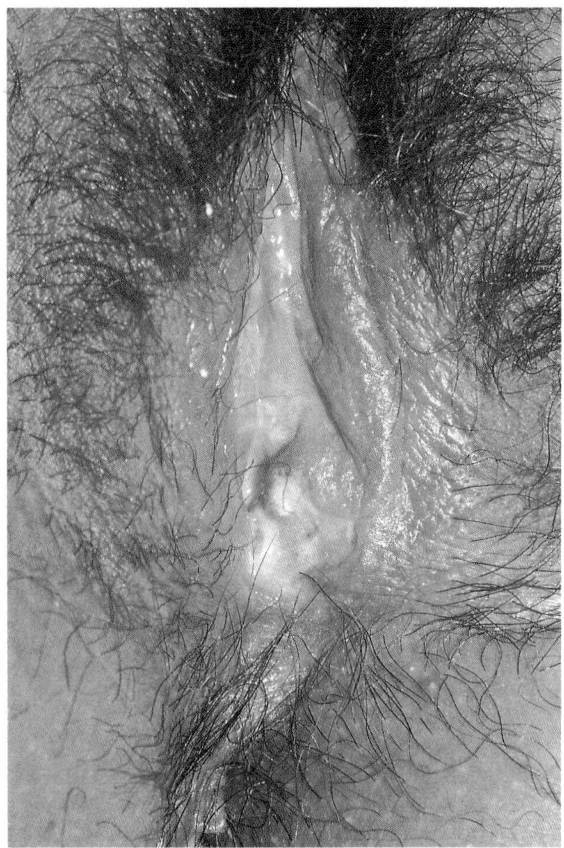

Fig. 18-1. Well-demarcated chronic aphthous ulcer associated with small oral ulcerations.

Ulcers due to malignancy and granulomatous disease are identified on biopsy. Because the diagnosis of aphthae is most often made on the basis of exclusion, biopsy should be performed in almost all instances.

Course and Prognosis

Individual ulcers heal in 2 to 4 weeks, but even as one ulcer is healing another new one may be developing. Most patients have "bursts" of activity during which many ulcers form and resolve. This active period may then be followed by a variable interval during which the frequency of ulcer formation is markedly reduced. Resolution of the ulcers most often occurs without scarring, but scarring is possible when the lesions are very large and deep. The frequency with which ulcers appear seems to decrease gradually after the fifth decade. Patients with aphthosis major sometimes experience fatigue and malaise when lesions are present, but evolution into full-blown Behçet's disease does not seem to occur with much frequency.

Pathogenesis

The cause of aphthae is unknown. The fact that oral lesions occur in such a large proportion of the population suggests that the etiology is likely to be multifactorial. Immunologic factors may be important since in vitro the mucosal cells of patients are attacked by their own lymphocytes. Likewise, mucosal cells of patients can cause DNA synthesis and mitotic activity of their own lymphocytes. Genetic factors may also play a role since some patients have a positive family history for similar lesions. Aphthous

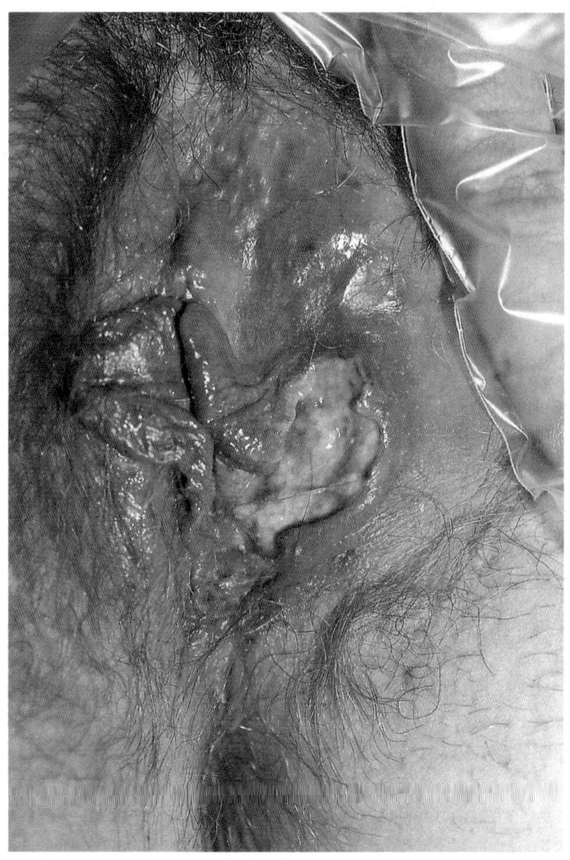

Fig. 18-2. Sharply demarcated aphthous ulcer with yellow/white fibrin base that healed completely in 3 weeks with oral prednisone therapy. (Courtesy of Gerald N. Goldberg, M.D.)

ulcers tend to develop in the mouth during periods of stress and anxiety. It is possible that psychological factors operate in the pathogenesis of genital lesions also.

Treatment

Small lesions that are not too symptomatic can be left untreated. Those associated with modest discomfort can be locally treated with lidocaine; Xylocaine ointment (5 percent), jelly (2 percent), or viscous solution (2 percent) can be applied several times a day by fingertip or a cotton-tipped applicator. This approach is particularly useful prior to urination and defecation. Alternatively, a silver nitrate stick can be touched to the base once every day or so by either patient or physician. Care must be taken when using silver nitrate sticks, as overly generous use may result in a greater than desired degree of tissue necrosis.

Larger, more symptomatic lesions can be intralesionally injected with 0.1 to 0.3 ml of triamcinolone acetonide (Kenalog 10) prepared in a concentration of about 5 mg/ml. While this approach avoids any significant systemic steroid effect, it is understandably quite painful. For this reason most physicians prefer oral prednisone administered as 40 mg a day for 5 to 10 days. This type of "burst" treatment can be repeated, if necessary, as often as once every 10 to 12 weeks.

Even with the use of systemic steroids, some lesions will not respond or will recur very quickly. For these patients longer term treatment with a variety of anti-inflammatory agents such as tetracycline, Dapsone, colchicine, Plaquenil (hydroxychloroquine), oral contraceptives, or even azathioprine may be required. The use of all of these agents is discussed in Chapter 3 in the sections on intralesional and systemic treatment.

BEHÇET'S DISEASE

Behçet's disease was defined more than 50 years ago as a triad of oral ulcers, genital ulcers, and ocular inflammation. In the interval since then, many additional components have been added to the description. For practical purposes Behçet's disease encompasses a spectrum of symptoms and signs ranging from the sole presence of oral and genital ulcers (aphthous major), as described in the section above, to that of a rarely encountered process involving multiorgan severe systemic disease.[1] The diagnostic criteria currently used are those of the International Study Group for Behçet's Disease. The criteria include the presence of oral aphthae plus any two of the following: aphthous type genital ulceration, defined eye disease, defined skin lesions, or the presence of a pustule at the site of intracutaneously injected saline (skin pathergy).[2]

Behçet's disease as it is recognized in Western Europe and North America includes oral and genital ulceration, but this variant is associated with less severe systemic disease than that described in Eastern Europe and Japan. Specifically, "Western" Behçet's disease is more common in women and is associated with collagen-vascular disease-type symptoms, whereas "Eastern" Behçet's disease is more comon in men and is most often associated with significant central nervous system (CNS) disease and with ocular disease severe enough to cause blindness.[3]

Clinical Presentation

Oral ulcers of the aphthous type occur in essentially all patients with Behçet's disease. Anogenital aphthous ulcers (see Aphthous Ulcers above) are found in about 90 percent of affected patients (Fig. 18-3). Ulcers in both locations vary in severity, number, and duration; they may or may not occur concomitantly. Inflammation of either the anterior or posterior portion of the eye occurs in approximately 75 percent of patients. In addition, patients may develop several or all of the following problems: gastrointestinal symptoms (primarily diarrhea simulating Crohn's disease), arthritis, thrombophlebitis, psychiatric problems, and various types of neurologic disease. Additional cutaneous problems include erythema nodosum, erythema multiforme, and pustular lesions occurring at the site of trauma (pathergy).[4] Recently Sweets syndrome has been reported as occurring in association with Behçet's disease,[5] and a group of patients with relapsing polychondritis and ulceration of the mouth and genitalia has been described.[6]

Histology

As indicated in the section on aphthous ulcers, the microscopic appearance of material from the edge of ulcers, whether genital or oral, is fairly nonspecific.

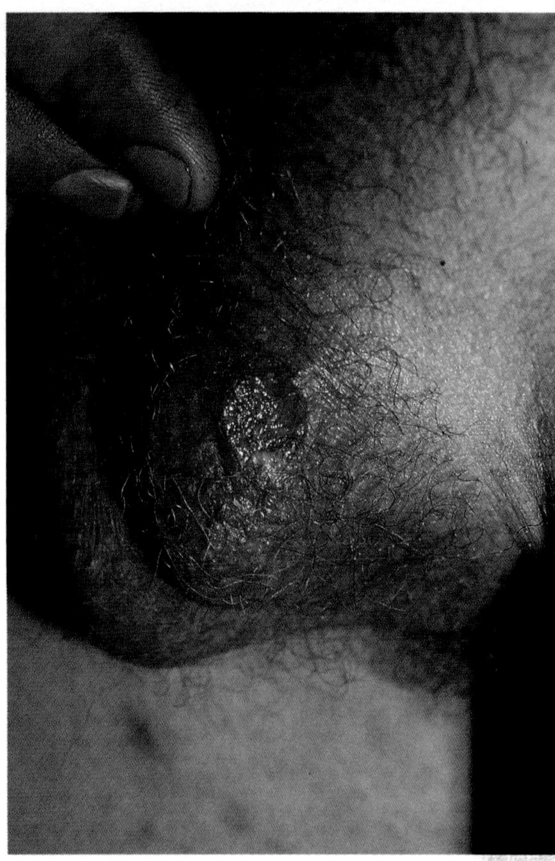

Fig. 18-3. Round ulceration of Behçet's disease in a typical location on the scrotum. (Courtesy of Gerald N. Goldberg, M.D.)

Inflammatory changes in the form of either leukoclastic or lymphocytic vasculitis are generally present.[7]

Differential Diagnosis

The major ulcerative diseases of the genitalia to be considered include chancroid, Crohn's disease, and genital herpes, especially when the latter occurs in immunosuppressed individuals. The term *aphthosis major* or complex aphthosis should be used for patients who present with only oral and anogenital disease; Behçet's disease should only be diagnosed when the criteria of the International Study Group for Behçet's Disease (see above) are met.

Course and Prognosis

The course of the mucocutaneous ulcerative disease is described in the section on aphthous ulcers. The other symptoms and signs may also have an intermittent course, although usually one or another of the problems is present on a more continuous basis. Inflammation of the posterior eye can lead to the development of blindness. CNS disease, when severe enough, can result in a clinical picture suggesting meningoencephalitis or stroke.

Pathogenesis

Many aspects of Behçet's disease suggest the possibility of an infectious etiology. Most speculation has revolved around a possible role for the herpes simplex virus or streptococcal bacteria, but the data remain unconvincing. As indicated in the section on aphthae, immunologic factors seem to be important in the development of the mucocutaneous ulcers. Circulating immune complexes and enhanced neutrophil chemotaxis are frequently identified; leukocytoclastic vasculitis seems to explain the development of the disease in some, but not all, sites.[8] Even though only a few familial cases have been reported, genetics are also probably involved, based on the high proportion of patients with the Eastern form of the disease who have the HLA-B5 and -B51 haplotypes. A hormonal influence might explain the marked female preponderance in the Western variant of Behçet's disease.

Treatment

Treatment of the mucocutaneous ulcers is described in the section on aphthae. The systemic medications mentioned in that section would be appropriate for the systemic manifestations of Behçet's disease. Many patients with severe forms of the disease require indefinite administration of systemic steroids or cytotoxic agents, or both.

CROHN'S DISEASE

Involvement of the anogenital region with Crohn's disease occurs in two forms: contiguous, in which there is direct extension from involved intestine, or noncontiguous, in which "metastatic" disease occurs at a distant site. Contiguous involvement of the perianal region is quite common, occurring in as many as

30 percent of all patients with the disease and in 80 percent of those patients with disease of the colon. Genital involvement in the form of noncontiguous disease is distinctly rare. Fewer than 25 cases of vulvar Crohn's disease have been reported, although one review suggests that 2 percent of women with Crohn's disease have associated vulvar involvement.[9] Only a few cases of male genital involvement are known.[10] The incidence of Crohn's disease in men and women is approximately equal, so the discrepancy in genital involvement is unexplained. The disease occurs most commonly in young adulthood, but genital lesions have been reported in women ages 11 to 70.

Clinical Presentation

Lesions in the perianal area, reflecting extension from involved bowel, occur primarily as anal abcesses or draining fistulae, whereas noncontiguous lesions of the vulva appear as labial swelling,[11] nodules (Fig. 18-4), abcesses, ulcers, fissures, and occasionally fistulae. A very distinctive finding, if present, is the tendency for linear fissures to develop within intertriginous folds (Fig. 18-5). This finding has sometimes been termed the "knife cut" sign.

Most of the patients with genital involvement had had recognized Crohn's disease prior to the appearance of the genital lesions. However, in at least three instances the genital lesions were recognized sometime before the gastrointestinal involvement occurred.[11] In all probability this sequence occurs more frequently but is not reported because of hesitancy in making the diagnosis when no gastrointestinal involvement is present.

Patients with Crohn's disease of the gastrointestinal tract will almost always have associated features of abdominal pain, diarrhea, and sometimes low-grade fever, although it is possible to develop mucocutaneous disease at a time when the gastrointestinal involvement is clinically quiescent.

Other histologically nonspecific mucocutaneous lesions are also known to occur with some frequency in patients with Crohn's disease. These include aphthous ulcers, cutaneous pustules, erythema nodosum, and pyoderma gangrenosum.

Histology

The diagnosis of noncontiguous Crohn's disease of the genitalia depends on biopsy. In most cases fairly characteristic granulomatous changes can be identified, but in some instances a rather nonspecific inflammatory reaction is all that is seen.

Differential Diagnosis

Diseases to be considered when granulomatous changes are present in biopsy specimens include hidradenitis suppurativa, sarcoidosis, genital Melkers-

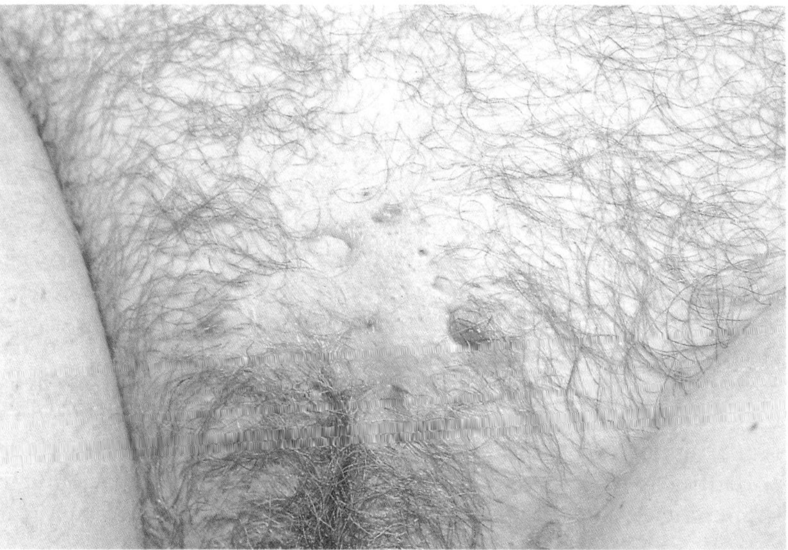

Fig. 18-4. Fleshy, pink, lobular papules of Crohn's disease.

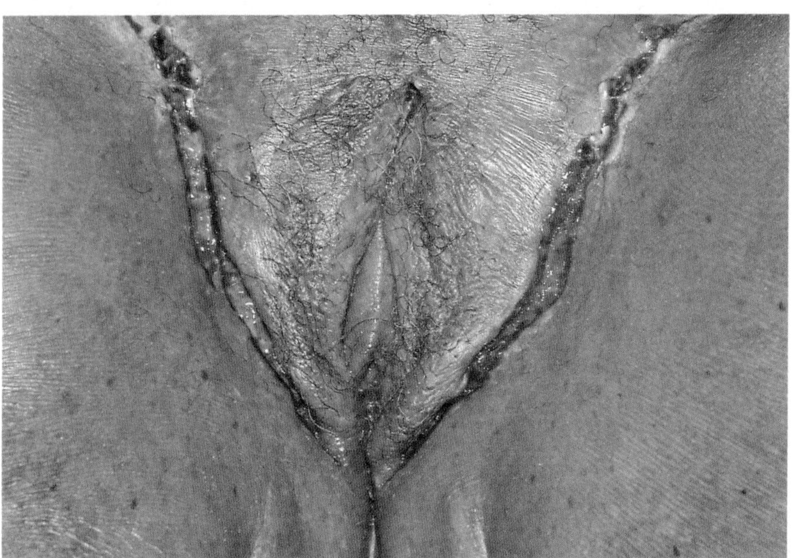

Fig. 18-5. Linear ulcerations along skin creases of the genital area are a classic finding for Crohn's disease.

son-Rosenthal disease, granuloma inguinale, and granulomatous fungal and mycobacterial infection. Of these, granuloma inguinale is the one most likely to be confused clinically since it often presents with deep linear fissures like those of Crohn's disease.

Course and Prognosis

Anogenital disease persists for long periods of time with little evidence of spontaneous remission, but it does tend to improve if active gastrointestinal disease can be brought under control. Because of the severity of the inflammatory reaction, healing of anogenital lesions generally occurs along with scarring, architectural damage to the labia, and persistent labial edema.

Pathogenesis

The cause of Crohn's disease is unknown. Periodically, evidence is presented suggesting that the granulomatous reaction occurs as the result of an unrecognized infectious agent, but at this point there is no proof of an infectious etiology. Another attractive hypothesis suggests that normal intestinal bacteria trigger an inflammatory reaction on the basis of "molecular mimicry." Immunologic factors may be important in the pathophysiology of the disease; the supporting data are similar to those presented in the section on aphthous ulcers. Genetics may also play a role inasmuch as familial cases occur in a significant minority of patients. Additional data suggesting a genetic predisposition include the high frequency of the HLA-B27 haplotype, the high incidence in Jews, and the low incidence in blacks. Psychological factors may serve as a precipitating event for the periodic exacerbations that characterize the disease.

Treatment

Treatment of anogenital Crohn's disease is primarily directed toward achieving the best possible control of the intestinal involvement. This includes provision of nutritional support and the use of orally administered sulfasalazine. Metronidazole may also be helpful, and in severe cases orally administered corticosteroids or azathioprine, or both, are often necessary. Specific information regarding dosage and duration of treatment can be found in a recent review on drug treatment of Crohn's disease.[12] A few patients will ultimately require bowel resection to control the process. Little is possible in terms of direct treatment of the mucocutaneous lesions themselves, although small lesions can be intralesionally injected with triamcinolone acetonide using 0.5 to 1.0 ml of the stock 10 mg/ml solution.

FACTITIAL DISEASE

Factitial disease is defined as a destructive modification of tissue that occurs as a direct result of an individual's actions. The variety of ways this is accomplished is most remarkable. One of the most frequently encountered forms of factitial disease is penile and vulvar piercing with subsequent placement of rings and other "jewelry." Another form of factitial disease, seen mostly in individuals from the Far East, occurs in the penis as a result of injection of various products[13] or the insertion of formed foreign bodies.[14] This type of manipulation is purported to enhance pleasure for the women during coitus. Use of the penis as a site of illicit drug injection has also led to cutaneous damage.[15] We have seen, mostly on a one-time basis, an array of other severe reactions such as penile necrosis due to the use of a rubber band as a form of contraception (Fig. 18-6), vulvovaginal ulceration following a kerosene douche, and a penile ulcer from picking and scrubbing (Fig. 18-7).

Related problems, which are not strictly speaking factitial, can occur accidentally. Penile necrosis has occurred following the medical use of condom drainage to prevent or relieve bladder distension.[16] Tourniquet-type constriction with subsequent necrosis can occur when hairs or fibers become tightly wrapped around the penile shaft.[17] Finally, iatrogenic damage to the genitalia has occurred due to the application of a variety of agents such as fluorouracil, podophyllin, trichloroacetic acid, and other similar products.[18] Less destructive similar problems are discussed in Chapter 5 in the section on contact dermatitis.

FISSURES

Fissures most often occur in the genital area from infection, neurodermatitis, and, in women, inadequate estrogen (see also Ch. 7). Fissures are occasionally encountered in the intergluteal fold. These linear ulcers extend posteriorly from the anus along the gluteal cleft for 2 to 3 cm, and similar linear fissures may occur on the vulva in the interlabial skin folds. These fissures occur in two settings. The first is that of infection, especially intertriginous candidiasis. Characteristically the skin at the lateral margins of the fissure is markedly inflamed. Other signs of candidiasis (pustules and satellite papules) may or may not be present. Similar fissures can be seen in the inguinal genital folds, the infragluteal folds, and the interlabial folds. These candidal fissures are analogous to the fissures of angular cheilitis occurring at the mouth. Possibly other infectious agents such as streptococcal bacteria can cause similar fissures. The second setting is that of chronic atopic/neurodermatitis (lichen simplex chronicus). In this situation the lateral margins of the fissure are white and thickened

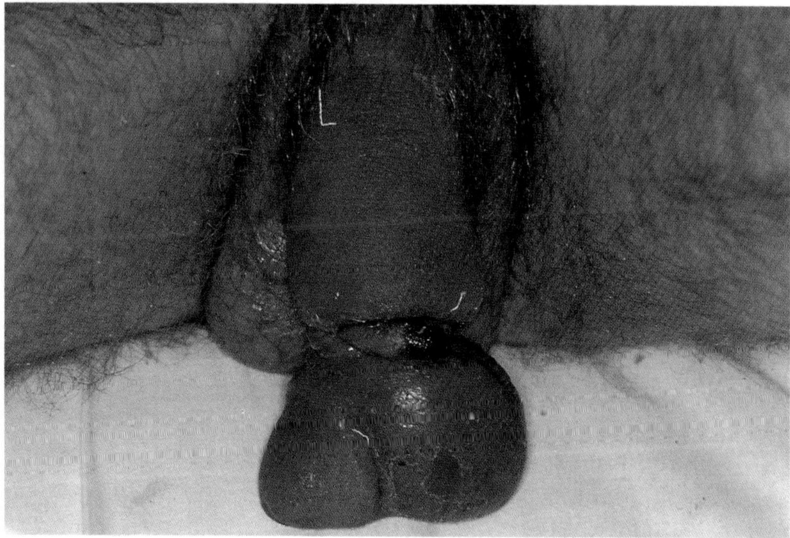

Fig. 18-6. Inflammation and edema from a rubber band wrapped around the penis as a contraceptive measure and inadvertently left on afterward.

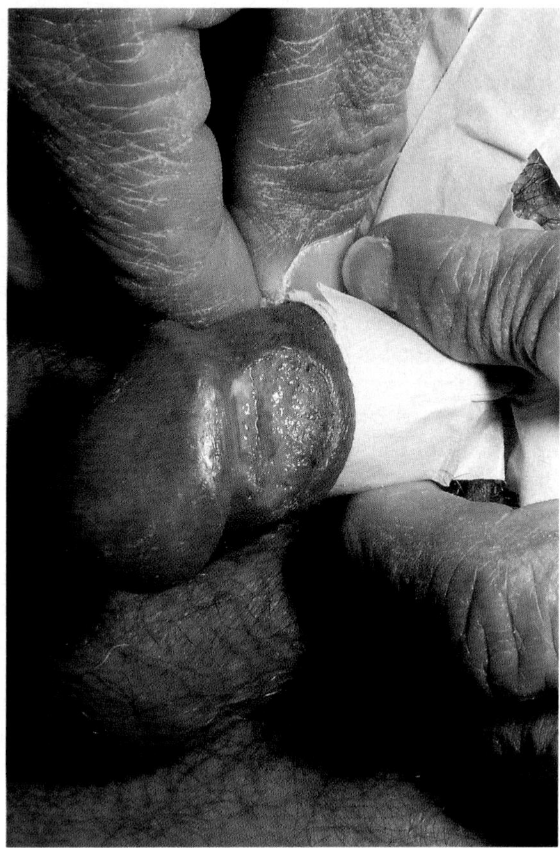

Fig. 18-7. A clean, perfectly round factitial ulcer that showed no evidence of infection or primary inflammation on biopsy and cultures. The elaborate taping by the patient that extended over the mons and lower abdomen and very frequent washing with various harsh agents were measures that he felt would facilitate healing.

(Fig. 18-8). Usually other evidence of chronic atopic/neurodermatitis such as lichenification or excoriation, or both, will also be present (see Ch. 5). These fissures occur because a thickened stratum corneum has reduced flexibility and tends to crack when it is flexed or bent, analogous to the cracking of callused heels.

Treatment requires the use of anticandidal agents for the former and the use of drugs that will ameliorate the itch-scratch cycle for the latter. The differential diagnoses include the linear fissures that sometimes occur in Crohn's disease and in granuloma inguinale.

An entirely different type of fissure is sometimes found in the vulvar vestibule at the posterior fourchette. In that location, the posterior portions of the labia minora unite, forming a fold of skin that marks the posterior portion of the vestibule. In some women the fold is both prominent and taut. During coitus, as a result of thrusting trauma, this fold can tear. Approximately 5 to 10 percent of women with vulvodynia will experience this painful condition. Treatment is difficult. Sometimes the provision of additional lubrication during intercourse is sufficient, but in most cases surgical intervention is necessary. One can sometimes simply surgically snip the fold, which relaxes the tissue tension across it. More often a modified perineoplasty, as described in the section on vulvodynia in Chapter 21, will be required. Simi-

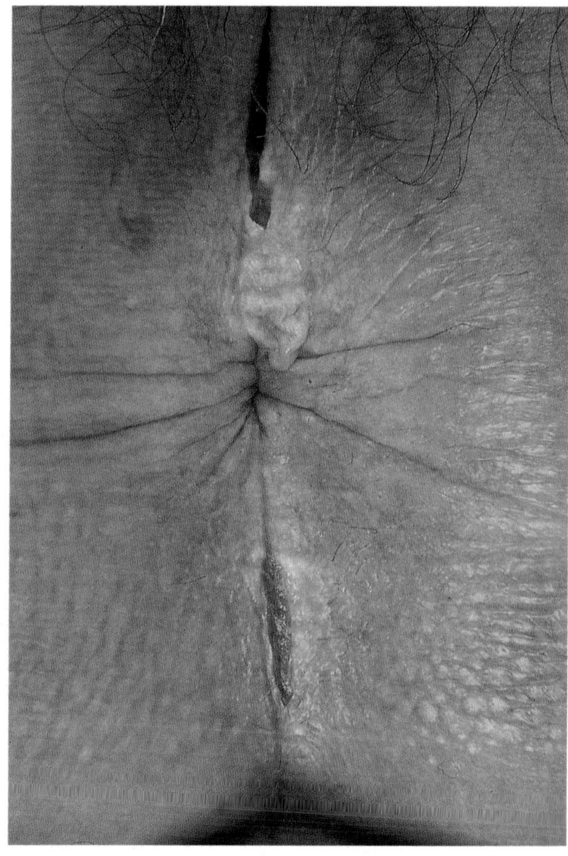

Fig. 18-8. Shiny, lichenified skin of lichen simplex chronicus from rubbing, with fissures in the hyperkeratotic midline skin.

lar fissures may also develop in the presence of inadequate tissue estrogen levels (e.g., when oral contraceptives are used and in the postpartum and postmenopausal setting). Topically applied estrogen products (Estrace or Premarin vaginal cream) can be used effectively.

REFERENCES

Aphthous Ulcers

1. Jorizzo JL, Taylor RS, Schmalstieg FC et al: Complex aphthosis: a forme fruste of Behçet's syndrome? J Am Acad Dermatol 13:80, 1985

Behçet's Disease

2. International Study Group for Behçet's Disease: Criteria for diagnosis of Behçet's disease. Lancet 335:1078, 1990
3. O'Duffy JD: Behçet's Syndrome. N Engl J Med 322:326, 1990
4. Ozarmagan G, Saylan T, Azizlerli G et al: Re-evaluation of the pathergy test in Behçet's disease. Acta Derm Venereol (Stockh) 71:75, 1991
5. Cho KH, Shin KS, Sohn SJ et al: Behçet's disease with Sweet's syndrome-like presentation—a report of six cases. Clin Exp Dermatol 14:20, 1989
6. Orme RL, Nordlund JJ, Barich L, Brown T: The MAGIC syndrome (mouth and genital ulcers with inflamed cartilage). Arch Dermatol 126:940, 1990
7. Chun SI, Su WP, Lee S: Histopathologic study of cutaneous lesions in Behçet's syndrome. J Dermatol 17:333, 1990
8. Jorizzo JL, Hudson RD, Schmalsteig FC et al: Behçet's syndrome: immune regulation, circulating immune complexes, neutrophil migration and colchicine therapy. J Am Acad Dermatol 10:205, 1984

Crohn's Disease

9. Donaldson LB: Crohn's disease: its gynecologic aspect. Am J Obstet Gynecol 131:196,1978
10. Levine N, Bangert J: Cutaneous granulomatosis in Crohn's disease. Arch Dermatol 118:1006, 1982
11. Werlin SL, Esterly NB, Oechler H: Crohn's disease presenting as a unilateral labial hypertrophy. J Am Acad Dermatol 27:893, 1992
12. Peppercorn M: Advances in drug therapy for inflammatory bowel disease. Ann Intern Med 112:50, 1990

Factitial Disease

13. Foucar E, Downing DT, Gerber WL: Sclerosing lipogranuloma of the male genitalia containing vitamin E: a comparison with classical "paraffinoma." J Am Acad Dermatol 9:103, 1983
14. Norton SA: Fijian penis marbles: an example of artificial penile nodules. Cutis 51:295, 1993
15. White WB, Barrett S: Penile ulcer in heroin abuse: a case report. Cutis 29:62, 1982
16. Steinhardt G, McRoberts JW: Total distal penile necrosis caused by condom catheter. JAMA 244:1238, 1980
17. Novick NL, Gribetz ME: Annular constriction of the glans penis. J Am Acad Dermatol 15:351, 1986
18. Fisher AA: Unique reactions of scrotal skin to topical agents. Cutis 44:445,1989

SUGGESTED READINGS

Aphthous Ulcers

Hutton KP, Rogers III RS: Recurrent aphthous stomatitis. Dermatol Clin 5:761, 1987

These two articles describe only apthous ulceration of the mouth. Nevertheless, many of the data presented are applicable to genital aphthae as well.

Porter SR, Scully C: Aphthous stomatitis—an overview of aetiopathogenesis. Clin Exp Dermatol 16:235, 1991

Behçet's Disease

Arbesfeld SJ, Kurban AK: Behçet's disease. New perspectives on an enigmatic syndrome. J Am Acad Dermatol 19:767, 1988

This article provides a complete review of all aspects of Behçet's disease, but there are no photographs of the mucocutaneous lesions.

Schreiner DT, Jorizzo JL: Behçet's disease and complex aphthosis. Dermatol Clin 5:769, 1987

This article sets out the points to be used in differentiating the more benign complex aphthosis from Behçet's disease.

Crohn's Disease

Glanz S, Maceyko RF, Camisa C, Tomecki KJ: Mucocutaneous presentations of Crohn's disease. Cutis 47:167, 1991

Scully RE, Mark EJ, McNeely WF, McNeely BU: Case records of the Massachusetts General Hospital. Case 26-1989. N Engl J Med 320:1741, 1989

19 Ulcerated Nodules and Plaques

Basal Cell Carcinoma

Squamous Cell Carcinoma

BASAL CELL CARCINOMA

Basal cell carcinoma (BCC) (basal cell epithelioma) is, in light-skinned individuals at least, the most common type of human malignancy. It is usually considered to be a sunlight-induced tumor because nearly all of the lesions develop on sun-exposed skin. Nevertheless, lesions do develop elsewhere, including the genitalia and perianal skin. Overall, BCC makes up 2 to 4 percent of all vulvar carcinomas and accounts for a somewhat smaller percentage of penile and scrotal carcinomas. The male to female ratio for BCC of the genitalia appears to be about 1 : 4. The age range is that of mid- to late adult life. Only a few black patients (either male or female) have been reported with genital BCC.[1]

Clinical Presentation

Basal cell carcinomas of the genitalia generally present as skin-colored, nonscaling, dome-shaped nodules 1 to 2 cm in diameter (Fig. 19-1). Some are smooth-surfaced, but most are ulcerated. Small lesions are generally asymptomatic, although mild itching or irritation can occur. Large ulcerated lesions are associated with slight discharge and subsequent staining of the underwear.

In women BCC is usually located on the hair-bearing skin of the labia majora. A few lesions, however, have been reported on the labia minora and clitoris. In men the location of BCC is about evenly divided between the penis and the scrotum. A few instances of perianal BCC have been reported.[2]

BCC of the genitalia is almost always solitary; only a few patients have been reported to have multiple genital lesions.[3,4]

Although the appearance of BCC, especially if ulcerated, is quite distinctive, biopsy is required for definitive diagnosis. Nonulcerated lesions are easily confused clinically with cysts and other types of both benign and malignant tumors.

Course and Prognosis

The average size of BCC found on the genitalia is somewhat larger than those that occur on the head and neck. This is probably due to the relatively hidden location and subsequent long period of growth prior to identification. In spite of this, metastases to regional nodes, or elsewhere, is rarely found at the time of diagnosis. A few cases of metastatic disease have been reported, but on review, elements of squamous cell carcinoma were found, suggesting that these may have been "mixed" tumors.[3] Overall, it is believed that the likelihood for occurrence of metastases in genital BCC is no higher than for tumors located elsewhere. Recurrence rates following excision of genital BCC are higher than for lesions on sun-exposed skin,[5] but these recurrences can be satisfactorily retreated either with a second conventional excision or with Mohs micrographic surgery.[6]

Pathogenesis

It is not known why BCC develops on the genitalia. Ultraviolet light exposure is the most important etiologic factor for BCC appearing on sun-exposed skin;

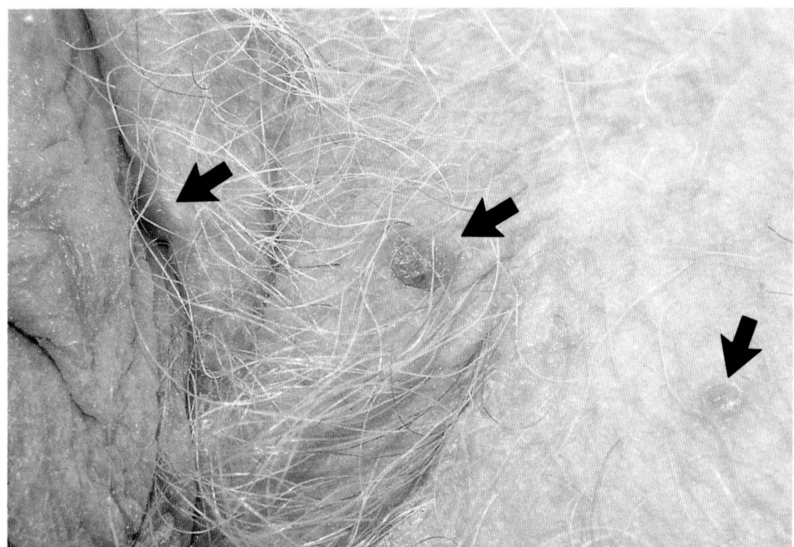

Fig. 19-1. Slightly pink and skin-colored translucent vulvar basal cell carcinomas *(arrows)*. Some areas of hyperpigmentation are present within the larger lesion.

clearly this cannot be the explanation for genital lesions. Possibly other predisposing factors such as previous radiation treatment could play a role,[4] but in most instances these are not identifiable. Smoking[7] and wart virus infection play a role in the development of genital squamous cell carcinoma but, regarding the latter, human papillomavirus (HPV) DNA has not been found in the few cases of genital BCC so far investigated.[8]

Treatment

The treatment of choice is surgical removal. Previously rather radical procedures were carried out, but now most authorities recommend local excision with fairly narrow margins. Mohs micrographic surgery, in which frozen section control is used for each small horizontal slice of tissue removed, would appear to be particularly well suited for treatment of these lesions.[6] Basal cell carcinomas are radiosensitive, and thus radiation treatment can be used quite effectively. Laser treatment, because margins can not easily be determined, would seem to be less preferable. Treatment of metastatic disease falls outside the scope of this textbook.

SQUAMOUS CELL CARCINOMA

Squamous cell carcinoma in situ (SCCIS) is discussed in Chapter 6; this section describes squamous cell carcinoma of the invasive type.

Clinical Presentation

Penile and Scrotal Squamous Cell Carcinoma

Invasive squamous cell carcinoma (SCC) of the penis occurs infrequently, and the incidence with which it is seen appears to be decreasing. Currently it accounts for less than 1 percent of all types of malignancy in men. The average age at diagnosis is 55 to 65 years, but it can occur in the fourth or fifth decade. A few instances of onset in childhood have even been described. Almost all penile SCC is found on the glans, coronal sulcus, or prepuce. Not infrequently, the early lesions are undetected because associated phimosis interferes with adequate examination by both the patient and the physician.

The clinical morphology of penile SCC is extremely variable. Some lesions appear identical to the in situ lesions described earlier: pink, red, or brown flat-topped papules and plaques.[9] In these cases, invasion is not suspected clinically and is only recognized when excised lesions are examined histologically. In general, however, in situ disease is an infrequent precursor for invasive SCC.

More typically, invasive SCC presents as ulcerated nodules and plaques that range in size from 1 cm to several centimeters in diameter (Fig. 19-2). The base of the ulcer is usually crusted and often bleeds easily because of the presence of unevenly growing, friable granulation tissue. The margins of the ulcer are slightly heaped up and may or may not have overlying scale. The shape (configuration) of the ulcer is circular in early lesions but is often quite irregular in well-established tumors. When ulcers have lasted for many years, destructive ulceration ("rodent ulcer") leads to autoamputation of the distal penis.

Less frequently, invasive SCC presents as a verrucous, hyperkeratotic nodule without clinical evidence of ulceration. These latter lesions are similar in appearance to the HPV-induced Buschke-Loewenstein tumors described in the section on genital warts.[10]

Scrotal SCC of the invasive type is similar in appearance to the penile lesions described above, but the lesions tend to be more distinctly circumscribed and are less destructive of involved tissue.

Vulvar Squamous Cell Carcinoma

Invasive SCC of the vulva is an uncommon disease. It accounts for no more than 5 percent of female genital tract malignancies and occurs about 8 to 10 times less frequently than cervical cancer. Most vulvar squamous cell carcinomas develop after 60 years of age, but onset has been reported as early as the second decade.

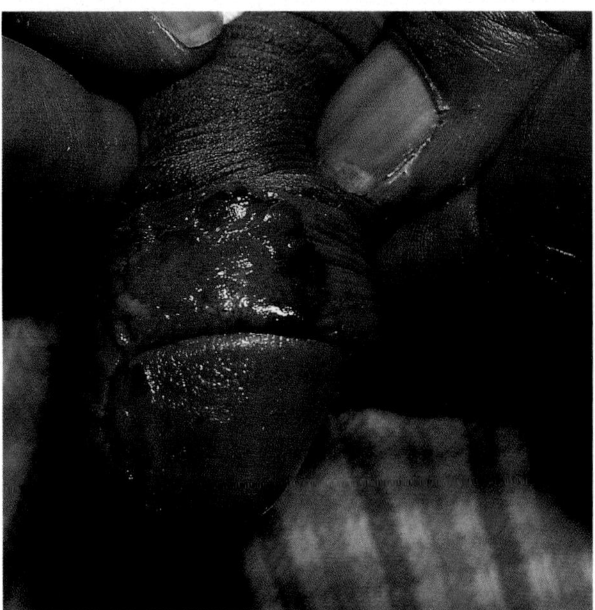

Fig. 19-2. Ulcerated squamous cell carcinoma of the glans and shaft of the penis. (Courtesy of Ronald C. Hansen, M.D.)

The morphologic appearance of these lesions is highly variable. A small (but increasing) percent of invasive carcinomas arises from one or more foci of carcinoma in situ.[11] These patients will present with flat-topped papules and plaques that are pink, red, or white in color. The lesions are generally not eroded or scaling; most will be multifocal. The invasive nature of the process is not apparent until microscopic examination is carried out on a biopsy specimen.

Most invasive SCC still, however, arises as such in a unifocal manner. These lesions may be nodular or ulcerated. The nodules are generally 1 to 2 cm in diameter and may have either a hyperkeratotic or eroded surface. In a few cases the nodule appears distinctly verrucous. The ulcerated carcinomas more often appear as red or white infiltrated plaques with one, or multiple, focal areas of erosion or deeper ulceration. Some of these latter tumors can be appreciated as arising from underlying areas of lichen sclerosus.[12]

The posterior fourchette, labia minora, labia majora, and interlabial folds are the most common sites for invasive SCC. The clitoris is involved less often. Pruritus occurs in about half of the patients and is the most common symptom reported. Mild pain and easy bleeding occur in a smaller proportion of cases.

Anal Squamous Cell Carcinoma

Invasive SCC can arise from either the anal canal or the anal margin. The latter area is loosely defined as the tissue extending from the dentate line out as far as 5 cm beyond the anal verge. Carcinomas occurring in this region may arise multifocally from one or more sites of carcinoma in situ or as unifocal primary tumors. Those arising from sites of carcinoma in situ appear as flat-topped papules that are either dusky red or gray-brown in color. The invasive nature of these lesions is not apparent until microscopic examination of a biopsy specimen is carried out.[13]

Unifocal primary carcinomas usually present as nodules or plaques with varying degrees of hyperkeratosis or ulceration. These lesions range in size from 1 to 5 cm or more in diameter. Itching, discomfort, or bleeding may be present.

Course and Prognosis

Discussion of the course and prognosis of invasive carcinoma of the anogenital region lies outside the scope of this textbook. Material on this subject can be found in standard gynecologic and urologic textbooks.

Pathogenesis

The cause of anogenital squamous cell carcinoma is only poorly understood. Clearly infection with HPV plays an important role, especially for those tumors that begin as papules and plaques of carcinoma in situ (see Anogenital Warts in Ch. 9 and Carcinoma In Situ in Ch. 6). Overall, HPV DNA can be found in about 30 percent of invasive squamous cell carcinomas.[14] Other infectious agents (especially herpes simplex virus) may also play a role, although evidence to support this possibility is much less well developed. It has long been recognized that age at first intercourse and number of sexual partners play a role in the development of cervical carcinoma. This observation is probably related to the increased likelihood of acquiring HPV and other sexually transmitted infections in these circumstances.

Of the remaining factors, cigarette smoking has been the best studied. Nearly every publication on the subject has shown a linear relationship between the amount and duration of smoking and the subsequent development of SCC.[15] The mechanism through which this occurs is not known, but in the case of cervical cancer, tar products have been shown to be present in significant concentrations at that site.

Unifocal invasive SCC of the penis, for all practical purposes, exists only in uncircumsized men. It is believed that the presence of an intact foreskin traps smegma and other products that might then incite chronic low-grade inflammation. Support for this hypothesis is derived from the fact that phimosis, which interferes with good hygiene of the preputial sac, is often an associated finding.

Carcinoma of the scrotum has been related to a number of environmental causes. The best recognized are exposure to chimney soot, asbestos, tars, and related petroleum products.[16] More recently, ultraviolet light, administered medically in the form of psoralen and ultraviolet light (PUVA) treatment, was shown to result in the development of carcinoma.

Immunosuppression plays a critical role. Transplant patients[17] and individuals infected with the human immunodeficiency virus (HIV) develop anogenital cancers at an earlier age and more frequently than would otherwise be expected. In all probability immunosuppression also confers a poorer prognosis for a given tumor size and stage.

Several dermatologic diseases of the anogenital region have been related to subsequent development of SCC. Lichen sclerosus of the vulva and penis is the best recognized of these,[12,18] but there is probably also an increased risk for those with lichen planus.[19] Interestingly, the presence of lichen sclerosus in men is very common in those with phimosis, which is in turn a risk factor (see above).

Treatment

The treatment of invasive SCC lies outside the scope of this book. Suffice it to say that Mohs micrographic surgery is playing an increasingly important role in the excisional removal of these lesions.[20] Additional material on the staging and treatment of SCC can be found in standard gynecologic and urologic sources.

REFERENCES

Basal Cell Carcinoma

1. Greenbaum SS, Krull EA, Simmons EB: Basal cell carcinoma at the base of the penis in a black patient. J Am Acad Dermatol 20:317, 1989
2. Espana A, Redondo P, Idoate MA et al: Perianal basal cell carcinoma. Clin Exp Dermatol 17:360, 1992
3. Goldberg DJ: Multiple basal-cell carcinoma of the vulva. J Dermatol Surg Oncol 10:615, 1984
4. Stiller M, Klein W, Dorman R, Albom M: Bilateral vulvar basal cell carcinomata. J Am Acad Dermatol 28:836, 1993
5. Kharfi M, Mokhtar I, Fazaa B et al: Vulvar basal cell carcinoma. Eur J Dermatol 2:81, 1992
6. Brown MD, Zachary CB, Grekin RC, Swanson NA: Genital tumors: their management by micrographic surgery. J Am Acad Dermatol 18:115, 1988
7. Hellberg D, Valentin J, Eklund T, Nilsson S: Penile cancer: is there an epidemiological role for smoking and sexual behavior? Br Med J 295:1306, 1987
8. Nahass GT, Blauvelt A, Leonardi CL et al: Basal cell carcinoma of the scrotum. Report of three cases and review of the literature. J Am Acad Dermatol 26:574, 1992

Squamous Cell Carcinoma

9. Schwartz RA, Janniger CK: Bowenoid papulosis. J Am Acad Dermatol 24:261, 1991
10. Schwartz RA: Buschke-Loewenstein tumor: verrucous carcinoma of the penis. J Am Acad Dermatol 23:723, 1990
11. Barbero M, Micheletti L, Preti M et al: Biologic behavior of vulvar intrepithelial neoplasia. J Reprod Med 38:108, 1993

12. Leibowitch M, Neill S, Pelisse M et al: The epithelial changes associated with squamous cell carcinoma of the vulva: a review of the clinical, histological, and viral findings in 78 women. Br J Obstet Gynaecol 97:1135, 1990
13. Scholefield JH, Hickson WGE, Smith JHF et al: Anal intraepithelial neoplasia: part of a multifocal disease process. Lancet 340:1271, 1992
14. Crum CP: Carcinoma of the vulva: epidemiology and pathogenesis. Obstet Gynecol 79:448, 1992
15. Daling JR, Sherman KJ, Hislop TG et al: Cigarette smoking and the risk of anogenital cancer. Am J Epidemiol 135:180, 1992
16. Castiglione FM, Selikowitz SM, Dimond RL: Mule spinner's disease. Arch Dermatol 121:370, 1985
17. Penn I: Cancers of the anogenital region in renal transplant recipients. Analysis of 65 cases. Cancer 58:611, 1986
18. Pride HB, Miller III OF, Tyler WB: Penile squamous cell carcinoma arising from balanitis xerotica obliterans. J Am Acad Dermatol 29:469, 1993
19. Bain L, Gernemus R: The association of lichen planus of the penis with squamous cell carcinoma in situ and with verrucous squamous carcinoma. J Dermatol Surg Oncol 15:413, 1989
20. Brown MD, Zachary CB, Grekin RC et al: Genital tumors: their management by micrographic surgery. J Am Acad Dermatol 18:115, 1988

SUGGESTED READINGS

Squamous Cell Carcinoma

Fraley EE, Zhang G, Sazama R, Lange PH: Cancer of the penis. Prognosis and treatment plans. Cancer 55:1618, 1985

Frost DB, Richards PC, Montague ED et al: Epidermoid cancer of the anorectum. Cancer 53:1285, 1984

Lifshitz S, Savage JE, Yates SJ et al: Primary epidermoid carcinoma of the vulva. Surg Gynecol Obstet 155:59, 1982

Narayana AS, Olney LE, Loening SA et al: Carcinoma of the penis. Analysis of 219 cases. Cancer 49:2185, 1982

Norman RW, Millard OH, Mack FG et al: Carcinoma of the penis: an 11 year review. Can J Surg 26:426, 1983

Wilkinson EJ, Rico MJ, Pierson KK: Microinvasive carcinoma of the vulva. Int J Gynecol Pathol 1:29, 1982

VII Pruritus and Pain

20 Anogenital Pruritus

PRURITUS

The sensation of itching (pruritus) is carried from mucocutaneous tissue by means of thin, nonmyelinated sensory spinal nerve fibers. These nerve fibers cross to the contralateral portion of the spinal cord and ascend from there by way of the spinothalamic tract to the thalamus and sensory cortex. Originally specialized nerve endings were thought to be responsible for the various types of sensation, but it is now known that most sensation, including that of itching, starts in free nerve twigs that terminate within the epithelium of hair follicles, mucous membranes, and surface skin.

Triggering of these free nerve endings by any stimulus sends an impulse of either light pain or itching along the nerve axon. It is not known why, in some circumstances, itching rather than pain is conveyed. In an attempt to explain this dichotomy, some authors have proposed that the difference between pain and itching is just a matter of degree; in this scenario itching is simply subliminal pain. Today most authorities disagree and postulate that there are *qualitative* differences between pain and itching and that these differences might be due to the nature of the stimulus, the chemical mediators present in the skin, or the receptors triggered at the cortical level.

Pruritus occurs in four settings. First, itching can occur as a reflection of internal disease such as hematopoietic malignancy, liver dysfunction, renal dysfunction, and so forth. Itching caused by systemic disease is generalized and thus is not important in the context of itching limited to the anogenital region. Second, itching can occur because of physiologic changes in the skin that are easily missed such as sweat retention and excess dryness (xerosis). Third, itching can occur as the result of factors occurring at the level of the central nervous system; these are primarily psychological factors such as anxiety and depression. The second and third categories are discussed together in the following section on essential pruritus. The fourth category, pruritic dermatoses and infestations, concludes the chapter.

ESSENTIAL PRURITUS

Pruritus, as described above, is found as a component of many of the diseases described in this book. In addition, pruritus can occur in the absence of any visibly detectable disease; this is generally termed *essential* or *idiopathic pruritus.* In the specific setting of the anogenital region, terms for essential pruritus include *pruritus vulvae,*[1] *pruritus scroti,* and *pruritus ani.*[2] The nature of pruritus in each of these areas is similar in presentation, cause, and treatment; for this reason they are discussed together.

Clinical Presentation

The onset of essential pruritus may either be insidious, with no recognized precipitating factor, or it may occur as the result of a "trigger" that may or may not be recognized by the patient. However, it is important to understand that the triggering event often is no longer playing a role by the time the patient seeks medical attention. Three of the most important triggers include candidiasis, sweat retention, and xerosis secondary to overly vigorous hygiene. In each of these settings the patient's presenting history is that of paroxysms of itching superimposed on a background of constant low-grade pruritus.

In most instances, patients state that they experience relatively little itching during the busy portion of the day but that the problem becomes severe in the evening and at night. Because of this, and because of the interference of clothing and the embarassment of scratching in public, most patients do not scratch much during the day. Almost always, though, there is a history of nighttime scratching, often to the point that sleeping is difficult for a bed partner.[3] On awakening, the patient sometimes even finds flecks of blood on the sheets and under the fingernails. Patients are often unaware of this nighttime scratching because it generally occurs during the lighter stages of sleep.

Findings on examination of patients with anogenital pruritus are unpredictable. In some cases the involved area appears completely normal, whereas in others there is evidence of scratching (excoriations) or rubbing (lichenification), or both. By definition, no other clearly identifiable disease is present.

Course and Prognosis

Essential pruritus is a chronic disease. Usually by the time the patient first seeks medical attention, the process has been in place for many months and thus the itch-scratch cycle (see Ch. 5) is well established. In this setting the scratching that occurs, no matter how minimal, is sufficient to constantly stimulate the nerve endings of the skin such that the mind commands the scratching to continue. In effect, a habit of scratching is present that is hard to break. No serious consequences of chronic scratching occur, although essential pruritus can lead to the development of full-blown atopic/neurodermatitis (lichen simplex chronicus).

Pathogenesis

The cause of essential pruritus is unknown. A reasonable hypothesis suggests that some individuals have a genetic predisposition to experience pruritus, having inherited the atopic diathesis. Probably those with essential pruritus are genetically atopic even when the clinical phenotype for atopy is not otherwise expressed. However, even if one assumes that there is a genetic predisposition for itching, it is not clear whether it is expressed peripherally (at the level of the skin and nerve endings) or whether it is a problem of "overinterpretation" at the level of the cortex. Additional discussion regarding the definition and recognition of atopy can be found in the section on atopic/neurodermatitis in Chapter 5.

Many factors can act as triggers to initiate episodes of itching. The three most common, candidiasis, sweat retention, and xerosis, were mentioned above. In addition, the clinician has to be a detective to identify other triggers that may apply in an individual situation. Examples of less commonly encountered factors include soilage (anal or vaginal), contact irritants, contact allergens, and pinworms.

The role played by psychological factors in essential pruritus is controversial. Even when such factors are identified, it is difficult to determine whether psychological abnormalities cause itching, or result from it. Nevertheless, type-A behavior, obsessive-compulsive traits, generalized anxiety, and varying degrees of depression are found with considerable frequency.[4,5]

Treatment

Chronic idiopathic pruritus is quite difficult to treat. Trigger factors should be identified and modified or removed when possible. However, all too often by the time the patient seeks medical care the initiating factor is no longer playing any ongoing role. Attention to environmental factors is crucial. Every effort should be made to reduce the retention of sweat. Thus loose cotton blend clothing should be worn, air conditioning should be used if available, wicker car cushions should be placed over leather and vinyl upholstery, and so forth.

Bathing after sweat-inducing activities is desirable as long as the water temperature is not too hot and the use of soap is avoided or minimized. Lubrication after bathing is very helpful, but otherwise all cosmetic products used in the anogenital region should be discontinued. Cleaning after defecation and urination is important, but the techniques used should not be so harsh or vigorous as to irritate the tissue. Plain water on a folded pad of toilet tissue works well, as does a rubber bulb syringe filled with tap water. Some like the use of medicated cleansing pads (e.g., Tucks) but these can cause a worsening of the problem in some patients. During menstrual flow, the use of tampons generally proves less irritating than pads and panty liners. In the case of pruritus ani, avoidance of spicy foods may prove helpful.

Most physicians will feel obligated to try a variety of topically applied medications. Any corticosteroid used should be nonfluorinated and of low potency; 1 percent hydrocortisone cream or ointment applied twice daily represents a good choice. If improvement is not noted within 2 weeks, longer use of topical steroids is unlikely to help. Topical analgesics such as lidocaine (Xylocaine) ointment and anti-itch products such as pramoxine (Prax) cream sometimes give relief for a very short period but most often they are totally ineffective.

In the long run, most patients with well-established essential pruritus of the anogenital region will require the use of systemically administered antihistamines or psychotropic agents, or both.[6] Such treatment is useful in breaking up the itch-scratch cycle and allows reestablishment of "microscopic normalcy" to the involved mucocutaneous tissue. Information regarding specific drugs and their dosages can be found in Chapter 3.

Unfortunately, because of the recurring nature of the process a new episode of itching may require reinstitution of treatment. It is important to treat these recurrences quickly to obtain relief before the itch-scratch cycle once again becomes established.

PRURITIC DERMATOSES

Many factors are responsible for itching associated with dermatologic disease. The first relates to the nature of the disease, that is, some diseases are inherently pruritic, while others are not. The second relates to the location. Any condition occurring in a warm, moist area such as the anogenital region is more pruritic than the same disease occurring elsewhere. The third relates to the innate constitution of the individual experiencing the disease; those who are genetically atopic experience itching in many more circumstances than do those who are nonatopic. Each of these features is discussed below.

Some diseases of the anogenital region (most notably scabies and lice) cause pruritus in almost everyone who acquires the disease (see below). Other diseases are associated with pruritus in most, but not all, affected individuals. These include lichen sclerosus (women only), tinea cruris, candidiasis, rectal fissures, pinworms (children only), Fox-Fordyce disease, contact dermatitis, atopic/neurodermatitis, and squamous cell carcinoma (women only). Each of these diseases is discussed separately elsewhere in this book.

Some diseases are not generally pruritic unless they occur in warm, moist areas. Thus psoriasis rarely causes itching when it occurs on the trunk but is commonly associated with pruritus when it develops on the scalp or in the anogenital region. Nearly all the other diseases covered in this book can cause some degree of itching at one time or another, simply because of their location in the anogenital region.

About 20 percent of the population is atopic. These individuals are identified on the basis of a personal or immediate family history of hay fever, asthma, or atopic dermatitis. Other characteristic features are covered in the section on atopic dermatitis, but one of them is important to this discussion: atopic individuals are inherently itchy people. This fact is undisputed, while the reason is unknown. Such itchiness most likely occurs because of the biochemical makeup of atopic skin, its nerves, and the presence of various inflammatory mediators. However, the possibility also exists that there are differences in processing of sensory nerve signals at the cortical level. Regardless of the explanation, anything that triggers peripheral nerves in atopic individuals (cutaneous disease, xerosis, sweat retention, and so forth) generally leads to itching and subsequent scratching in these individuals. For example, psoriasis may be quite pruritic in atopic individuals, whereas it is not associated with itching in the rest of the population.

The combination of all these factors can help to explain why so many patients with anogenital disease complain of itching and why so many pages in this book are devoted to this important subject.

INFESTATIONS

Infestations are often confused with essential pruritus because the responsible organisms are frequently not seen due to their small size. Early lesions are usually removed by scratching fingernails, so that nonspecific excoriations predominate. However, a high index of suspicion and a careful examination generally yield the correct diagnosis.

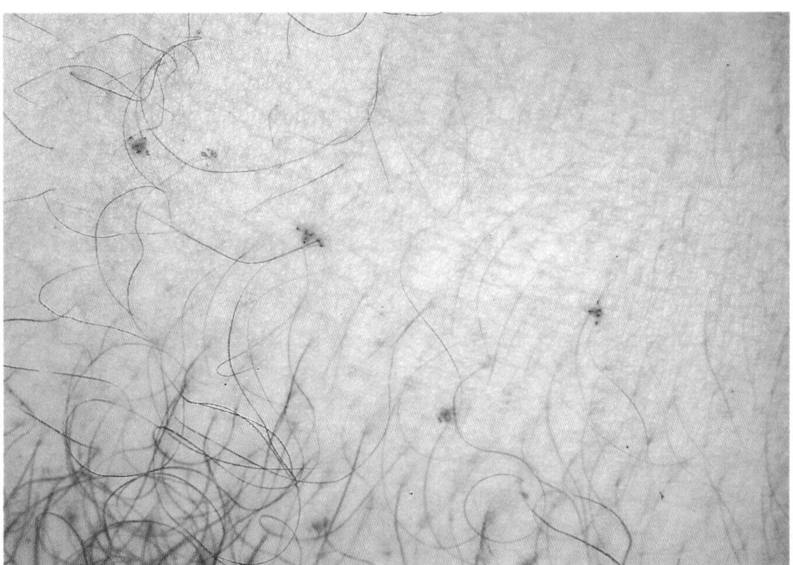

Fig. 20-1. Brown specks at the base of hair shafts can be identified on careful inspection as pubic lice.

PUBIC LICE

Infestation with pubic lice (pediculosis pubis) is a relatively common disease. It occurs in males and females with equal frequency and is most commonly encountered in teenagers and young adults.

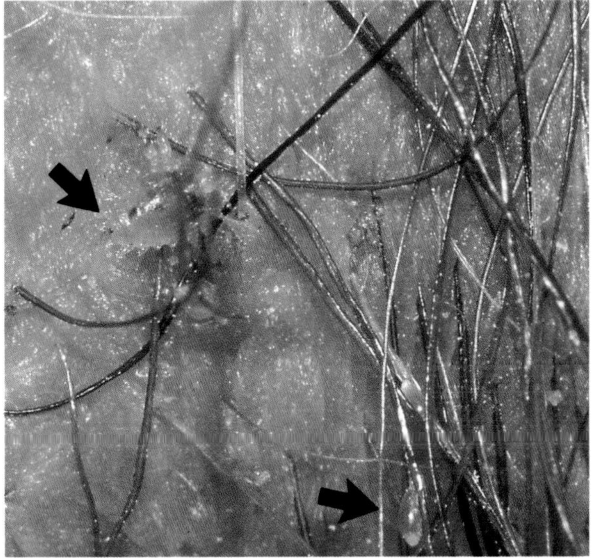

Fig. 20-2. Pubic lice *(arrows)*, clinging to hair. Several nits are also present.

Clinical Presentation

Generally, itching or slight irritation brings the condition to the attention of the patient. Pubic lice are only about 1 to 2 mm long and are therefore easily missed on clinical examination by both the patient and the physician. For this reason, not all patients are aware of the nature of their problem at the time they present for medical attention. The astute physician will not only note the mobile tan to brown specks representing the mites (Figs. 20-1 and 20-2) but will also recognize the nits, which are attached to the lower portion of pubic hair shafts. Rarely, the infestation will also be noted on axillary, eyebrow, and eyelash hairs; the scalp, however, is never involved. Historically, gray-blue macules (maculae caeruleae) were described as occurring on the skin in affected locations; they are rarely if ever found today.

Course and Prognosis

The pubic louse does not carry any other risk of disease and for this reason infestation can be viewed more as a nuisance than as anything more serious. Immune response to the insect does not seem to occur, which allows reinfestation to occur easily on subsequent exposure; failure to treat all appropriate contacts all too often leads to "ping-pong" reinfection.

Pathogenesis

The insect responsible for the infestation is the blood sucking insect *Phthirus pubis.* These lice are shorter than they are wide and have clawlike extremities that allow them to grasp hair shafts easily (Fig. 20-3). This anatomic feature also accounts for the colloquial name of the disease: "crabs." Acquisition of this ectoparasite almost always occurs during sexual activity, but it can also be transferred via contaminated clothes, towels, and bed linen. Once in place the female lays eggs that are cemented to hairs, where they appear as white or lightly pigmented accretions called nits. Hatching occurs a week or so later. The larvae reach adulthood through a series of molts, after which they continuously feed on human blood.

Treatment

Treatment is easily accomplished. Gammabenzene hexachloride (lindane, Kwell) is applied and left in place overnight or for about 8 hours. Alternatively, over-the-counter products such as pyrethrins (RID) and permethrins (NIX) can be used as soaps or shampoos. These are applied and left in place for 10 to 15 minutes before being rinsed off. Controversy exists as to the degree to which any of these products are ovicidal. For this reason historically the involved hairs were shaved or the nits were picked off with a tweezer. This approach does not seem to be necessary; most infestations will respond to one or two chemical treatments as described above.

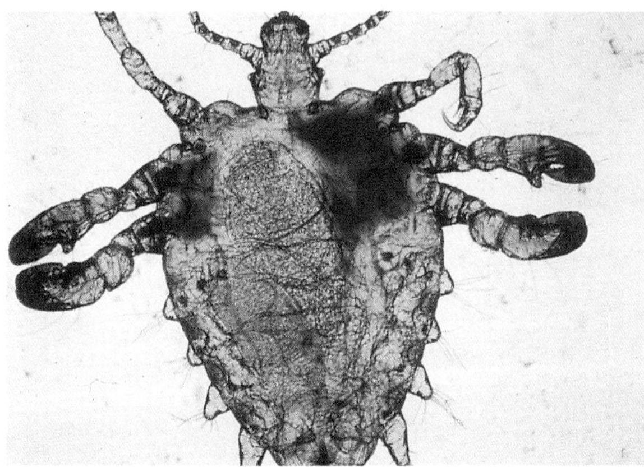

Fig. 20-3. Low-power microscopic view of *Phthirus pubis,* the causative agent of pubic lice.

SCABIES

Scabies is a common disease that occurs in both children and adults. Girls and boys are affected equally, but in adult life (as is true for many sexually transmitted diseases), men outnumber women. Epidemics of infestation occur in periodic cycles, suggesting that some degree of herd immunity develops to end one cycle and then wanes to allow the start of a new one. For reasons not understood, the disease is rarely encountered in blacks.

Clinical Presentation

Strictly speaking, scabies is a vesicular disease, but the intensity of the itching and the inflammation engendered by the immunologic reaction to the organism generally results in a presentation that is papular or eczematous in morphology. Most often, excoriated and crusted lesions, together with a few smooth-surfaced papules, are found. However, on the hands and elbows, a few intact vesicular burrows may also be noted.

The most common sites of infestation include the digital web spaces, elbows, axillary folds, and buttocks. In women the breasts and inframammary folds are commonly involved, whereas in men lesions are often noted on the glans and shaft of the penis (Fig. 20-4). Depending on the level of hygiene, duration of the infestation, and level of immunocompetency,[7] the number of lesions present varies from 10 to several hundred. Occasionally papular and nodular lesions persist for weeks to months after treatment (Figs. 20-5 and 20-6). These latter lesions do not contain live mites but rather represent immunologic reactions to retained fragments of mite protein.

Suspicion that scabies is present should occur whenever an eczematous disease presents primarily with papules rather than with plaques. A history of contagion should then be sought. A suspected diagnosis can be confirmed through the microscopic examination of material scraped from an intact burrow. Since the ability to do this represents an acquired skill, it is tempting to employ a trial of treatment as a diagnostic test. There are times when this is un-

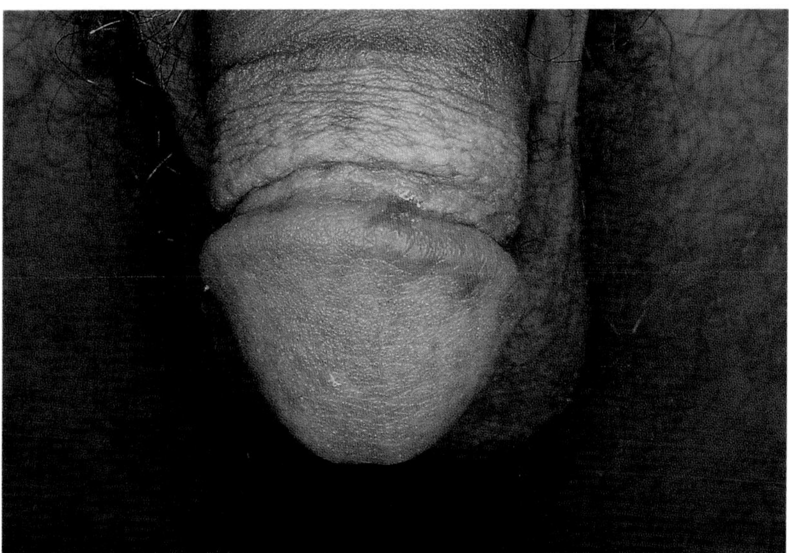

Fig. 20-4. Firm, pink, pruritic papules of scabies in a patient with multiple distant excoriations, vesicles, and scale.

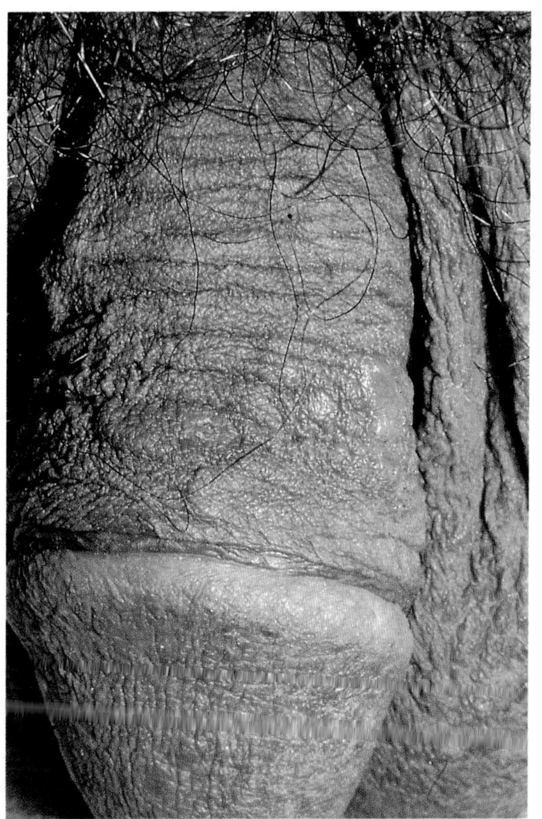

Fig. 20-5. Pruritic nodular scabies remaining on the penis after therapy cleared evidence of scabies elsewhere.

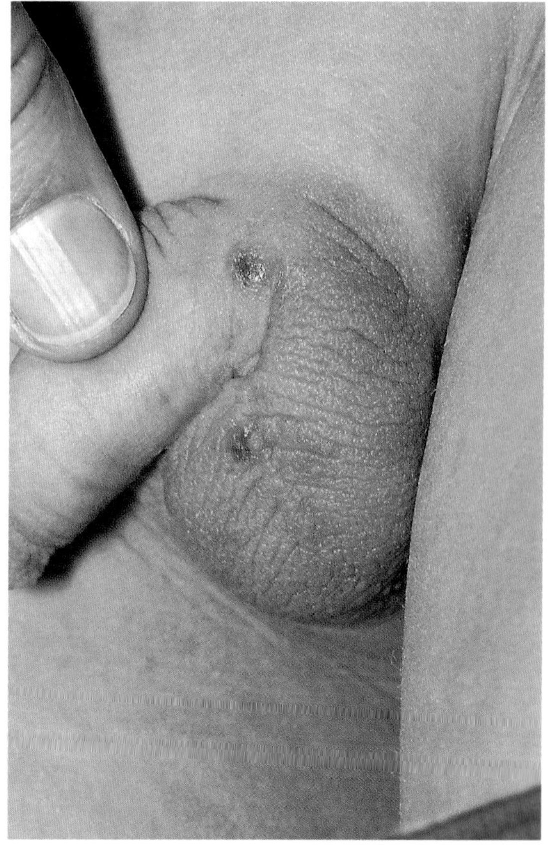

Fig. 20-6. Excoriated nodules of scabies.

doubtedly the most practical approach, but keep in mind what it means to the patient's friends, family, and psyche when a diagnosis of scabies is made. Preferentially, in a situation of clinical uncertainty, it is better to carry out a biopsy. Histologically, even if mites are not located, the nature of the eosinophilic inflammatory reaction is characteristic enough to make the diagnosis.

Course and Prognosis

When scabies is treated, pruritus disappears quickly, and clinical evidence of infestation is generally lost within 2 weeks. However, in some patients the itch-scratch cycle has become well established, and eczematous disease, pruritic papules, or both remain. Scabies, if left untreated, persists for years. This accounts for the older, colloquial name of the disease: "the seven-year itch."

Pathogenesis

Scabies occurs as a result of infestation with the human variety of the mite *Sarcoptes scabiei* (Fig. 20-7). Female mites burrow into the stratum corneum, where they deposit eggs. Several weeks later the eggs hatch and mature into adult mites. The scabetic mite is very small and at best, without a hand lens, it can be seen only as a dark red, minute dot located at the end of an intact burrow.

Transmission of the disease in both children and adults occurs as a result of close personal contact. A large proportion of infestations in adults occurs as a result of sexual activity, but the disease can also be acquired by other types of personal contact and also through contact with infected fomites.

Treatment

Historically scabies has been effectively treated with gammabenzene (lindane, Kwell). More recently, concerns about absorption and consequent toxicity, especially in infants and pregnant women, has led to its replacement with 5 percent permethrin (Elimite). Both products are used in the same manner.[8] Application is carried out from chin to toes, including all the skin folds. The medication is left in place for about 8 hours and is then washed off. All known personal contacts are treated similarly. Recently used clothing and bed linen should be washed in a normal fashion.

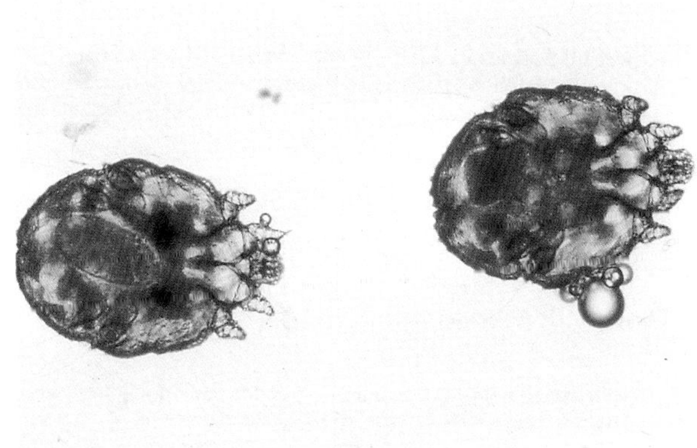

Fig. 20-7. *Sarcoptes scabiei,* with characteristic dark brown globules of feces seen within the mite, and a large ovum in the mite on the left.

A single treatment will be effective for 90 percent of those affected. The others will require retreatment because of poor compliance or reinfection. A small number of patients will have developed a well-established itch-scratch cycle. These individuals continue to experience itching after adequate treatment and require treatment of their eczematous lesions with topical steroids, lubricants, and oral antihistamines.

REFERENCES

Essential Pruritus

1. Pincus SH: Vulvar dermatoses and pruritus vulvae. Dermatol Clin 10:297, 1992
2. Hanno R, Murphy P: Pruritus ani. Classification and management. Dermatol Clin 5:811, 1987
3. Aoki T, Kushimoto H, Hishikawa Y, Savin JA: Nocturnal scratching and its relationship to the disturbed sleep of itchy subjects. Clin Exp Dermatol 16:268, 1991
4. Hatch ML, Paradis C, Friedman S et al: Obsessive-compulsive disorder in patients with chronic pruritic conditions: case studies and discussion. J Am Acad Dermatol 26:549, 1992
5. Sheehan-Dare RA, Henderson MJ, Cotterill JA: Anxiety and depression in patients with chronic urticaria and generalized pruritus. Br J Dermatol 123:769, 1990
6. Wahlgren CF, Hagermark O, Bergstrom R: The antipruritic effect of a sedative and a non-sedative antihistamine in atopic dermatitis. Br J Dermatol 122:545, 1990

Scabies

7. Orkin M: Scabies in AIDS. Semin Dermatol 12:9, 1993
8. Orkin M, Maibach HI: Scabies therapy—1993. Semin Dermatol 12:22, 1993

SUGGESTED READINGS

Essential Pruritus

Denman ST: A review of pruritus. J Am Acad Dermatol 14:375, 1986

This review article, with 142 references, covers the pathophysiology, associated systemic diseases, evaluation, and treatment of itching.

Pubic Lice

Elgart ML: Pediculosis. Dermatol Clin 8:219, 1990

This article contains a complete review of infestation with all types of lice, including pubic lice.

Scabies

Elgart M: Scabies. Dermatol Clin 8:253, 1990

This is a good review paper covering all aspects of scabies infestation.

21 Anogenital Pain

VULVAR PAIN SYNDROMES

Vulvodynia (burning vulva syndrome) refers to symptoms of vulvar burning or raw sensations not adequately explained by observable physical findings. Until recently, vulvodynia was felt to be an uncommon manifestation of depression, anxiety, or psychosexual dysfunction. In 1982, the International Society for the Study of Vulvovaginal Disease (ISSVD) appointed a task force to study this issue. Largely as a result of the work of interested members, this condition has achieved recognition in the medical and lay literature. As clinical trials and beneficial therapies are reported, vulvar burning is becoming accepted as a treatable, albeit poorly understood, symptom that is likely a final common manifestation of any inflammation or neuropathy, although psychological factors play a major role in some patients.

The presenting complaint is burning, although some patients describe rawness, irritation, soreness, stinging, pin pricks, or a sensation of "paper cuts". An occasional patient vehemently denies pain, even though their burning may be life-ruining ("I don't hurt, I burn"). Itching is normally absent but is a minor symptom in some women. Patients have often consulted multiple physicians, usually without encountering one who is familiar with the evaluation and management of these symptoms. Women with vulvodynia have generally used multiple topical anticandidal preparations, topical and oral antibiotics, and topical corticosteroids, usually without improvement. In fact, many patients report burning with application of some creams and overall worsening of symptoms. Vulvodynia usually interferes with sexual function. Pain during or following intercourse is common. Even in those rare patients without dyspareunia, simply the presence of unexplained burning or rawness is sufficiently anxiety-producing and damaging to self-esteem and sexual identity that coitus is almost always unsatisfactory and thus avoided. The resulting guilt and interference with interpersonal relationships worsens anxiety already present as a result of ongoing discomfort, the lack of a diagnosis, and unresponsiveness to therapy. Additional discussion of psychological factors can be found below (Penile and Scrotal Pain). The physical examination, by definition, is basically normal. However, a very careful evaluation of the vulva and vagina sometimes shows minor abnormalities such as mild erythema normally insufficient to cause the severity of symptoms described and sometimes even present in asymptomatic women.

There is no known unifying cause of vulvodynia (Table 21-1). These symptoms can be produced by known but unusually subtle skin diseases or infections. Pain of neural origin sometimes occurs in the absence of any objective clinical findings. Often, multiple or sequential minor abnormalities are identified, none of which adequately explains the degree of symptoms experienced by the patient. Finally, in many patients, no abnormalities that would cause burning can be identified. In an attempt to categorize, understand, and treat this last group of women with vulvodynia, clinical subsets determined by the pattern of burning, types of exacerbating factors, minor physical findings, and response to therapy have been described.[1] These include vulvar vestibulitis, dysesthetic vulvodynia, and cyclic vulvodynia. Most

Table 21-1. Diagnoses in Vulvar Pain

Diagnoses
Specific etiologic or exacerbating factors
Dermatoses: Lichen sclerosus, lichen planus, immunobullous diseases, contact dermatitis
Vulvar fragility/fissures due to estrogen deficiency, superficial bacterial, or *Candida*
Yeast infection
Vaginitis/vaginal discharge of any cause
Genital wart virus infection
Herpes simplex infection, postherpetic neuralgia
Pudendal neuralgia
Patterns
Vulvar vestibulitis—also associated with yeast, human papillomavivus, any vaginal discharge; or may be idiopathic
Dysesthetic ("essential") vulvodynia
Cyclic vulvitis

patients do not fall neatly into one subset but rather show features of several. However, these subsets help to guide therapy and bring organization to a poorly understood disorder or group of disorders.

The evaluation of patients with vulvodynia includes the careful examination for the presence of and possible role for any abnormality that could be a factor in the symptoms of vulvodynia. Each of the causes, exacerbating factors, and subsets discussed below should be considered in each patient. The clinician should be aware that vulvar erythema, pain to palpation in the vestibule with a cotton-tipped applicator (the Q-Tip test, not to be confused with the Q-Tip test to evaluate incontinence), and a biopsy that exhibits nonspecific chronic inflammation are all common findings in asymptomatic women and may not represent pathologic abnormalities. The details of management are discussed at the end of this section, since distinctions among the different causes and subsets may be subtle, many patients exhibit manifestations of more than one entity, and some treatments are useful for all clinical patterns.

Specific Diagnoses

Lichen Sclerosus

Although the hallmark symptom of lichen sclerosus is pruritus, this condition is also well known to produce irritation, rawness, and burning, especially in association with erosions resulting from mild trauma in the fragile skin of advanced disease (see also Ch. 11). These patients are not usually a diagnostic problem because their disease is obvious. However, an occasional patient is symptomatic from subtle disease.

All areas of the vulva should be examined carefully, and at each visit, since visible signs may vary with time, lighting, and the clinician's index of suspicion. Any area of hypopigmented skin should be biopsied, and a negative biopsy should not dissuade the physician from the possible existence of the disease. Sometimes, several biopsies over time are needed to yield a positive diagnosis.

Lichen Planus and Other Causes of Desquamative Vulvovaginitis

Lichen planus of the vulva often occurs in the vagina and proximal vestibule without obvious external lesions. A purulent vaginal discharge resulting from erosive lichen planus of the vagina, especially when superinfected, often produces vulvar pain. The vagina should be examined carefully since rugae may hide erosions from a casual inspection. Erythema and erosion of the vestibule may be the only signs of vulvar lichen planus, but these can certainly produce burning pain and a sensation of rawness. An examination of the mouth usually shows mucous membrane lesions, either classic reticulate white papules, or erosions of the buccal mucosa with or without gingival or tongue lesions. When accompanying lesions are nonspecific, a biopsy may help to distinguish lichen planus from other causes of erosive vulvovaginitis.

Other blistering and erosive diseases that cause vulvar erosions or vaginal desquamation with an irritating purulent discharge can produce sensations of burning or rawness. These conditions are extremely uncommon causes of burning without obvious clinical findings, although early vestibular erosions may be subtle. These diseases usually declare themselves within a few weeks as multiepithelial diseases with very prominent findings in other areas so that diagnosis is not difficult. Cicatricial pemphigoid is the most likely to present with painful, indolent mucous membrane disease that may be undiagnosed if other mucous membranes are not carefully examined (see also Chs. 6, 7, and 16).

Contact Dermatitis

A chronic or mild allergic or irritant contact dermatitis sometimes produces symptoms of vulvodynia, often with minor erythema representing the only clinical abnormality (see also Ch. 5). An irritant contact dermatitis produced by any vaginal discharge is a very common cause of burning, and there is one case report of burning associated with alkaline urine containing a high concentration of oxalate.[2] In addition, most patients with vulvodynia have used multiple medications, lubricating agents, local anesthetics, soaps, wipes, or pads. At best, some of these are irritating, are likely to exacerbate symptoms, and at worst may be the underlying cause. If the correction of abnormalities of irritating body fluids and the discontinuation of all topical agents, including frequent washing, does not improve symptoms, patch testing for allergic contact dermatitis may be indicated.

Vulvar Skin-Fold Fissures

In addition to rawness or burning, patients sometimes describe recurrent fissures in the skin that look and feel like "paper cuts." Examination of the vulva shows mild, usually unimpressive, shininess, erythema, and scale of the modified mucous membrane portion of the vulva. Small, superficial fissures that lie along skin folds, especially at the crease between the labia majora and labia minora can sometimes be seen on careful examination but may be intermittent. Candidiasis is a common culprit. In the absence of yeast, a bacterial culture often reveals growth of group A β-hemolytic streptococcus and sometimes other bacteria as well, including *Staphylococcus aureus.* Other bacteria may be identified on vaginal cultures. It is likely that this condition is analogous to perianal streptococcal disease and, like this condition, can be stubborn and recurrent (Fig. 21-1). When vaginal involvement is absent, mupirocin ointment and a low-potency (hydrocortisone 1 percent) or midpotency (triamcinolone 0.1 percent) corticosteroid ointment often ameliorates symptoms. Otherwise, oral antibiotics as determined by culture results are indicated, maintaining vigilance for the possible development of a yeast infection, and recurrence of disease with discontinuation of therapy. Neurodermatitis can cause these fissures, sometimes assisted by superinfection, but surrounding skin changes show characteristic signs of that disease (see also Ch. 18).

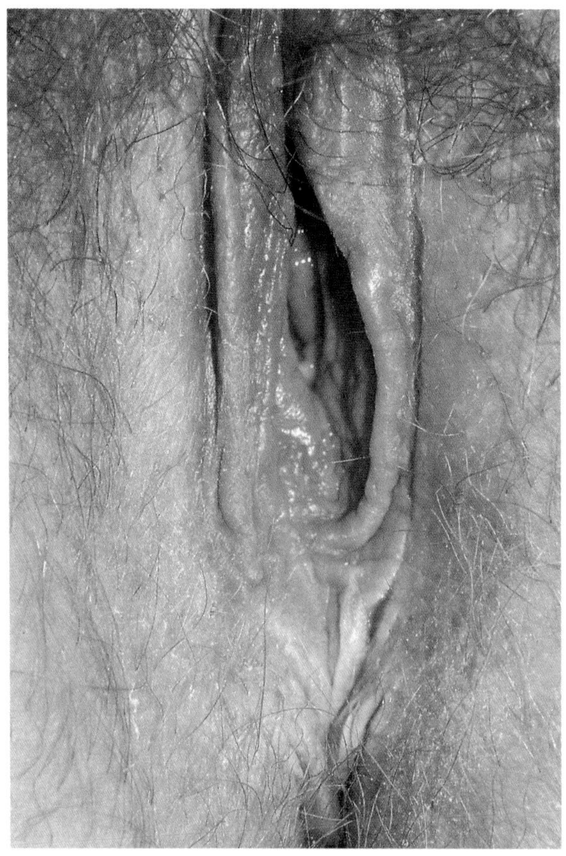

Fig. 21-1. Erythema, shininess of skin, and linear fissures of skin folds are characteristic of this streptococcal vulvitis, but they can also be seen with a Candidal infection; therefore, clinical correlation, cultures, and potassium hydroxide preparations are indicated.

Posterior Fourchette Fissure

Some patients describe burning or soreness in association with fragility and a recurrent painful fissure at the posterior fourchette of the vulva, usually precipitated by coitus. The fissure is not always visible on clinical examination, since the abnormality is episodic. This painful abnormality is often a result of estrogen deficiency. The usual setting is a patient on oral contraceptives or a patient who is postpartum, breastfeeding, or postmenopausal without estrogen replacement therapy. Discontinuation of oral contraception or breastfeeding is beneficial, but this alone requires many months for recovery. Likewise, women who are estrogen deficient as a result of natural or surgical menopause and who are then treated with oral or transdermal estrogen replacement can also expect very slow improvement. However, in all of these patients, topical conjugated estrogen cream (Premarin) 0.625 mg/g applied intravaginally and over the posterior fourchette nightly for 3 weeks and then twice a week usually effects improvement within weeks; therapy may then be further tapered to the most infrequent dosing that maintains healthy skin. For patients who experience irritation with application of the cream, estradiol cream (Estrace) 0.01 percent may be better tolerated, especially if the patient pretreats with triamcinolone ointment 0.1 percent twice daily for several days initially to decrease inflammation. Pregnant women and many women with breast cancer should not receive estrogen therapy in any form. Those patients refractory to estrogen therapy usually benefit from a perineoplasty: the posterior fourchette is surgically excised and the vagina is undermined and advanced to cover this excised area (see also Ch. 18).

Candida

Women often present to the physician convinced that they have burning and other nonspecific constitutional symptoms resulting from chronic or systemic yeast infections and allergies to yeast. Some have read the popular lay literature on yeast and have patterned their lives around yeast-free and sugar-free diets, yogurt douches, microwaved underwear, and oral *Lactobacillus* capsules. Whether or not this syndrome exists at all, yeast plays an important role in a significant minority of women with vulvar burning or irritation despite multiple courses of appropriate topical and sometimes oral therapy. Sometimes local therapy has not totally cleared the infection, and patients describe short-term improvement with medication. In other women, non-*Candida albicans* yeast forms are present but are extremely difficult to identify on potassium hydroxide (KOH) smears and sometimes require prolonged culture time not routinely performed for detection and identification, particularly when the inoculum is small. These infections not only are more likely to be undiagnosed, but also are more resistent to therapy, sometimes requiring both topical therapy and lengthy courses of oral ketoconazole or fluconazole. Occasionally, a vaginal yeast infection has been recognized and treated, but vulvar involvement was not appreciated and therefore not treated. These patients generally have recognizable skin changes on the vulva, but on rare occasions these changes are so subtle that a high index of suspicion is required to perform the confirmatory tests needed.

Every patient with vulvodynia should be evaluated for yeast with a potassium hydroxide preparation at each visit. At the first visit, a vaginal culture is indicated if the smear is negative. The physician should alert the laboratory that organisms may be few or that less common yeast forms such as *Torulopsis (Candida) glabrata, Candida tropicalis, Candida parapsilosis,* or *Saccharomyces cerevisiae* may be present. Some cultures may require up to a month of culture time and great care for detection.

Those patients with vulvodynia and a yeast infection usually have already been treated for yeast so that a standard course of a topical anticandidal medication generally does not provide adequate therapy. Sometimes prolonged treatment with a topical agent provides permanent relief, but many patients experience burning with application of the medication because of the alcohol-containing vehicle. This route has the advantage of safety and lower cost, but affected women are often coping poorly with their disease, their experiences with multiple physician visits, and unhelpful medications. In these patients with chronic symptoms, a month-long course of oral ketoconazole at 200 mg a day, or fluconazole at 100 to 200 mg a day is more effective and efficient than topical agents. Women should be advised of the expense, side effects, and alternatives. Depending on the patient's response, some women benefit from longer courses of medication or, occasionally, ongoing oral therapy. Intravaginal boric acid 600 mg bid has been reported useful in some patients with refractory non-*Candida albicans* yeast.[3] Some patients experience permanent resolution of their symptoms after successful therapy, but many experience only a significant lessening of irritation or burning. It is important to warn patients of this possibility and the likelihood of multiple factors so that they view this diagnosis as a partial answer rather than simply another in a long list of dead ends. Many of these patients require chronic anticandidal therapy either topical or oral to remain comfortable, sometimes as seldom as twice weekly, even though yeast can no longer be identified (see also Chs. 5 and 7).

Non-Candida Vaginitis

Any vaginal discharge can be a vulvar irritant. The vagina of every patient with vulvodynia should be thoroughly evaluated, including a measurement of pH both for the diagnosis of a vaginal infection and for the identification of an unusually alkaline and therefore irritating discharge. A saline preparation (wet preparation, hanging drop test; see also Ch. 2) should be examined microscopically and a vaginal culture performed. Infections should be treated, but in most patients with chronic symptoms this treatment improves but does not alleviate the burning. Occasionally a purulent vaginal discharge cannot be ascribed to a specific infection. This idiopathic discharge may be due to an erosive vaginitis with recurrent superinfection or inflammation, to cervicitis, or possibly to human papillomavirus (HPV) infection. These patients deserve colposcopy and thorough examination of the entire vagina for genital wart infection, erosions, or other lesions potentially diagnosable on biopsy and treatable. Purulent secretions may clear with an accompanying improvement in symptoms if treated with a broad-spectrum antibiotic such as amoxicillin, amoxicillin/clavulanate potassium, or clindamycin even in the absence of a specific infection. This improvement is often either incomplete or temporary, but nonetheless may provide some relief, although the patient should be warned of the possibility of developing an intercurrent yeast infection.

Cervical secretions that increase the vaginal pH sometimes occur in those with a wide transition zone, resulting in an increased number of secreting mucous glands, or in multiparous patients with a patulous cervix and an exposed endocervical region that again secrets mucus with a basic pH. These patients with sterile cervical secretions resulting in a significant vaginal discharge and/or a high vaginal pH sometimes improve with cryotherapy of the cervix (see also Ch. 7).

Human Papillomavirus Infection

Although genital wart virus infections are usually asymptomatic, some patients, especially those with extensive warts, experience irritation and itching. Occasionally, even clinically inapparent disease is associated with vulvar burning, particularly in the pattern of vulvar vestibulitis.[4]

Many women who do experience pain on the basis of genital wart virus infection have obvious involvement of the vagina, with a thick, white, and irritating vaginal discharge composed of keratin debris from the hyperproliferative infected epithelium. Others have little evidence of genital wart virus infection even with a very careful examination of both the vulva and vagina. Colposcopy and biopsies may be useful in some patients, but the physician should be aware that an acetic acid application nonspecifically whitens any area of hyperkeratosis or inflammation, and biopsies from these lesions, seen microscopically, are often erroneously interpreted as HPV infection (see also Ch. 9).

Herpes Simplex Infection

Frequently recurrent herpes simplex virus (HSV) infection may cause episodic burning, but patients are usually already very aware of their diagnosis, or clinical findings support the diagnosis. Theoretically, minor skin changes or subclinical outbreaks can be accompanied by significant pain, and long-lasting nerve pain, especially pudendal neuralgia, can occur. Also, cervical HSV infection can produce an irritating purulent vaginal discharge. A patient with a history suggestive of past or present HSV infection may benefit from a long-term trial of oral acyclovir at 200 mg three to five times a day for several months. In addition, low-dose oral amitriptyline or desipramine as for postherpetic neuralgia may be useful (see also Ch. 15).

Pudendal Neuralgia

A neuropathy may produce genital sensations of burning or rawness and should be considered in the absence of more specific physical abnormalities. Although the sensory nerve supply derives from several nerves, the pudendal nerve is the predominant source for this area.

Patients with pudendal neuralgia describe spontaneous, constant burning, sometimes associated with deep aching or episodic, sharp, shooting pain. Even light contact with substances including clothing and water often precipitates or worsens burning, so that coitus is painful or impossible. Some patients complain of dysuria and frequency. However, spontaneous, short-lived remissions of all symptoms may occur. These symptoms may be present anywhere in the distribution of the pudendal nerve, which encompasses the entire genital area, from the anus to the mons pubis, and extending laterally to the proximal, inner thighs.

On physical examination, there are no characteristic, visible, physical findings. There is no evidence of skin disease, or vulvovaginal infection. Burning pain may be elicited by a delicate touch with cotton or a normally painless light pin prick, although sometimes hypoesthesia is present. Hypersensitivity, particularly to a repetitive stimulus, or a delay in perception with lingering sensations may occur. Certain patients describe radiation of pain, especially down a leg. Sometimes scarring or thickening of the tissue (usually from an injury at delivery) in the area of pain can be seen during a pelvic examination. In some patients spasm of the sacrococcygeal muscle is present, which suggests a diagnosis of neuralgia.

Pudendal neuralgia can result from any damage to the pudendal nerve, including an obstetrical or surgical injury, tumor, trauma, degenerative disc disease, metabolic injuries such as diabetes, or infection, particularly with HSV.

The diagnosis is made by a careful examination to determine the location and nature of the pain and to rule out other causes. Evidence of scarring, tumor, or sacrococcygeal spasm suggests this disorder.

Therapy consists primarily of nonsteroidal anti-inflammatory agents, oral amitriptyline or desipramine, and Williams flexor exercises to increase tone to flexor muscles within the pelvis. Patients with evidence of HSV infection may be treated with chronic oral acyclovir at 200 mg tid or 400 mg bid to prevent acute worsening with outbreaks, although the chronic pain is generally unaffected. Recalcitrant cases may be treated with phenytoin at 300 to 400 mg a day, with results expected within 3 weeks, or carbamazepine at 100 mg a day, increasing in 100-mg increments every 2 days to a maximum dose of 600 mg.[4] The physician should be aware of the toxicities of these medications and follow patients appropriately.

SUBSETS OF VULVODYNIA

Some patients show no clinical findings consistent with the known entities discussed above. In an attempt to bring order and standardized nomenclature to confusing and unexplainable symptoms and generate a treatment plan, these women can be categorized according to patterns defined by aggravating and alleviating factors, setting, exact location of pain, physical findings, and their response to therapy. However, many patients do not fit neatly into one subset, but show features of several different ones. Also, a patient who originally presents with a clinical picture of one subset may evolve into a different pattern at a later visit as a result of normal fluctuations in symptoms, therapy, or new, superimposed factors such as infection.

VULVAR VESTIBULITIS

Some women complain of burning, irritation, or rawness that is always limited to the vulvar vestibule and is elicited by physical touch or pressure to the area. Patients with these symptoms that are corroborated on physical examination but not found to be due to a specific disease process are categorized as having vulvar vestibulitis. These patients, who are usually white premenopausal women, typically complain of pain with manipulation of the area during foreplay, as well as with vaginal penetration during intercourse. Using tampons, wiping the area with toilet tissue, wearing blue jeans that bind the area, and riding a bicycle are usually painful. Turner and Marinoff[5] have developed a grading scale to evaluate the severity of disease in these patients. Grade I vulvar vestibulitis causes discomfort but does not prevent intercourse, whereas grade III completely prevents intercourse.

A physical examination should include systematic exploration of the vulva for pain with a cotton-tipped applicator applied with moderate pressure. Patients with vulvar vestibulitis experience pain to this pressure in the vestibule only, without extension to other areas. This test should be performed at each visit, because many patients exhibit different painful areas at different visits. Otherwise, inspection of the vulva shows a variable degree of erythema of the vestibule (Fig. 21-2). Although many clinicians feel that inflammation may be so intense as to produce erosive disease, it is likely that these cases actually represent an undiagnosed but specific bullous or erosive disease (see also Chs. 7 and 16). Care should be taken in diagnosing vestibulitis solely from the presence of pain to Q-Tip pressure on an erythematous vestibule.

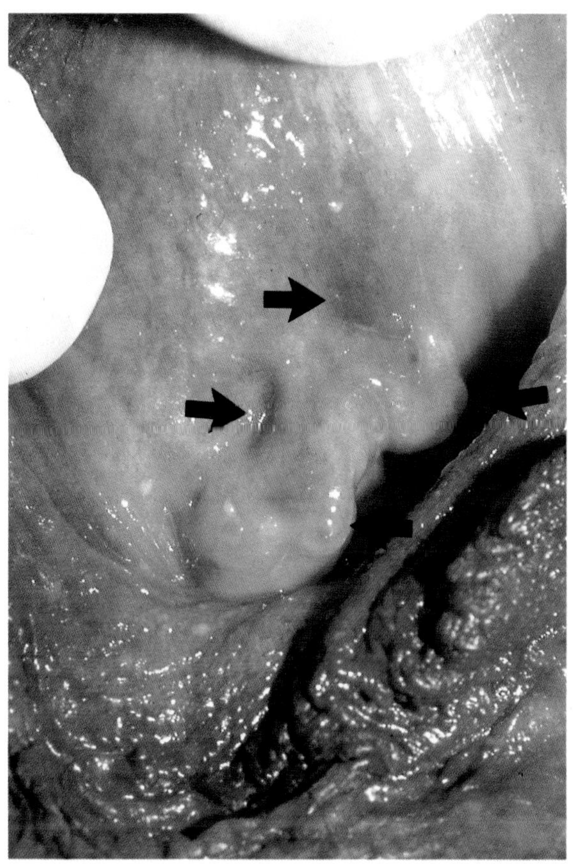

Fig. 21-2. Pits representing the ostia of the vestibular glands *(small arrows)* just distal to the hymeneal remnants *(large arrows)* show the erythema that is characteristic of vulvar vestibulitis.

Up to one-half of all premenopausal women exhibit this redness, and over a third of them are tender to direct pressure (Moyal-Barracco M et al, personal communication, 1993). A biopsy reveals only chronic nonspecific inflammation and is only useful when a specific, visible lesion is present that may reveal an identifiable skin disease.

The cause of vulvar vestibulitis is not known. Turner and Marinoff (personal communication, 1993) have postulated a role for reflex sympathetic dystrophy. The symptoms of vulvar vestibulitis are sometimes associated with subclinical HPV infection, candidiasis, or contact of the area with irritants, including alkaline vaginal secretions, destructive wart treatments, topical medications and cleansers, or an alkaline urine containing a high concentration of oxalate.

Management of this condition includes a careful evaluation at each visit for any of the known factors listed above that may cause or at least aggravate the symptoms. The specific treatments for vulvar vestibulitis are local α-interferon injections and surgical excision. These are discussed in more detail below. Symptoms are sometimes lessened with the use of tricyclic agents (see the section on treatment).

DYSESTHETIC VULVODYNIA

Dysesthetic vulvodynia (essential vulvodynia, idiopathic vulvodynia) is characterized by burning or rawness that is not limited to the vulvar vestibule and often includes the labia majora.[1] Common in older women or women who are estrogen deficient, this pain is often spontaneous and occurs even in the absence of pressure and friction. Sexual intercourse may not be painful, but symptoms are often worse for a variable time following intercourse. Clinical findings are limited to occasional erythema of the vulva and variable pain to pressure with a cotton-tipped applicator over the vulva. It is likely that this condition is often a manifestation of pudendal neuralgia.

The treatment for dysesthetic vulvodynia, in addition to evaluation for any aggravating or precipitating factors, is oral amitriptyline or desipramine. Topical lidocaine jelly 2 percent or lidocaine ointment 5 percent (with the latter preparation more likely to produce stinging on application) may be useful for short-lived relief of symptoms.

CYCLIC VULVITIS

Some patients with symptoms not limited to the vulvar vestibule describe exacerbations and improvement that correspond to the menstrual cycle.[1] Sexual intercourse may or may not be painful, but symptoms are often worsened following coitus. On physical examination, subtle erythema and scale may be present, but otherwise there are no specific findings. There may be pain on pressure with a cotton-tipped applicator.

Patients with a history and clinical findings of cyclic vulvitis are likely to respond to anticandidal therapy, especially oral ketoconazole or fluconazole, even in the absence of positive KOH preparations or cultures for yeast.

MANAGEMENT OF VULVODYNIA

Evaluation

The management of vulvodynia begins the moment the patient is seen for the first time (Table 21-2). These are not women who can be fit into a 15-minute appointment slot. A generous dose of listening, patient education, and sympathy is essential in the management of vulvodynia. All but those patients with the most recent onset of the mildest symptoms are anxious and frightened. Most have used multiple unhelpful therapies, and many have been told that "nothing is wrong." In addition to the burning, these women often are concerned that they may have an undiagnosed and untreated dangerous or sexually transmitted disease, especially cancer or acquired immunodeficiency syndrome (AIDS). They are often embarrassed by their symptoms and have not discussed them with family or friends except for their sexual partner, so that many patients are lacking their usual support systems. Finally, there are obvious repercussions for sexual relationships when women are unable to enjoy intercourse and sometimes cannot tolerate it at all, while physicians find no abnormalities.

Table 21-2. Management of Vulvar Pain

General:

- History with adequate time for patient to ventilate
- Physical examination: evaluation of skin, mucous membranes, vaginal secretions with smears and culture; mapping of pain at each visit
- Patient education regarding disease and prognosis
- Correction of any observed clinical abnormalities
- Discontinue previous topical medications, soaps, and so forth
- Topical lidocaine anesthesia
- Amiptriptyline or desipramine, 25–75 mg/day
- If no improvement
    - Topical midpotency corticosteriod ointment (e.g., triamcinolone 0.1%) twice each day
    - Consider oral ketoconazole 200 mg or fluconazole 100 mg/day for 2–4 months, tapering if beneficial

For Specific Subsets

- Vulvar vestibulitis
    - α-Interferon, 1 million units injected locally × 12
    - [illegible]
- Dysesthetic vulvodynia
    - Amitriptyline or desipramine, 25–75 mg/day
- Cyclic vulvitis
    - Ongoing topical antifungal medication, but if not tolerated or not beneficial, then
    - Ketoconazole 200 mg/fluconazole 100–200 mg/day for 2–4 months

A complete history is important only partly because of information needed to reach a diagnosis. Many patients have a real need to tell their story. They reasonably feel that if a physician would listen to all they have to say, a diagnosis might be possible. Also, most women need to confide, even if only once, to tell their fears of no diagnosis, no cure, ongoing pain, damage to their sexual identity, and stress and guilt in their sexual relationships. Tears and anger are common, but the patient who is listened to is then much more likely to believe that the physician is "on her side" and taking her seriously, so that trust remains even when a medication such as amitriptyline is prescribed.

Information useful for the evaluation of vulvodynia includes the location and quality of pain, exacerbating and ameliorating factors, a list of all medications used and their effects, hormonal status including oral contraception, and the possible existence of a cyclic nature of the pain. It is important to ascertain all topical medications, soaps, deodorants, douches, and so forth used in the area. A history of HSV or HPV infection is informative, as is one of back pain or injury.

A careful physical examination is extremely important since some possible physical findings are subtle, and multiple mild abnormalities may be present. Good lighting, adequate exposure, and close inspection are all mandatory. A common complaint of patients is that some physicians, especially dermatologists, keep their physical distance during an examination. These women then sometimes feel "untouchable" and inadequately examined. Manipulation of the vulva is important so that all areas of the inner labia majora and both sides of the labia minora can be inspected. The vestibule extending to the hymeneal ring should be examined. The patient should then point to the areas of discomfort, which should be recorded for comparison with future examinations that may show a different location of pain. The physician then lightly strokes the skin with a cotton wisp over the entire vulva and surrounding skin to assess the presence of dysesthesia suggestive of pudendal neuralgia. The Q-Tip test is essential: moderate pressure is applied systematically to the vulva with a cotton-tipped applicator to determine areas of sensitivity. Pain with pressure limited to the vestibule is characteristic of vulvar vestibulitis but can be seen in other diseases such as erosive lichen planus of the vestibule and candida vulvovaginitis, and even in some otherwise asymptomatic patients.

An examination of the vagina is essential. Physicians who deal at all with vulvar disease should have a small Pederson speculum in their office. This allows some visualization of the vagina with minimal discomfort in a woman with pain, although a regular Graves speculum or even vaginal colposcopy is needed if a high index of suspicion for epithelial vaginal disease exists, such as in patients with an unexplained recurrent purulent vaginal discharge. A pH determination, a vaginal culture, and an examination of both saline wet and KOH preparations should be performed. The oral mucosa should be inspected for subtle lesions.

Patient Education

Following the evaluation, a careful explanation of vulvodynia and what is and is not known should be given. The patient should be warned that hers is a chronic disease and that most patients do not experience a cure. However, significant improvement is common, and the goal is to relegate this symptom to one of minor aggravation with minimal burning and enjoyable intercourse. If the patient feels that the only acceptable goal is identification and cure of the specific etiology of her burning, she is likely to remain unhappy.

Treatment

Any abnormalities identified, such as a specific skin disease or vaginal infection, should be treated. However, women with long-standing vulvodynia and a specific physical finding that could account for their pain often continue to have burning and irritation even after therapy. Vulvodynia patients may exhibit a basic neurocutaneous abnormality that allows a common final pathway of burning with any irritating influences, including normal daily friction, sweat, and heat as well as vulvovaginal infections. These factors may simply be aggravating influences rather than underlying causes of burning, and careful attention to the alleviation of as many of these irritants as possible often significantly improves symptoms. Often, there are several concomitant or sequential factors. Patients may have more than one infection, or have symptoms aggravated by an irritant contact from the overwashing, topical medications, and so forth. Patients should discontinue everything except tepid water once or twice daily. Vegetable oil is useful for those who require lubrication during intercourse; unlike commercially available lubricants, it has the advantage of containing no allergens but has a soothing base without irritants. All abnormalities and possible irritating factors should be treated or removed. Topical lidocaine jelly 2 percent or lidocaine ointment 5 percent (with the latter preparation more likely to produce stinging on application) can make intercourse bearable to patients while waiting for the slower results of specific interventions.

For patients with an alkaline vaginal pH in the absence of a specific cause, correction is difficult but is sometimes helpful. Estrogen-deficient patients often acidify their vaginal secretions after estrogen replacement therapy is instituted. Dilute vinegar douches or the intravaginal use of a buffered acid jelly such as Aci-Jel twice a day are useful in some patients. Although the insertion of hydrogen peroxide–producing lactobacillus has been reported to be valuable, more recent evidence suggests that currently available forms do not repopulate the vagina. Cryosurgery of the cervix sometimes decreases the volume and alkalinity of vaginal secretions when the cervix produces unusually copious, sterile mucus, as discussed above.

Amitriptyline has been shown to be useful in the treatment of postherpetic neuralgia[6] and diabetic neuropathy, and desipramine and amitryptiline were recently found to produce equivalent pain relief that was unassociated with the alleviation of depression in patients with diabetic neuropathy.[7] Likewise, these two medications are extremely useful in the treatment of vulvodynia, whatever the diagnosis or pattern. Patients should be fully informed that these medications are classified as antidepressants although used in this instance for pain; otherwise, when they learn that they have been prescribed an antidepressant drug, they may feel tricked.

Many women with vulvodynia report that they are overly sensitive to medications. For that reason, and because amitriptyline is so important to their comfort, the starting dose should be so low as to ensure no adverse reactions during the first few days. Patients may be started on one half of a 10 mg tablet at bedtime, increasing as tolerated to a maximum necessary dose of 75 mg. Those women with significant psychological factors or depression sometimes benefit from higher psychotropic doses. Many patients do well by very slowly increasing the dose. Others tolerate this medication by taking it earlier in the evening to minimize morning drowsiness, or by dividing the dose during the day. In addition to the well-known side effects of sedation and dryness of eyes and mouth, patients should be aware of the relatively common increase in appetite that can occur with this medication. Although desipramine has also been found to be useful in pain syndromes and is less sedating than amitriptyline, more women with vulvodynia taking desipramine experience anxiety and jitteriness as a side effect. In those rare women who develop and cannot tolerate this side effect instead of the more common sedation, a medication that combines amitriptyline and chlordiazepoxide (Limbitrol) may be more acceptable. Women with vulvodynia should be warned at the outset that these medications represent their best and perhaps only source of meaningful therapy, so that they should make every attempt to reach therapeutic levels successfully.

Women who exhibit vulvar erythema or who experience itching sometimes benefit from a trial of a topical corticosteroid such as triamcinolone ointment 0.1 percent. Obviously, these patients require careful follow-up to monitor possible local adverse reactions.

Patients who are found on an objective examination to have a yeast infection occasionally improve only slightly or not at all with a topical medication for yeast, but experience dramatic improvement with oral ketoconazole or fluconazole over a 1- to 3-month period. An even smaller subset of patients respond to these oral anticandidal agents in the absence of documented *Candida* infection, perhaps by treating an atypical yeast form that is both difficult to detect and difficult to eradicate. Because some patients require ongoing oral therapy, these medications may treat chronic subclinical infection, or they may obliterate usually insignificant colonization that has nevertheless produced symptoms as a result of hypersensitivity. Finally, perhaps ketoconazole functions by its effect on steroid synthesis, including sex hormones and corticosteroids.

New experimental therapies include biofeedback and a low otalate diet. A significant minority of women have an enormous psychological component that should be addressed. A recent study evaluated the psychological profiles of 11 women with vestibular burning and no identified infectious or dermatologic cause.[8] In addition to personality profiles, specific evaluations for depression, self-esteem, hypochondriasis, and marital-sexual satisfaction were performed. Nine women were mildly and appropriately depressed for their degree of symptoms and dysfunction. Three patients were seriously disturbed, showing paranoia, histrionic personality, severe depression, and hypochondriasis. These patients were independently identified in the office as exhibiting inappropriate and excessively anxious behavior. Preliminary data from our questionnaire comparing the frequency of childhood sexual abuse and unpleasant first sexual experiences with those of controls does not suggest an increase of these events in patients with vulvodynia. This is particularly interesting because an increased frequency of sexual abuse has been demonstrated in women with chronic idiopathic pelvic pain.[9,10]

Although tears, anger, and frustration are common in women with vulvodynia, those patients with exaggerated dysfunctional behavior may benefit from professional psychological therapy. Also, many women (and often their sexual partners) who are normally psychologically well-adjusted but stressed from the emotional repercussions of vulvodynia should be referred for counseling to help them cope with their symptoms. Vigilant observation, especially during a flare of symptoms, for a new infection or process helps to keep patients as comfortable as possible.

In addition to the above interventions that may benefit vulvodynia of any cause, the subsets of vulvodynia have different treatment strategies that are sometimes beneficial.

Vulvar Vestibulitis

Approximately 20 percent of patients with vulvar vestibulitis enjoy long-term benefit from local α-interferon injections. Originally used on the assumption that these symptoms were caused by HPV infection, more sophisticated testing has not shown a disproportionate frequency of HPV infection in patients with vulvodynia. This regimen requires α-interferon, 1 million units, to be injected into the vestibule three times a week for 3 weeks for a total of 12 injections.[11] Most clinical trials have used recombinant α-interferon 2b, although some clinicians now use natural α-interferon because of the possibility of fewer side effects. The injections are placed around the edge of the vestibule, alternating from one side to the other so that eventually the entire periphery has been injected but no two places are injected twice. Patients should be premedicated with oral acetaminophen 650 mg to minimize the flulike side effects that are common after the first injection. A clinically insignificant decrease in white blood cell counts occurs in about 25 percent of patients, but laboratory testing is not necessary.

In those not controlled by conservative measures, a vulvar vestibulectomy is often beneficial. The success rate varies with the surgeon, length of follow-up, and patient selection, and ranges from 30 to 80 percent marked improvement or remission 1 year after surgery. The vestibule is excised to include the hymeneal ring, and the vagina is undermined and advanced to cover the area. Although the procedure seems straightforward, surgeon experience is important, and beneficial long-term responses are more common recently since techniques to retain the vaginal tissue over the vestibule have improved.

Dysesthetic Vulvodynia

The only known treatment for dysesthetic vulvodynia is tricyclic antidepressants, which are extremely beneficial for this subset, as outlined under general therapy. Most patients improve with a dose of 25 to 75 mg a day of either amitriptyline or desipramine, and many can discontinue medication after about 1 year and remain comfortable.[12]

Cyclic Vulvitis

Cyclic vulvitis, whether or not associated with an objective yeast infection, may respond to long-term anticandidal therapy.[1] Some patients can be managed with nightly topical medication, whereas other women either do not respond or experience burning with the application of cream and require oral ketoconazole at 100 to 200 mg, or fluconazole 100 to 200 mg each day for 4 to 6 months, occasionally requiring ongoing therapy often at lower doses.

PENILE AND SCROTAL PAIN

Penile and scrotal pain are at least partially analogous with vulvodynia, although they are appreciably less frequently encountered.

Very little has been published regarding this problem and for this reason most of the data presented in this section is derived from the personal experience of one of the authors (P.J.L.). Thirteen patients have been seen over the last 3 years. The average age of the patients was 50, with a range of 35 to 70 years. Five patients were married; the other eight were single and had never been married. These patients could be divided into two groups: a younger group (35 to 50 years old) of whom only two of nine were married and an older group (60 to 70 years old) of whom three of four were married.

Clinical Presentation

The onset of male genital pain can be insidious or can be related to a single precipitating event. Precipitating events, when present, were most often a sexual encounter which caused the patient some degree of guilt or anxiety, or both. Pain, once established, tended to be constantly present albeit at a fairly low level of intensity. Episodes of more severe pain were then superimposed on this background of constant pain. These episodes were provoked by a variety of factors such as attempts at sexual activity, exercise, rubbing of clothing, buildup of heat, and retention of sweat.

Pain was confined to the penis in nine patients and to the scrotum in two patients; two additional patients had pain in both areas. The glans was the major site of discomfort in all of the patients with penile pain, although two also experienced pain in the shaft of the penis. All of the patients stated that the involved areas were redder than normal and that the red color varied in intensity from moment to moment. Invariably the patients felt that the redness present at the time of examination was less remarkable than was usual. On examination, the degree to which redness was present was usually within normal limits, although several patients (all of whom were using topical steroids) did seem to have more redness than would be otherwise expected.

A diagnosis of idiopathic genital pain is made only after careful evaluation for the presence of associated disease. Testicular pain should be carefully differentiated from scrotal pain since the former is associated with a variety of significant medical problems. Specific dermatologic problems can usually be ruled out without difficulty. Evaluation for the presence of neuralgia, due either to herpetic infection or to other causes, is more difficult. In some instances, consultation with a neurologist may be helpful.

Course and Prognosis

Idiopathic male genital pain is a chronic process. Most patients had experienced discomfort for months to years. About half thought that it was slowly getting worse with the passage of time. In the others the pain remained at a relatively stable level. None of the patients had had, nor did they develop, evidence of dermatologic or sexually transmitted disease even though several of the patients expressed concern over the possibility that they may have "caught something" that the doctors were not able to find.

Pathogenesis

The cause of penile and scrotal pain is unknown. As noted, careful examination of the patients described above failed to reveal any evidence of underlying sexually transmitted disease. Except for the slight degree of redness, which presumably was related to poststeroid changes, no other dermatologic diseases were present. Biopsies were carried out in a minority of patients; they were reported as normal or as showing minimal inflammatory changes.

Psychological factors seem to play an important role in these patients. Those in the younger group often seemed to be sexually dysfunctional. Seven of the nine younger unmarried patients also had never been in a long-term heterosexual relationship and generally were relatively inactive sexually. The sexual activity they had experienced occurred mainly after alcohol use or in a commercial setting. Four of the five patients in the older group were married and all lacked evidence of sexual dysfunction; they were, however, relatively inactive sexually. Patients in both groups stated that their sexual inactivity occurred as a result of the pain that they were experiencing.

Depression was unarguably present in 5 of the 13 patients; most of the others had some features of depression but were functioning reasonably well in everyday life. Only two patients were entirely "normal" as judged by the lack of sexual dysfunction and the absence of overt depression.

The role of psychological factors identified in this series of patients, notably the history of sexual dysfunction, the subconscious use of pain to avoid sexual activity, and the presence of varying degrees of depression, is similar to that often present in vulvodynia[13] and fits the experience of others who have published on this subject.[14,15] Overall, these genital pain problems seem to fit well within the spectrum of other chronic pain syndromes.[16]

Treatment

All of these patients had been seen by several physicians, and the usual topical remedies such as antifungal and antiinflammatory agents had been unsuccessfully tried. Likewise, oral analgesics had provided no relief. Several patients were taking antidepressants for reasons unassociated with their genital pain; these individuals felt that the pain had decreased somewhat since the treatment began. Others were started on antidepressants (doxipen or amitriptyline) because of their pain. The starting dose was 25 mg taken 2 hours before bedtime. This was gradually increased; some improvement of symptoms was usually noted on a dose of about 75 mg a day. No patients were completely relieved of their pain. It is not known whether the improvement related to the use of tricyclics is due to an effect on depression or whether it occurs through other mechanisms. The fact that these drugs are helpful in postherpetic pain and in other forms of neuropathy suggests that the latter may be the correct explanation.[17]

ANAL PAIN

Little can be said of anal pain that has not already been covered in the sections on vulvodynia and male genital pain above. Suffice it to say that it occurs in both men and women, usually in mid- to late adult life. Not surprisingly, sexual dysfunction, as found in many of those with genital pain, is not present. However, the frequency with which depression is identified seems, if anything, even higher.

REFERENCES

Vulvar Pain Syndromes

1. McKay M: Vulvodynia: diagnostic patterns. Dermatol Clin 10:423, 1992
2. Solomons CC, Melmed MH, Heitler SM: Calcium citrate for vulvar vestibulitis. A case report. J Reprod Med 36:879, 1991

3. Redondo-Lopez V, Lynch M, Schmitt CA et al: Torulopsis glabrata vaginitis: clinical aspects and susceptibility to antifungal agents. Obstet Gynecol 76:651, 1990
4. Turner MLC, Marinoff SC: Pudendal neuralgia. Am J Obstet Gynecol 165:1233, 1991
5. Marinoff SC, Turner MLC: Vulvar vestibulitis syndrome. Dermatol Clin 10:435, 1992

Management of Vulvodynia

6. Watson CP, Evans RJ, Reed K et al: Amitriptyline versus placebo in postherpetic neuralgia. Neurology 32:671, 1982
7. Max MB, Lynch SA, Muir J et al: Effects of desipramine, amitriptyline, and fluoxetine on pain in diabetic neuropathy. N Engl J Med 326:1250, 1992
8. Turner ML: Chair's summary: vulvar diseases p 1948. In Burgdorf WHC, Katz SI (eds): Dermatology Progress & Perspectives. Parthenon, New York, 1993
9. Walker E, Daton W, Harrop-Griffiths J et al: Relationship of chronic pelvic pain to psychiatric diagnoses and childhood sexual abuse. Am J Psychiatry 145:75, 1988
10. Reiter RC, Shakerin LR, Gambone JC, Milburn AK: Correlation between sexual abuse and somatization in women with somatic and nonsomatic chronic pelvic pain. Am J Obstet Gynecol 165:104, 1991
11. Horowitz BJ: Interferon therapy for condylomatous vulvitis. Obstet Gynecol 73:446, 1989
12. McKay M: Dysesthetic ("essential") vulvodynia. Treatment with amitriptyline. J Reprod Med 38:9, 1993

Penile and Scrotal Pain

13. Lynch PJ: Vulvodynia: a syndrome of unexplained vulvar pain, psychologic disability and sexual dysfunction. J Reprod Med 31:773, 1986
14. Coterill JA: Dermatological non-disease: a common and potentially fatal disturbance of cutaneous body image. Br J Dermatol 104:611, 1981
15. Koblenzer CS: Psychogenic pain syndromes. p. 131. In: Psychocutaneous Disease. Grune & Stratton, Orlando, FL, 1987
16. Dworkin SF, Von Korff M, LeResche L: Multiple pains and psychiatric disturbance. Arch Gen Psychiatry 47:239, 1990
17. Watson CP, Evans RJ, Reed K et al: Amitriptyline versus placebo in post herpetic neuralgia. Neurology 32:671, 1982

SUGGESTED READINGS

Vulvar Pain Syndromes

Friedrich EG Jr: Vulvar vestibulitis syndrome. J Reprod Med 32:110, 1987

A report of the clinical characteristics and outcome of 87 patients with vestibulitis.

Lynch PJ: Vulvodynia: a syndrome of unexplained vulvar pain, psychologic disability and sexual dysfunction. J Reprod Med 31:773, 1986

A complete survey of the characteristics of pain, physical examination, and demographics of 37 consecutive patients with vulvodynia with suggestions for the etiology and treatment that reflect the opinion that this is a psychological disease.

Marinoff SC, Turner MLC: Vulvar vestibulitis syndrome. Dermatol Clin 10:435, 1992

The authors review different possible etiologies for this pattern of pain and discuss medical and surgical therapy.

McKay M: Vulvodynia: diagnostic patterns. Dermatol Clin 10:423, 1992

Different causes of burning vulvar pain that has no obvious, identifiable etiology are discussed. This experienced author divides patients into subsets depending upon morphology, setting, and response to treatment with an easily understood, organized table.

Peckham BM, Maki DG, Patterson JJ, Hafez GR: Focal vulvitis: a characteristic syndrome and cause of dyspareunia. Features, natural history, and management. Am J Obstet Gynecol 154:855, 1986

This early article detailed the clinical characteristics, laboratory findings, and responses to therapy of 67 patients with vulvar vestibulitis.

Turner MLC, Marinoff SC: Pudendal neuralgia: Am J Obstet Gynecol 165:1233, 1991

The authors discuss the anatomy, symptoms, physical findings, diagnosis, and therapy of pudendal neuralgia.

VIII Special Issues

22 Pediatric Problems

NORMAL GENITALIA AND CONGENITAL ABNORMALITIES

The normal labia minora of newborn girls appear large, and the vagina exhibits a thick, white, occasionally bloody, vaginal discharge as a result of maternal estrogen. In newborn boys, the penis and foreskin are usually fused, at least ventrally, and the foreskin cannot be retracted without force. The foreskin is retractable in up to half of 1-year-olds, and most are retractable by school age. Parents should avoid forcible retraction for cleaning. Circumcision has been an extremely controversial procedure, and medical recommendations have varied over time. Circumcision is painful, associated with occasional complications, and is performed without patient consent in newborns. Recent studies have shown an increase in urinary tract infections in uncircumcised boys. At this time there seems to be no absolute answer on this topic.

Normal newborn term boys show descended testes with a pendulous scrotum covered with rugae. The testes are undescended in 3 to 6 percent of boys, and only about 1 percent are cryptorchid at 1 year.[1] Treatment for cryptorchidism should be instituted at about 1 year of age to enhance future fertility, decrease the risk of malignancy, and minimize psychic impact. Physicians who cannot palpate testes in the scrotum or inguinal area should consider the diagnosis of congenital adrenocortical hyperplasia causing androgen excess with male external genitalia in a female infant, or other "intersex" conditions (see below).

Older prepubertal girls show normal clinical findings that are sometimes mistaken for disease.[2] As in adults, over half of children exhibit erythema of the vestibule. Also found in about half of young girls are periurethral bands of tissue that are usually bilateral, extending from the urethral orifice to, most often, the anterior vestibule. From one third to one half of girls develop labial adhesions, although many are only appreciated with a very careful examination under magnification. Most girls have asymptomatic adhesions between the clitoris and prepuce until the age of 7 years. There are multiple normal morphologies of the hymen, depending on the individual child, age, and method of examination.

HYDROCELE

One of the most common congenital abnormalities is a hydrocele, or fluid trapped in the processus vaginalis, the tract through which the testes descend. Most often, the proximal processus vaginalis is obliterated so that there is no communication; the resulting mild swelling of the scrotum is stable and gradually resolves. The scrotum should be transilluminated with a flashlight to confirm this diagnosis. If the swelling is due to fluid, the scrotum transilluminates brightly, but an inguinal hernia does not. Occasionally the fluid occurs as a result of a patent canal, and the hydrocele persists or fluctuates in size. These children often have an associated indirect inguinal hernia.

PENILE HYPOSPADIAS

Another common abnormality occurring in about 0.8 percent of boys is penile hypospadias, in which the urethral opening is displaced ventrally. This can result in very slight displacement without a significant functional impediment, or in a meatus located as proximally as the perineum. The displaced meatus is associated with a variable deficiency of other normal penile tissue, including the corpora cavernosa and corpus spongiosum. Most often, the foreskin is incomplete, functioning as a dorsal hood over the glans with an absence of the ventral portion.

CHORDEE

Chordee, a ventral curvature of the penis, is usually present in association with hypospadias; it results from a deficiency of ventral tissue distal to the abnormally placed meatus and fibrous tissue. Occasionally, chordee occurs without hypospadias. The incidence of other urinary tract abnormalities in children with hypospadias is about double that of unaffected boys. These children should not undergo circumcision because the foreskin can be used in the surgical repair. This can be performed at any age after about 6 months but is often done early to minimize psychological trauma.

AMBIGUOUS GENITALIA

Ambiguous genitalia requires immediate referral for evaluation. This abnormality can result from multiple causes, but of most immediate importance is the possibility of congenital adrenocortical hyperplasia, which can cause death from a salt-losing syndrome and cortisol deficiency. This condition results from an inherited enzymatic defect of steroid synthesis and usually is associated with an increase in androgen production, producing girls with ambiguous genitalia. Other causes include maternal use of androgens, end-organ insensitivity to androgen stimulation, genetic genital tissue abnormalities, and the presence of functioning ovarian and testicular tissue in the same individual. The assignment of gender should be postponed and is less determined by karyotype than by the child's potential for future reconstructive surgery, sexual functioning, and fertility.

LABIAL ADHESION

Over one third of prepubertal girls develop fusion of the labia minora, particularly at the vulvar posterior fourchette[3] (Fig. 22-1). The cause is unknown, although some physicians have postulated irritation from poor hygiene as one factor (like phimosis), and others believe sexual abuse may play a role. Usually, adhesions are minor and spontaneously reverse by puberty, but occasionally agglutination produces difficulty with urination and retention of vaginal secretions. If labial adhesions are minor and asymptomatic but treatment is desired, simple lubrication and mild manual traction by the mother will often separate the labia. In more significant fusion, topical estrogen cream applied once or twice daily for several weeks allows gentle manual separation, again followed by lubrication. Traumatic severing of the labia should be avoided.

URETHRAL PROLAPSE

Urethral prolapse occurs in girls and consists of extrusion of the distal urethra mucosa, producing an annulus of friable, deeply erythematous tissue surrounding the meatus. Because of edema, the urethral orifice may be difficult to detect, and differentiation from a tumor may be difficult clinically.

Urethral prolapse occurs most often in black children and at about the age of 5 years. Although bleeding is the most common complaint, urinary symptoms and pain may be present. The cause is unknown, but the restriction of this condition to prepubertal children and postmenopausal women suggests that estrogen deficiency plays a role.

Treatment includes sitz baths, local care of erosions and secondary infections, and estrogen creams.

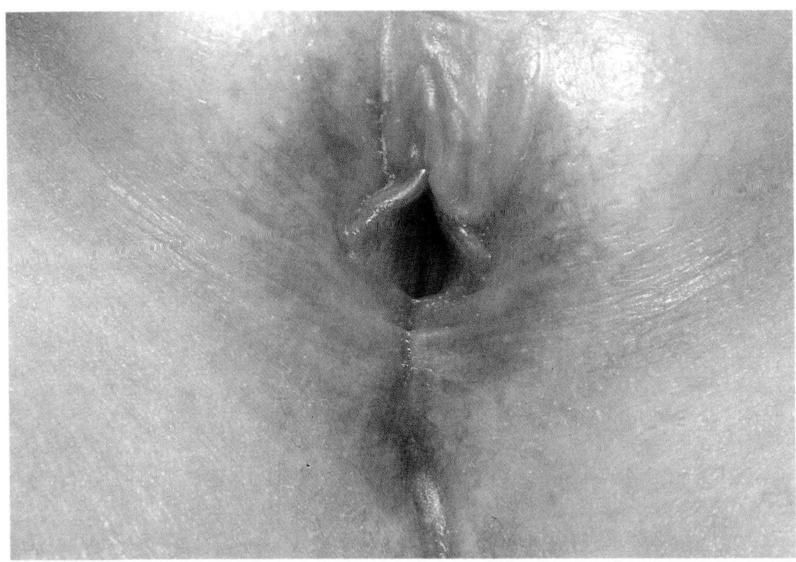

Fig. 22-1. Agglutination of the labia at the posterior fourchette in a small child.

When these measures fail, surgical excision or ablation of the tissue with cryotherapy or cauterization is usually curative.

DIAPER DERMATITIS

Diaper dermatitis (diaper rash, napkin dermatitis) refers to any dermatitis occurring in the diaper area. All children develop diaper dermatitis at some time, usually due to the expected maceration and secondary *Candida albicans* infections that occur on genital skin in an environment of incontinence, friction with a damp diaper, and occlusion. This irritant contact dermatitis, sometimes with *Candida* infection, represents the most common type of diaper dermatitis.

Clinical Presentation

This irritant consists of red, scaling plaques concentrated over the convex areas in direct contact with the diaper, including the mons, labia majora, scrotum, penis, buttocks, and inner thighs. The crural creases and other intertriginous areas protected by skin folds from urine, diaper friction, and feces are spared. When *Candida* plays a major role, the bright-red eruption is accentuated rather than decreased in the crural crease, and satellite pustules are often present. Occasionally, severe irritant diaper dermatitis results in exudation, and even less often punched-out ulcerations or ulcerated papules may occur (referred to as Jacquet's diaper dermatitis [see also Granuloma Gluteale Infantum below]). Postinflammatory hypo- or hyperpigmentation is common following diaper dermatitis in children with naturally darker skin color.

Diagnosis

Other skin eruptions may begin in the diaper area, or be accentuated there, and these should be considered in the event of atypical or recalcitrant irritant diaper dermatitis. Seborrheic dermatitis often occurs in the genital area, but usually appears first in the scalp and affects other intertriginous areas such as the axillae (see below). Other diseases easily confused with irritant diaper dermatitis include atopic dermatitis, which is generally associated with eczema of the extensor surface of extremities and the cheeks, and psoriasis, which usually also affects the scalp and is characterized by sharply demarcated plaques. However, both of these diseases may first appear in the diaper area and may only be diagnosed correctly as the course of the disease supplies clues. Herpes simplex virus infection and bullous impetigo also occur in the diaper area and usually can be recognized by the lesional morphology. Langerhans cell histiocytosis and zinc deficiency (acrodermatitis enteropathica) are very rare diseases that classically affect the diaper area but are also present elsewhere.

Treatment

The treatment of diaper dermatitis includes changing the local environment as well as using specific medication. Diapers should be left off entirely as much as possible to minimize chafing, to allow the area to dry, and to prevent urine and feces from being held against the skin. More practical is changing the diapers very frequently, as soon as they become soiled. Many of the baby wipes contain alcohols, irritating cleansers, and perfumes that are painful to inflamed skin, so these should be avoided. The area should be gently cleaned only with a soft, damp cloth, avoiding soaps, and the area patted dry. Zinc oxide paste, or the popular zinc oxide paste compound Desitin, may be applied in a thick layer to a mild or moderate eruption during each diaper change; it serves as a protective film against irritating excrement. When the dermatitis is severe and exudative, zinc oxide paste may only increase maceration. Hydrocortisone cream 1 percent (or ointment when the skin is broken or especially inflamed) enhances healing of irritant dermatitis, but if a yeast infection is present, then the area should also be treated with one of many topical anticandidal agents, such as clotrimazole or miconazole (over the counter), sulconazole nitrate, ketoconazole, haloprogin, ciclopirox olamine, and so forth (see also the sections on antifungal medications in Ch. 3). Mycolog II is often used for diaper dermatitis because it combines a corticosteroid and nystatin, an anticandidal agent. However, the potency of the corticosteroid, triamcinolone, is higher than necessary and may cause local steroid side effects if used for more than a brief period, and nystatin is less effective than the newer antifungal medications. Lotrisone also combines a midpotency corticosteroid and the antifungal medication clotrimazole, again with the disadvantage of containing a more potent steroid than needed. In general, from the choices available in the United States, the use of hydrocortisone 1 percent and a separate antifungal agent when indicated provide the most benefit with the least risk of adverse reactions.

GRANULOMA GLUTEALE INFANTUM

Granuloma gluteale infantum consists of nodules that occur in the setting of diaper dermatitis treated with potent topical corticosteroids. First reported in 1971, this disease is extremely uncommon and may be a new entity affected by new habits such as topical corticosteroids or disposable diapers and plastic pants.

Granuloma gluteale infantum consists of one to several dusky, violaceous and sometimes oval nodules on the inner thighs or perineum, often lying parallel to skin lines (Fig. 22-2). They occur on the convex surfaces of the skin covered by the diaper and

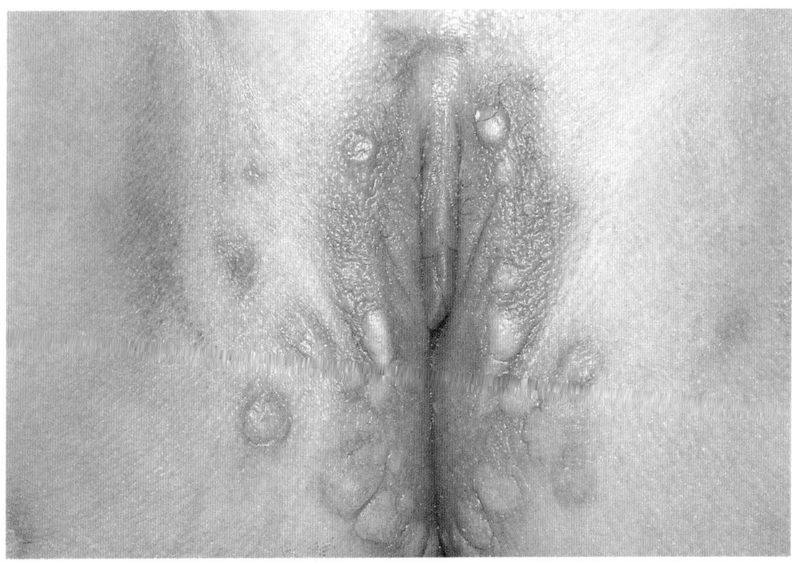

Fig. 22-2. Granuloma gluteate infantum. Irritant papules resembling genital warts from diaper dermatitis.

may reach up to 3 cm in size. Clinically, these may mimic lymphoma, and a biopsy may be required. Histologically, they show an intense inflammatory infiltrate reaching to the deep dermis and consisting of lymphocytes, neutrophils, histiocytes, and eosinophils.

There is no specific treatment other than control of the diaper dermatitis and discontinuation of corticosteroids. Diaper granulomas resolve spontaneously, although scarring may occur.

SEBORRHEIC DERMATITIS

Seborrheic dermatitis of infancy is a condition of unknown etiology characterized by red, scaling papules and plaques. Occurring in infants in the first 6 months of life, seborrheic dermatitis shows a predilection for the scalp, face, and diaper area but may extend to involve the skin surface generally. The first area of involvement is usually the scalp but may be the diaper area (Fig. 22-3). The erythema, scale, and poorly demarcated nature of the individual lesions may make differentiation from an irritant diaper dermatitis and atopic dermatitis impossible. However, the scale of seborrheic dermatitis is more likely to exhibit a yellowish color, and intertriginous areas are most involved rather than relatively spared. Some clinicians feel that the presence of linear fissures in the interlabial cleft of the vulva is characteristic of seborrheic dermatitis. Postinflammatory hypo- or hyperpigmentation is common following seborrheic dermatitis in children with naturally darker skin color. Langerhans cell histiocytosis is often said to mimic seborrheic dermatitis, although the former disease displays infiltrated papules, often with petechiae, that are not seen in seborrheic dermatitis.

Treatment consists of removal of scale, especially thick, adherent scale over the scalp, by soaking and gentle scrubbing. Hydrocortisone cream 1 percent applied twice a day to the affected genital area and attention to any secondary infection provide rapid improvement.

CAPILLARY HEMANGIOMA

A capillary hemangioma is a vascular tumor occurring in about 10 percent of infants and often arising in the anogenital area.

Clinical Presentation

This benign neoplasm may be present at birth or (more often) may appear in the first few weeks of life. The first visible lesion in newborns is a pale patch with telangiectasias, or sometimes a uniformly erythematous macule or patch. The hemangioma usually grows rapidly to become nodular, soft, and smooth or lobular (Fig. 22-4). Although usually single, several lesions are not uncommon, and dissemi-

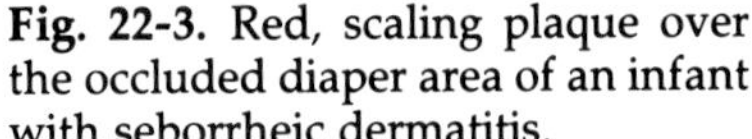

Fig. 22-3. Red, scaling plaque over the occluded diaper area of an infant with seborrheic dermatitis.

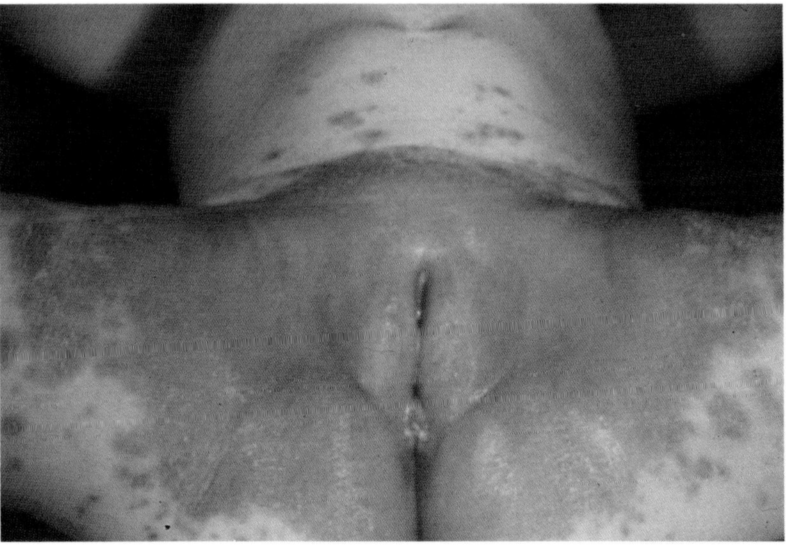

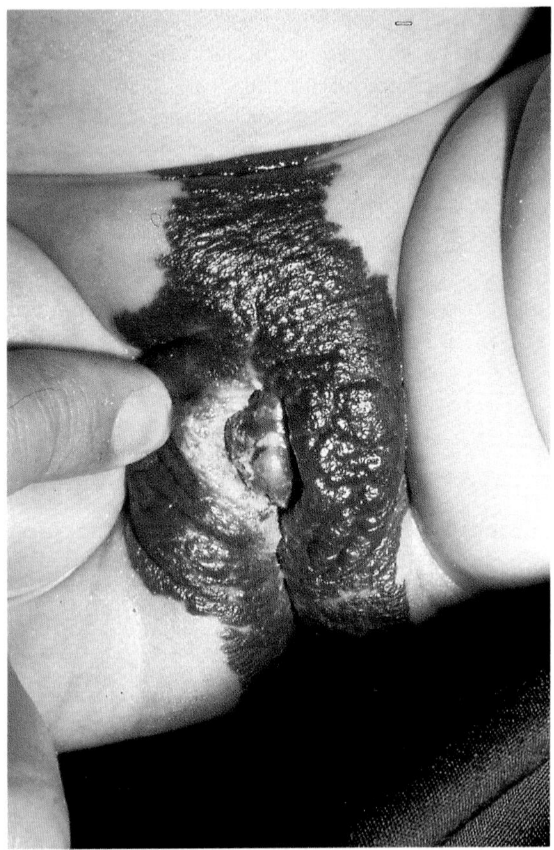

Fig. 22-4. Bright-red, shiny, nodular capillary hemangioma encompassing the vulva in an infant.

nated angiomas with or without life-threatening visceral involvement may occur rarely. Most capillary hemangiomas reach several centimeters in size within about 6 months, stabilize, and ultimately involute, causing medical problems only if the size and location interfere with necessary functions. Regression, sometimes with scarring, occurs by age 7 years.

Although hemangiomas are most common on the face and neck, the anogenital area is often affected, especially the labia majora. Genital hemangiomas most often cause difficulty when an orifice is obstructed or the tumor erodes and superinfection occurs by virtue of proximity to fecal material and diaper occlusion. Chronic ulceration of the tumor may produce bleeding, although significant bleeding is surprisingly uncommon. Other possible complications are intractable pain of ulcerated lesions and (rarely) thrombocytopenia and a consumption coagulopathy called Kasabach-Merritt syndrome. This syndrome is generally associated with large tumors, but mild cases occasionally are seen even with small tumors. Any of these complications in the genital area may require intervention, although most hemangiomas are handled best by allowing spontaneous regression.

When a hemangioma, or any cutaneous lesion in early infancy, occurs on the dorsal midline, the physician should be alert to the possibility of an associated neural abnormality. Lumbosacral capillary hemangiomas are sometimes associated with spinal dysraphism, in which there is incomplete closure of the midline embryonic structures. This can be manifested by the tethered cord syndrome. The physician should recognize and investigate this possibility early, since irreversible neurologic deficits may occur after spontaneous regression of the hemangioma.

Diagnosis

The diagnosis of a capillary hemangioma is generally made on clinical grounds without histologic confirmation because of the risk of bleeding with a biopsy. Occasionally a biopsy must be performed when there are atypical features and other tumors are considered.

Treatment

Treatment is usually limited to local care of any erosions or local infection. Parents require reassurance, but surgical removal during infancy or early childhood should be discouraged. General anesthesia is required, and a better cosmetic result follows spontaneous regression than surgery. Some physicians have recently suggested earlier removal than was previously accepted, using only laser ablation or combinations of laser and excision. Studies are in progress evaluating these approaches.

For those capillary hemangiomas that require treatment by virtue of obstruction, bleeding, pain, or consumption coagulopathy, oral corticosteroids at a dose of prednisone 1 to 2 mg/kg is the most dependable treatment although corticosteroid side effects are well-known and worrisome. High-dose intralesional corticosteroid treatment is sometimes used, although these doses produce systemic levels of medication. Cryotherapy has been beneficial in some cases, but the resulting ulceration may produce bleeding and the cosmetic outcome is inferior to that produced by spontaneous regression. Systemic α-interferon also has induced involution in infants with health-threatening hemangiomas. Although most children do well without specific intervention, some eventually require surgery to remove remaining hemangioma when the entire lesion does not regress, or when excess overlying skin persists.

CONGENITAL NEVI

About one percent of newborns have a pigmented nevus (congenital melanocytic nevus, congenital pigmented nevus), a hamartoma of melanocytes. Although pigmented nevi appearing after birth are common and usually of no consequence, congenital nevi carry an increased risk of malignant melanoma.

Clinical Presentation

Congenital nevi are brown lesions that exhibit some degree of surface change. Although some are small and exhibit sharp borders, they tend to be larger than the 5-mm diameter of acquired nevi. Congenital nevi also may be quite large, such as the so-called bathing trunk nevi that encompass the area normally covered by bathing trunks. The larger nevi are characterized by more irregular borders, irregular color, and an irregular surface. Both large and small congenital nevi often involve the genital area, and medium-sized or larger congenital nevi that are infiltrated may be disfiguring. Although congenital nevi do not enlarge except proportionately with growth of the skin, at puberty the nevi become thicker and darker. Small nevi are at minimal risk for malignant transformation, and this event occurs after puberty. However, large tumors carry a significant risk for the development of melanoma, which may develop early, including in utero.

Diagnosis

The diagnosis is usually made on the clinical examination, but sometimes the surface change is subtle and other diagnoses may be entertained. Mongolian spots are bluish in color with absolutely no surface change and often with indistinct borders. They are most common over the buttocks and backs of children of darkly pigmented races. Café-au-lait spots are evenly colored, light brown, sharply demarcated patches with no surface texture, most often distributed over the trunk rather than the genital area.

Treatment

The treatment of congenital nevi is controversial. Many pediatric dermatologists now recommend the removal of all congenital nevi because of the risk of melanoma. However, the removal of those large tumors at greatest risk of malignant transformation requires mutilating surgery performed during infancy. Because melanoma transformation occurs late in small nevi, these need not be removed until the child is old enough to tolerate removal under local anesthesia. Although the risk for melanoma in small congenital nevi is minimal and many are simply followed clinically, most of those occurring on the genitalia are relatively inaccessible to routine examination by the patient and probably should be removed.

PERIANAL STREPTOCOCCAL DERMATITIS

Perianal streptococcal disease (perianal streptococcal cellulitis) is a chronic, superficial (not cellulitic) perianal infection caused by group A β-hemolytic streptococcus. More common in boys, this condition is manifested by pain, especially with bowel movements, and pruritus. Feces may be streaked with blood, and although patients are not usually otherwise ill, streptococcus can also often be cultured from the pharynx. An examination reveals an erythematous, often well-demarcated, damp, perianal plaque without induration. Older lesions may show scale and fissuring. Streptococcal vulvovaginal infection with an accompanying vaginal discharge may also occur (see also Bacterial Vaginitis, below).

Other diseases that may be confused with perianal streptococcal disease include eczema, psoriasis, pinworms, and sexual abuse. The diagnosis is by the clinical examination and culture on 5 percent sheep blood agar. The treatment of choice is oral penicillin V, but recurrence is common. Recent evidence suggests that topical mupirocin ointment used concomitantly may decrease the recurrence rate.[4] Poor or incomplete response to therapy should alert the physician to possible underlying complicating factors such as lichen sclerosus.

IRRITANT DERMATITIS

Ordinarily well-tolerated contactants may cause genital inflammation (see also Ch. 5) in children, primarily girls. Well-known examples include bubble bath and soaps. Overly enthusiastic or frequent cleaning may produce irritation, and some children leak small amounts of urine during the night and experience a mild contact dermatitis. Feces, when trapped in the anal skin folds or vulva, may also cause pruritus and inflammation, as may sand not removed after a day at the beach or in the sandpile. This delicate skin is also more prone to injury and irritation with bicycle riding or bareback riding on a horse. With any evidence of trauma not adequately explained, the clinician should maintain a high index of suspicion for sexual abuse (see below).

The treatment for irritant vulvitis is removal of the precipitating factors and gentle tepid water flushes of the skin, without soaps, for cleaning. Hydrocortisone 1 percent ointment applied twice a day improves pruritus during healing. Occasionally, a topical estrogen cream may be needed in recalcitrant cases to thicken the skin temporarily and enhance healing.

CANDIDA VULVITIS

Although *Candida* infection (see also Ch. 5) occurs most often in diapered infants and postpubertal females, this infection also can affect the vulva of children. The skin exhibits red, moist or scaling plaques, often with satellite pustules or collarettes that show fungal elements on a potassium hydroxide examination or a positive culture of gently acquired skin scrapings. It can usually be treated with any topical anticandidal agent, although occasionally topical treatment applied to exudative skin produces burning. In this instance, or when vaginal involvement is suspected because of recurrence, discharge, and so forth, an oral agent such as ketoconazole or fluconazole may be indicated. The insertion of a vaginal cream or suppository in a prepubertal child may be physically and emotionally traumatic.

PINWORM INFECTION

The outstanding symptom of pinworm infection (enterobiasis vermicularis), an extremely common infestation, is perianal and vulvar pruritus. Children generally experience itching, especially during the night when worms migrate onto perianal and vulvar skin to lay eggs. Clinically, the perianal area, and sometimes the vulva, show only mild erythema. At times, secondary eczematous changes are present, showing prominent scale and excoriations. A vaginal discharge may develop as a result of migration of the parasite into the vagina.

The diagnosis is made by pressing the sticky side of clear cellophane tape to the perianal area in the early morning before eggs laid the night before have been removed by scratching, washing, or wiping. The tape is then examined under a microscope for the presence of adherent, easily identifiable ova. Occasionally the worm may be seen in the genital area in the night.

Treatment requires the oral administration to the patient and family members of mebendazole 100 mg, or pyrantel pamoate 11 mg/kg up to 1 g. One-time retreatment in 1 to 2 weeks is needed to kill worms that have hatched since the first treatment.

HERPES SIMPLEX

Herpes simplex (see also Ch. 15) can produce pruritus and pain of the genitalia in the pediatric age group. This disease is characterized by vesicles, round erosions, and exudation (Fig. 22-5). A viral culture should be performed to confirm the presence of this sexually transmitted disease, and sexual abuse should be carefully considered. Treatment of first-episode herpes simplex virus infection is with oral acyclovir at 250 to 600 mg/m^2/dose, given four to five times each day. If recurrences are significant, the immediate institution of acyclovir treatment may ameliorate the episode. When herpes simplex is frequently recurrent, low-dose suppressive daily administration of acyclovir can be considered.

CLITORITIS

Occasionally prepubertal children complain of clitoral irritation. The most common causes are trauma, secondary bacterial infection, and clitoral adhesions. Treatment depends upon the underlying causes.

VAGINAL DISCHARGE/VAGINITIS

Unlike many adults, children or their caretakers may not be able to differentiate between the staining on underwear from the exudate of vulvitis and a dis-

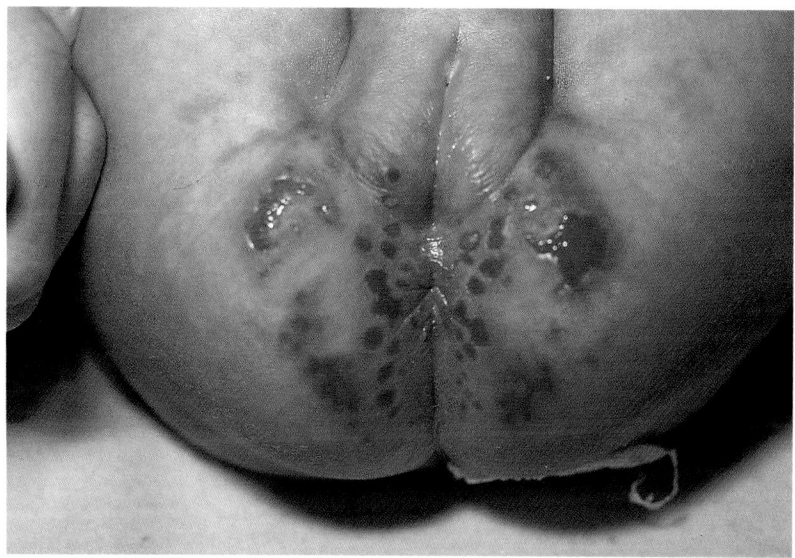

Fig. 22-5. Scattered round erosions with confluence into larger lesions with circinate borders in this child with herpes simplex infection whose blister roofs have eroded. Sexual abuse is a consideration in this child. (Courtesy of Gerald N. Goldberg, M.D.)

charge of vaginitis. Symptoms of pruritus or pain are most often associated with vulvitis, although a secondary vulvitis simply from contact with an irritating discharge is common.

When vulvitis is not present and it is clear that the discharge is not vulvar in origin, then the vagina must be evaluated. The evaluation of a vaginal discharge in prepubertal girls is similar to that in postpubertal women. However, there are qualitative differences between the thin, fragile, poorly estrogenized vulvar and vaginal epithelium of children and the glycogen-rich, estrogenized tissue of adults during child-bearing years. This difference is associated with an increased likelihood of particular conditions in childhood. Also, the inability of children to cooperate with a genital examination requires special knowledge and patience.

Children should be examined in the presence of a parent when possible, and the child should understand that this examination of their genital area is appropriate and condoned by the parent. If the child will not lie still for an examination, she can be placed in a parent's lap. If she is older or cooperative, she should support herself on her hands and knees, and then lower her chest to the examining table. This often allows the vagina to open to direct visualization. Often an otoscope with a nasal speculum can be used to assess the vagina better in infants, and a veterinary otoscope in older children. Because of the fragile character of the epithelium, the insertion of a cotton-tipped applicator to collect vaginal secretions produces pain. Hard or breakable instruments should also be avoided. Instead, a soft catheter attached to a syringe can be introduced more comfortably, but the end tends to be sucked against the vaginal wall when aspiration of vaginal secretions is attempted. Alternatively, one end of a section of intravenous butterfly tubing with the needle cut off and an attached syringe containing a small amount of saline at the other end can be inserted into a shortened 12-gauge urinary catheter.[5] The double catheter is inserted into the vagina, and a small amount of saline is injected and aspirated several times, until an adequate quantity of representative fluid is obtained for examination and culture. A pH measurement will not be accurate because of contamination with saline.

ECTOPIC URETER

When the discharge is copious and clear clinically and microscopically, an ectopic ureter opening into the vagina should be suspected. This can be confirmed with an intravenous pyelogram.

PHYSIOLOGIC LEUKORRHEA

Near menarche, girls may experience a dramatic but normal increase in vaginal secretions. This discharge is white or yellow and generally nonirritating.

A microscopic examination of secretions is normal and shows many squamous cells.

GONORRHEA

Most girls with gonorrhea (see Sexual Abuse, below) are symptomatic and exhibit an extremely purulent vaginitis. Any child with a vaginal discharge of unknown etiology should be cultured for gonorrhea. This is the most common organism obtained during the evaluation of a child for sexual abuse.

TRICHOMONAS, BACTERIAL VAGINOSIS

Although reported in prepubertal girls, trichomonas and bacterial vaginosis (see also Ch. 7) are extremely rare.

BACTERIAL VAGINITIS

Probably by virtue of the thin nature of prepubertal vulvovaginal epithelium, children are at increased risk for bacterial vaginitis. The discharge is purulent, and pruritus, pain, or dysuria may occur. A vaginal culture is most likely to show coliforms, β-hemolytic streptococcus, or coagulase-positive staphylococcus. Group A β-hemolytic streptococcal vaginitis resembles gonorrhea; both produce an unusually purulent vaginitis in prepubertal girls. Treatment is with oral antibiotics, and recurrence should alert the physician to the possibility of a foreign body. Some clinicians believe that occlusive clothing and poor hygiene and wiping techniques may predispose to bacterial vaginitis, but it is unlikely that these factors are of great importance. However, recurrent disease may be improved by the short-term use of a topical estrogen cream to thicken the vaginal mucosa.

FOREIGN BODY VAGINITIS

Retained foreign bodies can produce a purulent and malodorous vaginal discharge. The most common foreign body in prepubertal children is toilet paper; in postpubertal girls it is a retained tampon, but other common foreign bodies include toilet paper, sticks, coins, and safety pins. Usually there is no history of insertion of a foreign body. A culture of purulent vaginal secretions and treatment of any organisms may be instituted, but unresponsiveness to this treatment or recurrence should raise the suspicion of a foreign body. Because the vagina is difficult to examine in a child, the presence of a foreign body usually cannot be ruled out on inspection without general anesthesia or heavy anesthesia. With a double catheter (see section on Vaginal Discharge/Vaginitis, above), sometimes flushing of the vagina may remove the object, preventing the need for an examination under general anesthesia. Likewise, a rectal examination may reveal a foreign body by palpation, although this can sometimes be difficult with a frightened and alert child. Treatment consists of removal of the object.

SYSTEMIC INFECTIOUS ILLNESSES

Upper respiratory and gastrointestinal infections sometimes produce vulvovaginitis. *Shigella flexneri* and *Shigella sonnei* produce gastrointestinal symptoms in association with a bloody vaginal discharge that is often asymptomatic. Yersinia, varicella, and group A streptococcal infection also cause childhood vaginitis. Treatment is with oral antibiotics for bacterial infections.

LICHEN SCLEROSUS

Although lichen sclerosus (see also Ch. 11) is most often a disease of adult women, this condition also occurs in young boys and girls. Several studies have revealed it to be a common cause of phimosis requiring circumcision in boys, and lichen sclerosus is certainly well recognized in prepubertal girls. Boys often present with phimosis, and girls usually present with itching or pain (Fig. 22-6). Perianal involvement is common in girls, and occasionally a prominent symptom is painful defecation or constipation. Dysuria may also occur.

Clinical Presentation

Lichen sclerosus is characterized by white plaques most often over the glans and inner prepuce of boys; in girls the plaques encompass the mucous membrane and modified mucous membrane epithelium of the vulva, extending to the surrounding skin and often to the perianal area. Fine wrinkling and hyper-

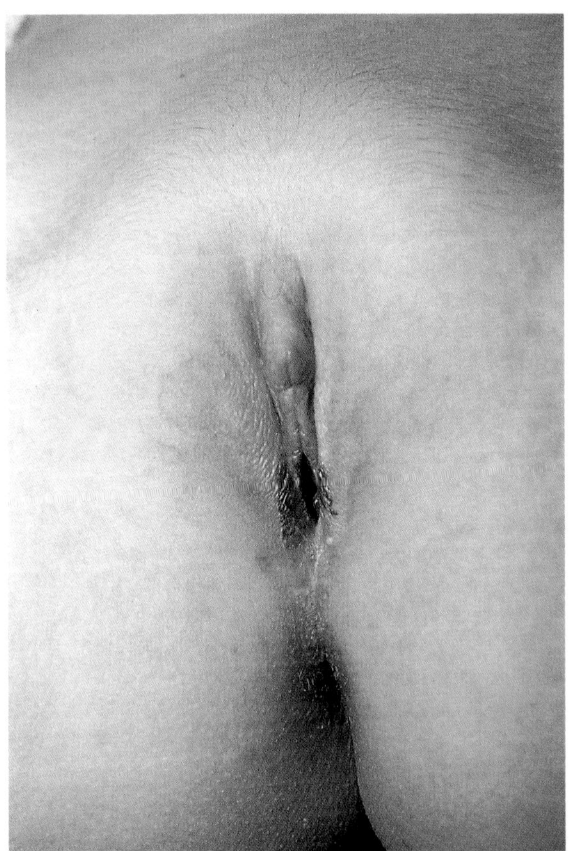

Fig. 22-6. A careful examination of this child with pruritus shows the typical sharply demarcated, white, fragile plaque of lichen sclerosus.

keratosis may be present but frequently are subtle. The presence of purpura is useful in making the diagnosis. The cutaneous changes of lichen sclerosus in childhood are occasionally difficult to see and require a high index of suspicion. The thin, prepubertal skin of the vulva, particularly when affected by lichen sclerosus, is unusually vulnerable to both bacterial or yeast infection, and girls may present with an exudative vulvitis that obscures the characteristic changes of lichen sclerosus. Only after the secondary process is treated is the lichen sclerosus appreciated.

Diagnosis

The fragility of the skin and frequent presence of purpura may lead to a misdiagnosis of sexual abuse. Erosions and purpura are to be expected with lichen sclerosus and should not arouse suspicion of abuse, although the presence of this disease obviously does not exclude childhood abuse. An evaluation of the hymen and vagina, which are always unaffected by lichen sclerosus, and a biopsy help to sort out this problem.

Treatment

The treatment of lichen sclerosus in childhood has been problematic in the past since the historic treatment of choice, topical testosterone propionate ointment, is absorbed and sometimes causes virilization. Now that corticosteroids are known not only to control the symptoms of the disease but also to reverse the skin changes, topical steroids are the preferred treatment. Usually a midpotency corticosteroid such as triamcinolone 0.1 ointment percent applied twice a day with careful follow-up to monitor the possible development of local adverse reactions provides rapid improvement. If the skin is exudative, an evaluation for infection is indicated. Treatment, including antibiotics for infection and corticosteroids for the lichen sclerosus, should be oral initially in these children until the skin begins to reepithelialize, since topical medications are both uncomfortable and less effective on weeping skin. Usually, within a week, topical medications can be substituted. In children with recalcitrant disease, a superpotent corticosteroid such as clobetasol propionate 0.05 percent as used for adults with this disease can be used. Extremely close follow-up is mandatory. When symptoms are controlled and the disease seems arrested, generally in 1 to 3 months, a low-potency corticosteroid such as hydrocortisone 1 percent can be substituted for the higher potency medications. Careful follow-up should continue to evaluate the skin for ongoing irreversible scarring, steroid atrophy, and (theoretically) the development of squamous cell carcinoma, although this appears to occur only in adults.

Although childhood lichen sclerosus has been generally thought to remit spontaneously, there have been no good prospective studies that examine this question. Most boys experience spontaneous resolution following circumcision, but many adult women with lichen sclerosus report symptoms since childhood. With proper treatment, children with lichen sclerosus should experience minimal scarring and future dysfunction.

GENITAL WARTS

Genital warts (see also Ch. 9) are well known to occur in infants and children. In addition to the multiple issues of transmission, treatment, latency, and carcinogenicity discussed elsewhere, there are additional considerations when genital warts occur in children.

In the past, genital warts were believed to occur nearly always as a result of sexual contact, so that affected children were felt to be victims of sexual abuse (Fig. 22-7). More recently, the long incubation periods for human papillomavirus infection, the ability of the virus to remain latent, and the possible roles of fomites and nongenital contact in transmission have been recognized. Also, careful evaluations of the social situations of affected children have shown that half or fewer children with genital warts have been sexually abused. This is especially true for children under the age of 3 years, many of whom were exposed to the wart virus in the birth canal during delivery. Still, a significant minority of children with genital warts *have* been abused, so that each patient deserves consideration of a report to child protective services and a thorough physical and social evaluation for other evidence of sexual or physical abuse.

The treatment of genital warts in children should be chosen not only to remove the warts, but also to minimize pain and overconcern with the genital area. Aggressive, destructive, and distressing treatment for the purpose of a cure is unreasonable in children because, as with adults, a virologic cure probably cannot be attained, treatment is often prolonged, and warts usually recur. Some asymptomatic patients can simply be followed and treated if symptoms occur or disease progresses significantly. Genital warts regress in some children, but the likelihood of this occurrence is not known. There have been no reported series of the natural course of this disease in untreated children, and many physicians and parents are not comfortable with observation alone as treatment. Podofilox, (purified podophyllotoxin; Condylox) is a relatively painless medication that can be applied at home by a trusted caretaker without undue attention and discomfort concentrated on the genital area by strangers. Children unresponsive to this treatment often tolerate well and respond to cantharidin (extract of blister beetle, purchased as Cantherone) applied without tape occlusion to warts on dry skin and 20 percent podophyllum resin in benzoin applied to moist warts. This treatment is repeated weekly or as soon as any erosions caused by treatment have healed.

Although an evaluation of the vagina and cervix is usual and is indicated in adult women with vulvar warts to assess both the extent of the infection and the presence of cervical dysplasia or cancer, this is not

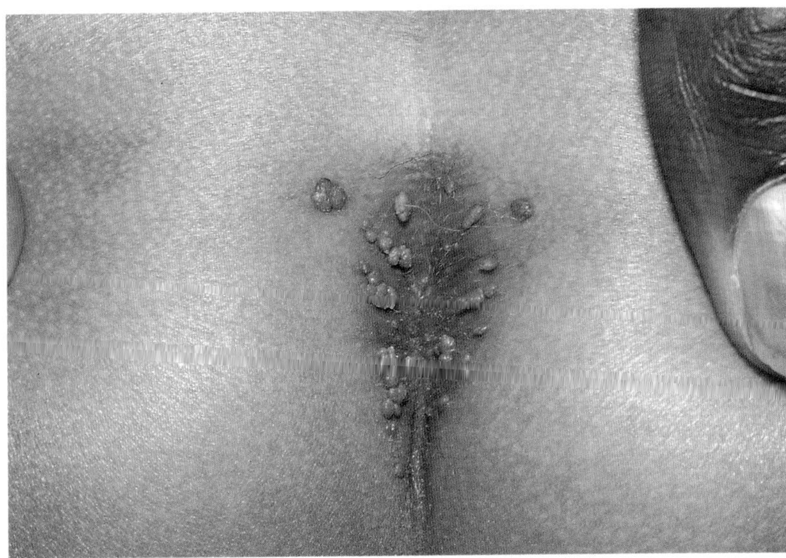

Fig. 22-7. Hyperpigmented, papular, and pedunculated genital warts in the very common perianal location of children. (From Edwards,[6] with permission.)

generally performed in children. This examination in a child would require general anesthesia and, although human papillomavirus-related carcinoma is certainly a theoretic risk, reports of cervical carcinoma in a prepubertal child are extremely rare. However, because the human papillomavirus cannot be eradicated, the patient, the parents, and the pediatrician should be aware of the future risk and need for careful follow-up.

SEXUAL ABUSE

Some diseases of the genitalia in children should alert the clinician to the possibility of sexual abuse. The consulting physician is in a position to recognize and identify diseases that confer an increased risk of abuse and to be knowledgeable about conditions that are not associated with a higher likelihood of abuse.

The diagnosis of sexual abuse is made by the identification of diseases that are only sexually transmitted (such as gonorrhea or syphilis), or by a careful psychological evaluation of the child and possible contacts in a setting in which physical findings raise a suspicion of sexual abuse. The physician should look for specific physical findings that suggest sexual abuse. Anal penetration may produce anal gaping, rectal fissures, ulcers or tears, and perianal scarring.[7] Erythema, skin tags, pigment changes, smooth areas of skin, or venous engorgement alone are found in normal children. Because the perianal area heals quickly in children following trauma, a normal examination does not rule out abuse. The vulva is difficult to examine for architectural changes resulting from trauma because of the wide range of normal variations, many of which are age dependent.[8] Obviously, lacerations, purpura, and scarring in the absence of lichen sclerosus are diagnostic of trauma. Hymeneal changes may occur, but subtle changes in the normally present notches, ridges, and bumps are difficult to assess since the normal variations at different ages are still poorly documented. Unfortunately, there is no single, specific test or physical finding diagnostic for sexual or physical abuse, so that any evaluation must take into account known normal anatomic genital variations, as well as a careful evaluation of the child's and family's history and environment.

Diseases that are at least sometimes associated with sexual abuse and should be reported to child protective services include any sexually transmitted disease. However, the physician should be aware that some child advocate professionals are not aware of the degree of risk that different diseases, particularly genital warts, bestow. When reporting the situation, it may be helpful to volunteer, for example, that fewer than half of children with warts have been abused. Molluscum contagiosum, even in the genital area, is generally not a sign of sexual abuse and need not be reported to child protective services unless other signs of abuse are present.

When a child presents with a disease or findings that suggest even a small possibility of sexual abuse, that case must be reported; the law provides immunity. The physician should tell the family that this condition has to be reported and why. Families can cope much better with this ordeal, and an adversarial relationship can usually be avoided if it is explained that the report is required by law for the protection of children who are in contact with a wide variety of people including many not under the control of or observation by the parents.

REFERENCES

Normal Genitalia and Congenital Abnormalities

1. Berkowitz GS, Lapinski RH, Dolgin SE et al: Prevalence and natural history of cryptorchidism. Pediatrics 92:44, 1993
2. McCann J, Wells R, Simon, Voris J: Genital findings in prepubertal girls selected for nonabuse: a descriptive study. Pediatrics 86:428, 1990

Labial Adhesion

3. McCann J, Wells R, Simon, Voris J: Genital findings in prepubertal girls selected for nonabuse: a descriptive study. Pediatrics 86:428, 1990

Perianal Streptococcal Dermatitis

4. Krol AL: Perianal streptococcal dermatitis. Pediatr Dermatol 7:97, 1990

Vaginal Discharge/Vaginitis

5. Pokorny SF: Pediatric vulvovaginitis. p. 55. In Kaufman RH, Friedrich EG Jr, Gardner HL (eds): Benign Diseases of the Vulva and Vagina. 3rd Ed. Yearbook Medical Publishers, Chicago, 1989

Genital Warts

6. Edwards L: Reiter's syndrome of the vulva. Arch Dermatol 128:812, 1992

Sexual Abuse

7. Berenson AB, Somma-Garcia A, Barnett S: Perianal findings in infants 18 months of age or younger. Pediatrics 91:838, 1993
8. Berenson AB: Appearance of the hymen at birth and one year of age: a longitudinal study. Pediatrics 91:820, 1993

SUGGESTED READINGS

Hydrocele, Penile Hypospadias, Chordee, and Ambiguous Genitalia

Churchill BM, McLorie GA: Ambiguous genitalia. p. 1916. In Gillenwater JY, Grayhack JT, Howards SS, Duckett JW (eds): Adult and Pediatric Urology. Year Book Medical Publishers, Chicago, 1987

Duckett JW: Hypospadias. p. 1880. In Gillenwater JY, Grayhack JT, Howards SS, Duckett JW (eds): Adult and Pediatric Urology. Year Book Medical Publishers, Chicago, 1987

Hensle T: Genital abnormalities. p. 1863. In Gillenwater JY, Grayhack JT, Howards SS, Duckett JW (eds): Adult and Pediatric Urology. Year Book Medical Publishers, Chicago, 1987

Congenital Nevus

From L: Congenital nevi—let's be practical. Pediatr Dermatol 9:345, 1992

A summary of the risks of melanoma versus surgery in children with congenital nevi is presented.

Perianal Streptococcal Dermatitis

Krol AL: Perianal streptococcal dermatitis. Pediatr Dermatol 7:97, 1990

The author presents the clinical manifestations and treatment of eight children with perianal streptococcal dermatitis and reviews the literature.

Lichen Sclerosus

Helm KF, Gibson LE, Muller SA: Lichen sclerosus et atrophicus in children and young adults. Pediatr Dermatol 8:97, 1991

The course of lichen sclerosus in 52 children and young adults was examined by telephone survey.

Ridley CM: Genital lichen sclerosus (lichen sclerosus et atrophicus) in childhood and adolescence. J R Soc Med 86:69, 1993

This extensive literature review discusses the prevalence, clinical appearance, natural history, and management of this disease in children.

Genital Warts

Cohen BA, Honig P, Androphy E: Anogenital warts in children. Arch Dermatol 126:1575, 1990

This article presents the physical findings in 73 children with anogenital warts, and virologic typing in 43 patients, as well as the results of a sexual abuse evaluation of all patients. They conclude that nonsexual transmission is the most common route of acquisition.

Obalek S, Misiewicz J, Jablonska S et al: Childhood condyloma acuminatum: association with genital and cutaneous human papillomaviruses. Pediatr Dermatol 10:101, 1993

The authors examined and typed anogenital warts on 25 children and discuss the routes of transmission in these children.

Sexual Abuse

Berenson AB, Heger AH, Hayes JM et al: Appearance of the hymen in prepubertal girls. Pediatrics 89:387, 1992

This article discusses normal variants of the hymen in 211 prepubertal girls between the ages of 1 month and 7 years, and should be useful for those who are called on to help evaluate children for sexual abuse.

General Pediatric Care

Pokorny SF: Pediatric vulvovaginitis. p. 55. In Kaufman RH, Friedrich EG Jr, Gardner HL (eds): Benign Diseases of the Vulva and Vagina. 3rd Ed. Yearbook Medical Publishers, Chicago, 1989

This chapter describes in detail an atraumatic and informative method for examining the vagina in small children. Normal variants, common skin diseases, and usual etiologies of vulvovaginitis in childhood are described and treatment discussed.

Williams TS, Callen JP, Owen LG: Vulvar disorders in the prepubertal female. Pediatr Ann 588, 1986

Although intended primarily for the care of females, this inclusive review of pediatric genital dermatology also discusses implications and presentation of diseases applicable to children of both sexes, including herpes simplex virus infection, molluscum contagiosum, condylomata acuminata, and atopic dermatitis.

23 Geriatric Problems

GERIATRIC ISSUES

Because of hormonal changes in the elderly, the increased incidence of incontinence, dementia, and depression, and the decreased ability to care for personal hygiene, older patients are likely to develop certain genital complaints. Although these conditions are generally not unique to the geriatric patient, they are often more prevalent and more difficult to treat. Many older patients expect aging to cause multiple physical disabilities, and they often minimize their symptoms. Astute and caring physicians listen to complaints and evaluate them carefully; they do not allow patients to pass off their symptoms as expected events of old age. Many diseases traditionally attributed to the normal aging process may be secondary to treatable disease, socioeconomic conditions, or depression.

Often, the dementia and depression that so often relate directly to genital symptoms must be addressed by the physician. Medication effects, congestive heart failure, dehydration, and other factors that produce or worsen dementia require attention both for the best care of the total patient but also to obtain optimal cooperation in the understanding and treatment of some conditions.

The physician should not overlook sexuality as an important issue to some elderly patients. These patients may not broach the topic because of embarrassment, but they respond readily to direct questioning about the effect of genital abnormalities on their sexual activities.

Geriatric patients are likely to be on multiple medications and to have difficulty with sight and hearing. The treatment of genital disease often includes several different interventions, including an alteration of usual genital care and the use of several medications. Some patients benefit from clear, written directions and careful follow-up either in the office or by telephone to ensure that directions are understood and are being followed correctly.

CONTACT DERMATITIS

Simple irritation (see also Ch. 5) of the genital skin is common in elderly patients. This condition manifests in symptoms of pruritus or pain with clinical findings varying from mild erythema with or without subtle scale to intense erythema and even erosion with exudation. Black patients exhibit more hyperpigmentation than erythema. There are several common causes of irritant contact dermatitis in older patients. These include urine or fecal material held against the skin within the skin folds themselves, particularly in obese patients, or by occlusive clothing or an adult diaper. Also, some patients become obsessed with cleanliness and wash the area with soap and water multiple times each day, causing irritation and xerosis. The more irritation that occurs, the more some patients clean, convinced that their symptoms are a result of poor hygiene or infection. As some patients lose their ability to think clearly, they may become fixated on symptoms and even use harsh cleansers. These patients may remain secretive and not report these habits.

Treatment is primarily one of reducing irritation. Incontinent patients should have feces and urine removed as soon as possible, and occlusive clothing or diapers should be changed frequently (see Diaper Dermatitis in Ch. 22). The skin should be cleaned gently with water, avoiding alcohol and other defatting cleansers. When incontinence is considerable, the application of zinc oxide paste to the affected area helps to protect it from excrement. A mild topical corticosteroid such as hydrocortisone 1 percent ointment helps to decrease inflammation, and any *Candida* infection should be treated. With severe dermatitis, empiric treatment for yeast is warranted, and this may require oral treatment to avoid further irritant effects from the alcohols in the creams. Other topical medications, deodorants, perfumes, and so forth should be discontinued, and the patient who is overwashing should be counseled to decrease the frequency, vigor of scrubbing, and harshness of the cleanser. Patients who are obsessive about using topical agents for cleanliness should be evaluated and treated for reversible causes of dementia or depression, or for worsening factors.

ATROPHIC VULVOVAGINITIS

Postmenopausal women not on estrogen replacement experience thinning of the vulvar and vaginal epithelium (see also Ch. 7). Patients may be asymptomatic, but many are aware of a sensation of dryness that sometimes makes intercourse uncomfortable. Regular coitus is somewhat protective and prevents some of the epithelial thinning and inelastic narrowing of the introitus and vagina. Some patients complain of dysuria, urgency, and frequency as a result of atrophic urethritis.

A physical examination reveals a wide spectrum of atrophic changes. Some patients without symptoms have minimal alterations, but most patients not receiving estrogen replacement treatment exhibit thinning of the pubic hair and smoothness and thinning of vulvar skin. The labia minora and labia majora lose substance and become more wrinkled; complete resorption of the labia minora occurs in some and may mimic the end stage of lichen sclerosus. The glycogen-poor vaginal epithelium also thins, and loss of vaginal rugae occurs. Vaginal secretions become more alkaline and provide a more hospitable environment for bacteria. Estrogen deficiency also increases the likelihood of a prolapsed bladder, uterus, rectum, or urethra. With protrusion of one of these structures into the vagina, hyperkeratosis or erosion of the vaginal wall may occur, producing inflammation, discomfort, and discharge. The net effect of these changes is to increase risk of inflammation secondary to tearing, erosions, fissures, and secondary infection of the fragile, atrophic epithelium.

The diagnosis of atrophic vulvovaginitis is by clinical examination, a history consistent with estrogen deficiency, and a vaginal wall maturation index.

Treatment should address both the estrogen deficiency and any secondary processes. In postmenopausal women, oral estrogen replacement confers the advantage of systemic benefits such as minimizing osteoporosis, vasomotor instability, and cardiovascular disease. However, adverse reactions include an increased risk of gallbladder disease. In addition, systemic estrogen treatment supports the growth of uterine fibroids, endometriosis, and fibrocystic disease of the breast, and it has a permissive effect on breast carcinoma. When used in a cyclic fashion with progesterone, the risk of endometrial carcinoma is minimized. Topical estrogen treatment provides benefit much faster and may produce better local effects. Concomitant administration of both oral and topical estrogen provides rapid improvement in symptoms until the systemic effects of the oral preparation take effect several months later. Topical conjugated estrogen cream (Premarin) 0.625 mg/g applied intravaginally and over the vestibule nightly for 3 weeks and then twice a week usually effects improvement within a month. Treatment may then be further tapered to the most infrequent dosing that maintains healthy epithelium. For patients who experience irritation with application of the cream, estradiol cream (Estrace) 0.01 percent may be better tolerated, especially if the patient pretreats with triamcinolone ointment 0.1 percent twice daily for several days to decrease inflammation. Some patients, however, may find any topical medication other than bland petrolatum irritating, and in those women oral treatment will be necessary when possible. A vaginal culture should be performed for those with a purulent discharge. Treatment of any secondary infections and the use of a vaginal lubricant such as Replens is useful in those with a complaint of dryness.

GENITAL AND RECTAL PROLAPSE

Estrogen deficiency, particularly in multiparous women, may cause relaxation of suspensory ligaments that support the bladder, urethra, uterus, and rectum. These structures may then protrude against the vaginal wall, mimicking a cystic tumor and producing excretory dysfunction and sensations of heaviness, tumor, or pain. Pressure and friction against the opposite vaginal wall may cause erosions or hyperkeratosis.

The mucosae of the rectum, vagina, or urethra may also prolapse through their respective openings; prolapse manifests through a red, glistening mass at the opening.

Presumptive diagnosis is by clinical examination, with a full evaluation by a gynecologist. Treatment can be aided by hormones and pessaries, but definitive treatment is surgical.

OTHER PROBLEMS

Pruritus and pain may occur more often in geriatric patients as a manifestation of depression. Sexual dysfunction is more common, resulting from dwindling hormones, depression, lack of opportunity, medication, prostate surgery, and diseases such as diabetes. Many benign tumors including cherry angiomas, seborrheic keratoses, and epidermal cysts are more common in older individuals. Dysuria and frequency occur more often in postmenopausal women due to atrophy of the urethral mucosa, and urinary frequency occurs in men as a result of benign prostatic hypertrophy.

24 Anogenital Problems in the Immunosuppressed

With the advent of the acquired immunodeficiency syndrome (AIDS), the widespread use of transplants, and the aggressive treatment of malignancies, immunosuppression has become a common occurrence. Immunosuppressed patients are at increased risk for some diseases, particularly infectious diseases and tumors, and many common diseases present atypically. Patients with AIDS also have a higher risk of some inflammatory skin diseases such as psoriasis, Reiter syndrome, and seborrheic dermatitis.

VIRAL INFECTIONS

Herpes Simplex Virus Infection

Infection with the herpes simplex virus (see also Ch. 15) is extremely common in patients with AIDS. Until proved otherwise, it should be assumed that a genital ulcer or erosion in these patients is due to herpes simplex infection. Chronic erosive herpes simplex virus infection is frequent in immunosuppressed patients in general, and the clinical appearance is often atypical.

The patient often describes a chronic ulceration rather than a recurrent lesion as occurs in immunocompetent patients. Vesicles are often not appreciated, but round erosions or ulcerations, often with larger confluent, arcuate borders are common (Fig. 24-1). With more chronic or superinfected disease, the characteristic round or scalloped borders may be lost and the depth of the ulceration may be impressive. Less often, herpes simplex virus infection on the non-hair-bearing portion of immunosuppressed skin manifests by white or yellow exudative papules with the characteristic round, arcuate margins (papular herpes) (Fig. 24-2). Finally, a herpes simplex infection in the setting of AIDS, when present on hair-bearing skin, occasionally consists of nondescript hyperkeratotic papules or plaques.

The diagnosis of herpes simplex infection under these conditions is made by the clinical appearance and culture and, when necessary for diagnosis or to rule out a second process, biopsy. A biopsy is usually characteristic of either herpes simplex or varicella zoster virus, but differentiation between these two infections is not possible on biopsy. A positive culture is definitive. A high index of suspicion for other infections such as *Candida* is also important, since multifactorial processes are common in the setting of immunosuppression.

The treatment of herpes simplex virus infection in the immunosuppressed patient often requires ongoing oral acyclovir. The starting dose is 200 mg five times a day, and many require this as a suppressive dose as well. Therapy is especially important for patients with AIDS, because chronic genital ulceration increases the likelihood of transmission in the sexually active patient. Also, there is evidence that inter-

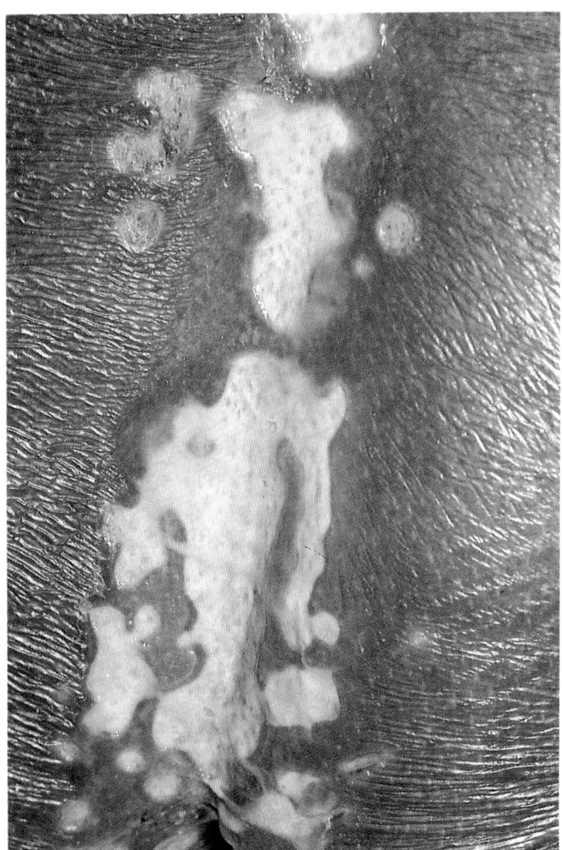

Fig. 24-1. Chronic enlarging confluent, arcuate ulcerations caused by herpes simplex virus infection in an immunosuppressed patient.

action between the herpes simplex virus and the human immunodeficiency virus (HIV) may potentiate the development of AIDS in HIV-infected individuals. The discontinuation of acyclovir is usually accompanied by a reactivation of the disease.

Immunosuppressed patients are at greater risk for the development of herpes simplex resistant to acyclovir. Patients on therapeutic doses of acyclovir who are culture positive for the virus are presumed to have a resistant virus infection. These patients may benefit from foscarnet treatment, but this medication is available for intravenous use only, and recurrence following discontinuation of treatment is common.

Varicella Zoster Infection

Immunosuppressed patients are at a markedly increased risk for the development of herpes zoster (shingles; see also Ch. 15), a localized recurrence of varicella zoster infection; unlike immunocompetent individuals, these patients may experience more than one episode. Similarly, AIDS patients with a history of childhood varicella sometimes develop a second clinical case of varicella.

The first episode of herpes zoster in a patient infected with HIV often occurs before the onset of AIDS and is clinically typical. Although the genital area is occasionally affected, the trunk and face are the most common sites of herpes zoster infection.

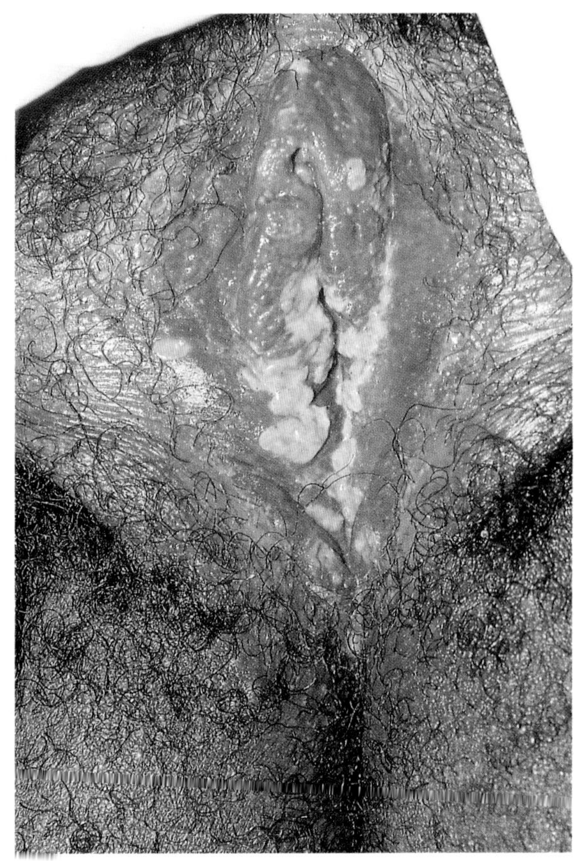

Fig. 24-2. Papular herpes simplex virus infection can be recognized because of its setting in immunosuppressed patients, its white macerated epithelium, and the coalescence of papules into a pattern similar to that of coalescing erosions.

Subsequent episodes are likely to arise after the onset of clinical AIDS, and these are more apt to be clinically atypical. Vesiculobullous lesions occur initially, but then are replaced by sharply demarcated erosions clustered in a dermatomal distribution. The lesions are often chronic and more necrotic than usual, and sometimes frank ulcers develop. Disseminated disease, with the generalized appearance of vesicles or necrotic ulcers, is more common in immunosuppressed patients, and some patients develop chronic, hyperkeratotic plaques.

The diagnosis is made on the basis of the clinical examination and culture. Treatment is with oral acyclovir at 800 mg five times a day or intravenous acyclovir 10 mg/kg every 8 hours. Anecdotally, many clinicians feel that postherpetic neuralgia is more common in patients with AIDS, compared with same-age nonimmunosuppressed patients.

Condylomata Acuminata

Reactivation or worsening of human papillomavirus infection in immunosuppressed patients is common (see also Ch. 9). Patients usually have a history of past genital warts and experience exuberant growth with immunosuppression. The warts sometimes attain a mass that interferes with intercourse, urination, or defecation. Sometimes trapped debris, heat, and perspiration may produce inflammation, pruritus, and resulting secondary infection. The usual concern for subsequent development of squamous cell carcinoma is increased as a result of the loss of the usual immunologic control of malignant degeneration. In addition, the common occurrence of herpes simplex virus in patients with AIDS and the possible synergistic role of this virus in the production of genital cancer may put those patients at particular risk.

The diagnosis is by clinical examination and, for any large or atypical lesions, by a biopsy to eliminate the possibility of a squamous cell carcinoma or atypia that would signify an increased risk of this occurrence.

Treatment is problematic. Eradication of the virus is not possible in the normal host, and control of the disease process in the immunosuppressed patient is even more difficult. The patient must be aware of the limitations of treatment and must help with decisions regarding aggressiveness of treatment. After the bulk of the disease is controlled, many patients do well with ongoing use of home-applied podofilox for chronic control, but concern exists because of the theoretical carcinogenicity associated with podophyllum resin. Ongoing reassessments for the development of a secondary squamous cell carcinoma should be performed.

Molluscum Contagiosum

Molluscum contagiosum (see also Ch. 9), an innocuous but aggravating, often sexually transmitted skin infection, is especially common and exuberant in patients with AIDS. The appearance is usually typical, although individual lesions may be larger than normally seen. However, because cryptococcal and histoplasmosis infection can mimic molluscum contagiosum, a representative lesion should be biopsied for histologic confirmation.

Treatment should aim for control rather than permanent eradication. Light curettage is effective but uncomfortable, and treatments that minimize bleeding are desirable in patients with AIDS. Light cryotherapy is also useful. Topical cantherone is effective but sometimes too irritating on thin genital skin and should be used carefully. Topical podofilox has been useful in some anecdotal reports, and Retin-A has been reported useful for ongoing control in other areas where the skin is less sensitive.

BACTERIAL INFECTIONS

Cutaneous bacterial infections are more common in immunosuppressed patients, but the most common etiologic agents remain *Staphylococcus aureus* and β-hemolytic streptococci. The clinical appearance is the same in these patients as in immunocompetent people.

FUNGAL INFECTIONS

Fungal infections of the skin (see also Ch. 6) are common and sometimes atypical in appearance in immunosuppressed patients. The most common fungal infections in the genital area are superficial dermatophyte infections and *Candida albicans.*

Tinea cruris in the immunocompromised host is common and is often characterized by thickened, scaling plaques that frequently lack the usual striking annularity with central clearing. The involved area often extends to the scrotum and penis. Patients with black skin often show striking hyperpigmentation rather than erythema. An examination of other body surfaces frequently reveals extension to the surrounding areas of the legs or trunk, and an associated infection of the feet.

Chronic or recurrent vulvovaginal candidiasis in women is common and often more severe and striking in appearance, with white papules and plaques on the skin surfaces, and sometimes erosive disease. Uncircumcised men may also have white papules, but occasionally these too erode, and differentiation from herpes simplex virus infection may be difficult. The gluteal cleft is often involved in both men and women.

The diagnosis of these diseases is by clinical appearance and potassium hydroxide preparation or culture. Treatment can be attempted with topical agents, but erosive, extensive, or hyperkeratotic disease may require oral treatment with griseofulvin for tinea infections and fluconazole for either tinea or *Candida* infection. Ketoconazole is generally avoided in patients with AIDS because of the increased incidence of gastric achlorhydria and the poor absorption of this medication in the absence of gastric acid. Ongoing treatment with a topical agent is usually needed for long-term control.

NONINFECTIOUS DISEASES ASSOCIATED WITH AIDS

Patients with AIDS have been found to be at risk of a number of inflammatory but basically noninfectious diseases that affect the genitalia. The recognition of these disorders helps to avoid unhelpful and unnecessary treatment.

Seborrheic Dermatitis

Clinicians reported early in their experiences with HIV disease the increased incidence and severity of seborrheic dermatitis (see also Ch. 5) in affected patients. In fact, unusually severe seborrheic dermatitis in a patient without neurologic disease should trigger a suspicion of AIDS. The clinical appearance is basically the same as in uninfected patients only more severe and often prominently affecting the face. Lichenification may occur, especially in black patients.

In AIDS patients, the differential diagnosis of genital seborrhea should especially include psoriasis, tinea cruris, candidiasis, and eczema.

Psoriasis

New onset (see also Ch. 6) or a sudden worsening of psoriasis is relatively common in patients with AIDS. The appearance of the disease is typical, with sharply demarcated, red, scaling plaques (Fig. 24-3), and the diagnosis is not usually difficult except for occasional confusion with tinea cruris or *Candida* in the genital area before generalized disease develops.

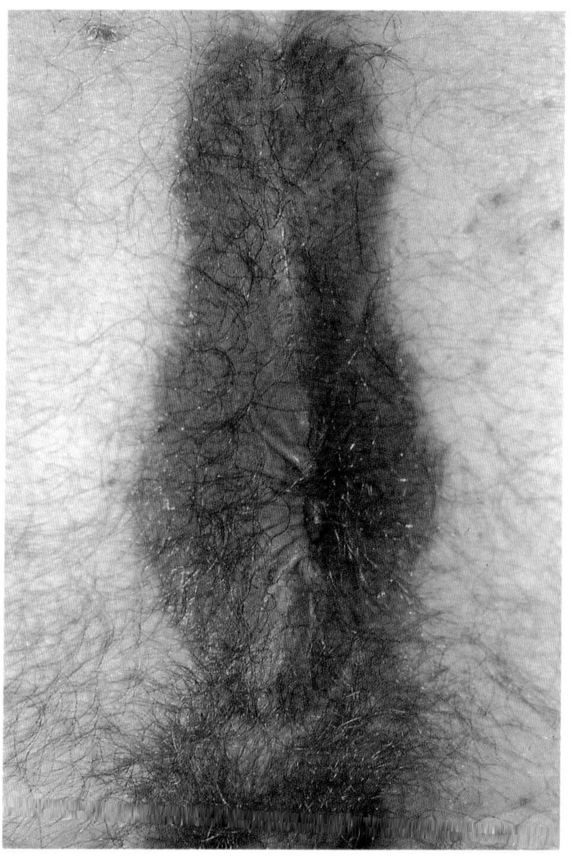

Fig. 24-3. Erythematous, thickened, well-demarcated plaque of psoriasis in a patient with AIDS who had been treated empirically for yeast for 2 months.

Although some recent reports suggest that AIDS-associated psoriasis is no more recalcitrant to treatment than that occurring in immunocompetent patients, some clinicians' experience indicates otherwise. It is known that the severity of the psoriasis parallels the course of the AIDS, and that zidovudine (AZT) improves psoriasis in patients with AIDS. The usual treatment is topical corticosteroids, despite the theoretic immunosuppressive side effects. Ultraviolet B light is also used, and most physicians are willing to use oral psoralens and ultraviolet A light (PUVA) in spite of the mild immunosuppression produced by this therapy.

Reiter Syndrome

Reiter syndrome (see also Ch. 6), existing on a spectrum with pustular psoriasis, is also more common in men with AIDS. The disease is similar in appearance to that occurring in immunocompetent patients, with red, crusting, well-marginated plaques prominent over the genital area, hands, and feet. The glans of uncircumcised males shows white annular papules that may become confluent into arcuate or serpiginous plaques. The other usual manifestations also occur in this setting, including urethritis, arthritis, and uveitis. Again, the differential diagnosis includes *Candida* infection, psoriasis, and (less often) tinea cruris.

Epidemic Kaposi's Sarcoma

Kaposi's sarcoma is a vascular tumor well known to occur with increased frequency in immunosuppressed patients, particularly homosexual men with AIDS. This neoplasm is multifocal rather than metastatic and occurs almost exclusively in those patients who contracted AIDS through sexual transmission.

Usually asymptomatic, these lesions present as red-brown, purple, or hyperpigmented papules or nodules and most often represent a cosmetic rather than a health-threatening problem. Patients are often extremely sensitive about the appearance of these lesions, which serve as a constant reminder of their underlying disease. Most patients gradually develop more lesions, and some develop visceral disease, although Kaposi's sarcoma is not usually the cause of death in affected AIDS patients.

The diagnosis is by clinical appearance with histologic confirmation to rule out less likely tumors or infection. Treatment is indicated for functional impairment caused by tumors, or in those patients who cannot tolerate these visible signs of disease. A limited number of lesions can be treated with intralesional vinblastine, 0.2 to 0.5 mg/ml using a volume sufficient to blanch the lesion.[1] Cryotherapy is useful in some patients. Patients with large numbers of lesions or health threatened by the tumors require systemic vinblastine or α-interferon, or local radiotherapy.

Pruritus

Patients with AIDS often experience generalized pruritus that may include the genital area. This may be associated with any specific skin disease including those discussed above as well as xerosis (dryness) or folliculitis. In addition, eczema produced by rubbing and scratching is often seen, and itching is often unaccompanied by any underlying skin abnormalities. Management includes the careful evaluation for treatable disease and correction of these abnormalities, oral antihistamines, sometimes in high doses, and emotional support. Extragenital sites may benefit from ultraviolet light.

Foscarnet-Induced Genital Ulcers

Foscarnet, an antiviral agent used primarily for cytomegalovirus retinitis and acyclovir-resistant herpes simplex virus infection, can induce vulvar and penile ulcerations in up to 20 percent of patients with AIDS.[2–4] Occurring from 7 to 27 days after medication is begun, the lesions may be initially bullous, erosive, or ulcerative. They occur in areas where pooling of urine is likely to occur, such as at the meatus, in the preputial sac, and on the scrotum where the tip of the penis rests. These are painful and may be associated with oral or esophageal ulcerations.

Biopsies have been nonspecific, usually showing no features of a fixed drug eruption. The ulcers are believed to be caused by local toxic effects of the urine, since 90 percent of the medication is excreted unchanged in the urine.[5]

The ulcers resolve with discontinuation of the medication, and meticulous rinsing of the area following urination may prevent the erosions.

REFERENCES

Epidemic Kaposi's Sarcoma

1. Bourdreaux AA, Smith LL, Cosby CD et al: Intralesional vinblastine for cutaneous Kaposi's sarcoma associated with acquired immunodeficiency syndrome. J Am Acad Dermatol 28:61, 1993

Foscarnet-Induced Genital Ulcers

2. Fergueux S, Salmon D, Picard C et al: Penile ulcerations with foscarnet (letter). Lancet 335:547, 1990
3. Evans LM, Grossman ME: Foscarnet-induced penile ulcer. J Am Acad Dermatol 27:124, 1992
4. Caumes E, Gatineau M, Bricaire F et al: Foscarnet-induced vulvar erosion (letter). J Am Acad Dermatol 28:799, 1993
5. Sjovall J, Karlsson A, Ogenstad S et al: Pharmacokinetics and absorption of foscarnet after intravenous and oral administration to patients with human immunodeficiency virus. Clin Pharmacol Ther 44:65, 1988

SUGGESTED READINGS

Herpes Simplex Virus Infection

Berger T: Herpes virus infections and HIV disease. Clin Dermatol 9:79, 1991

This review discusses the epidemiology of herpes simplex and varicella-zoster infection in HIV disease, including interactions between HIV and the herpes simplex virus, the clinical appearance of these diseases in patients with HIV infection, and management.

Safrin S, Crumpacker C, Chatis P et al: A controlled trial comparing foscarnet with vidarabine for acyclovir-resistant mucocutaneous herpes simplex in the acquired immunodeficiency syndrome. N Engl J Med 325:551, 1991

Noninfectious Diseases Associated with AIDS

Shupack JL, Stiller MJ, Haber RS: Psoriasis and Reiter's syndrome. Clin Dermatol 9:53, 1991

This article discusses psoriasis and Reiter syndrome in the setting of HIV disease, including possible pathogenesis and management approaches.

Pruritus

Buchness MR, Snachez M: HIV-associated pruritus. Clin Dermatol 9:111, 1991

The authors discuss an approach to the HIV patient who presents with pruritus, including a differential diagnosis of underlying causes and treatment for those with no specific skin findings.

Foscarnet-Induced Genital Ulcers

Evans LM, Grossman ME: Foscarnet-induced penile ulcer. J Am Acad Dermatol 27:124, 1992

This short article reviews in table form the presentation and course of foscarnet-induced genital ulcers reported in the literature.

Glossary

Acantholysis: Loss of adhesion between epithelial cells that creates an intraepidermal blister and rounded, detached keratinocytes within the blister.

Aceto-whitening: White discoloration of any hyperkeratotic epithelium when exposed to acetic acid; generally believed to be a sign of human papillomavirus infection but actually nonspecific.

Adhesion: Fusing of two epithelial surfaces by scar.

Agglutination: Coalescence of two epithelial surfaces with resorption of structures, as agglutination of the labia minora to the labia majora results in obliteration of any signs of the labia minora.

Atrophy: Thinning of skin, characterized by a smooth surface, fragility, and often telangiectasias visible through thin epithelium.

Balanitis: Inflammation of the glans penis.

Balanoposthitis: Inflammation of the glans penis and prepuce.

Bartholin's gland: Mucous-secreting glands located beneath the fascia at the vaginal introitus at about 5 and 7 o'clock, with ducts opening at these locations just distal to the hymen.

Clue cell: A vaginal epithelial cell covered with bacteria that provide a ragged appearance to the border of the cell; when found in the setting of an increased pH, odor, and a paucity of lactobacilli, it is pathognomonic for bacterial vaginosis.

Collarette: A circumferential rim of scale representing the peripheral remains of an unroofed blister; provides a clue to the underlying blistering nature of the lesion.

Colposcopy: Literally, examination of the cervix under magnification; practically, examination of any genital epithelial surface under magnification, usually for evaluation for the presence of human papillomavirus infection.

Crust: Dried serum or blood, often mixed with scale; indicates disruption of the epidermis by trauma (usually excoriation), prior blistering, or inflammatory erosive disease.

Desquamative: On mucous membranes, synonymous with erosive loss of epithelium; on keratinized skin, refers to superficial peeling from loss of upper layers of epithelium only.

Dystrophy: Outdated terminology referring to any skin disease of the vulva, usually lichen sclerosus (hypoplastic dystrophy) or neurodermatitis (hyperplastic dystrophy).

EMLA: Acronym for *eutectic mixture of local anesthesia,* a topical anesthetic that provides for nearly painless injected local anesthesia.

Erosion: Loss of epithelium with resulting exudation or crusting but with an intact underlying dermis.

Exocytosis: Presence of mononuclear inflammatory cells in the epidermis in association with intercellular edema.

Hart's line: Faint line of texture demarcation that separates the vulvar vestibule from the base of the labia minora.

Hyperkeratosis: Exaggerated degree of compact scale so that, when occurring on nonmucous membrane skin, the surface feels rough; histologically, thickening of the most superficial layer of the skin, the stratum corneum.

Hyperplastic dystrophy: Outdated term for skin disease of the vulva that exhibits squamous hyperplasia, most often referring to neurodermatitis, or chronic dermatitis.

Hypopigmentation: Lightening of the skin caused by a decrease in melanin production or distribution, as distinct from depigmentation (no melanin), or whitening from hyperkeratosis.

Hypoplastic dystrophy: Outdated term for lichen sclerosus.

Intertrigo: Skin fold such as axilla or crural crease, signifying an area with a predisposition to dampness, friction, warmth, and an increased permeability to medications, and therefore an increased likelihood of irritation and infection.

ISSVD: Acronym for *International Society for the Study of Vulvovaginal Disease,* a society of gynecologists, dermatologists, and pathologists dedicated to the understanding and treatment of vulvovaginal disease.

Köbner's phenomenon: Characteristic of some diseases in which injury precipitates the occurrence of a disease at the site of the injury; especially psoriasis, lichen planus, vitiligo, and probably lichen sclerosus.

Kraurosis vulvae: Severe, nonspecific scarring of the vulva producing introital stenosis and loss of normal architecture; usually refers to changes that are due to lichen sclerosus but may also occur with lichen planus or other erosive, scarring disease.

Lichenification: Thickening of the skin as a response to rubbing, often recognizable by accentuation of normal skin markings.

Marsupialization: Surgical treatment of a cyst, especially a Bartholin's gland duct cyst; the cyst is unroofed and the interior is exteriorized to provide a large and permanent opening to prevent recurrence.

Maturation index: Examination of vaginal epithelial cells to evaluate the estrogen effect as evidenced by their degree of maturity.

Modified mucous membrane: Clinically non-hair-bearing skin that is minimally keratinized; found over the glans penis, the inner aspect of the labia majora, and the labia minora.

Mucous membrane: Non-hair-bearing, unkeratinized epithelium that does not contain sweat glands or hair follicles; when used for genital tissue it lines the vagina and oral cavity; does not have to contain mucous-secreting cells.

Papillomatosis: Clinically, a surface consisting of confluent or closely set papillae; histologically, an epithelium that appears folded because of upward proliferation of the dermal papillae.

Paraphimosis: Inability to return the prepuce to its normal position after retraction; associated with scarring of the preputial opening and subsequent edema and engorgement of the glans from entrapment.

Paraurethral glands: Mucous-secreting glands that empty into the distal urethra, except for the most distal ducts (Skene's ducts), which open at or just outside the meatus.

Phimosis: Scarring of the preputial opening, so that retraction of the prepuce is difficult or impossible.

Posterior fourchette: Junction of the epithelium at the posterior vulvar vestibule, not to be confused with the posterior fornix of the vagina that lies posterior and caudal to the cervix.

Scale: Desquamated superficial, dead, keratinized stratum corneum with the visible amount generally increased, indicating greater turnover of skin or decreased release of old cells; often subtle on damp genital skin.

Scrotodynia: Scrotal pain, sometimes associated with penile pain, without a discernible objective etiology but usually with significant psychological factors.

Spongiosis: Epidermal intercellular edema.

Squamous hyperplasia: Skin disease characterized by thickening of the squamous epithelium (acanthosis).

Ulcer: Loss of epithelium and at least partial loss of dermis.

Verrucous: Warty.

Vesicle: Small blister.

Vestibular glands: Multiple mucous-secreting glandular invaginations in the vulvar vestibule, opening through the epithelium surrounding the hymen.

Vulvodynia: Burning vulvar pain without an obvious, objective etiology.

Whiff test: Test used for the diagnosis of bacterial vaginosis; when positive, potassium hydroxide added to vaginal secretions releases a fishy odor.

Index

Page numbers followed by f represent figures; those followed by t represent tables.

D

E

I

O

P